The Gut Microbiota in Health and Disease

The Gut Microbiota in Health and Disease

Edited by

Nimmy Srivastava
Amity University Jharkhand, India

Salam A. Ibrahim
North Carolina Agricultural & Technical State University, USA

Jayeeta Chattopadhyay
Amity University Jharkhand, India

Mohamed H. Arbab
Omdurman Ahlia University, Sudan

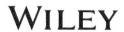

Contents

List of Contributors

Mahdi Hussein Abdelrazig
Omdurman Ahlia University
Sudan

Gholamreza Abdi
Persian Gulf Institute
Persian Gulf University
Bushehr
Iran

Sarah Adjei-Fremah
Winston-Salem State University
Winston-Salem
North Carolina
USA

Israrahmed Adur
Vellore Institute of Technology
Tamil Nadu
India

Nahid Akhtar
Lovely Professional University
Phagwara
Punjab, India

Muhammad Altaf
The Islamia University of Bahawalpur
Pakistan

Mohamed Hussein Arbab
Omdurman Ahlia University
Sudan

Usman Atique
Chungan National University
South Korea

Aparajita Bagchi
Vellore Institute of Technology
Tamil Nadu
India

Jutishna Bora
Amity University Jharkhand
Ranchi
Jharkhand
India

Shuvam Chakraborty
Vellore Institute of Technology
Tamil Nadu
India

Shahana Chowdhury
Department of Biotechnology
German University
Bangladesh

Inderpal Devgon
Lovely Professional University
Phagwara
Punjab
India

Ankita Dey
North Eastern Hill University
Shillong
Meghalaya
India

Rohan Dutta
Vellore Institute of Technology
Tamil Nadu
India

Sumitha Elayaperumal
JSS Academy of Higher Education
and Research
Mysore
Karnataka
India

Shakira Ghazanfar
Pakistan Agricultural Research Council
Islamabad
Pakistan

Md. Ayenuddin Haque
Bangladesh Fisheries Research Institute
Bangladesh

Richismita Hazra
Amity University Kolkata
West Bengal
India

Salam Ibrahim
North Carolina Agricultural and
Technical State Universit
Greensboro
North Carolina
USA

Anu Jacob
Karunya Institute of Technology
and Science
Coimbatore
India

Vishal Johar
Lovely Professional University
Phagwara
Punjab
India

Parneet Kaur
Shoolini University of Biotechnology and
Management Sciences
Solan
India

Khushboo
Lovely Professional University
Phagwara
Punjab
India

Saurabh Kulshreshtha
Shoolini University of Biotechnology
and Management Sciences
Solan
India

Kunal Kumar
Amity Institute of Biotechnology
Amity University Jharkhand
Ranchi
India

Jissin Mathew
Karunya Institute of Technology
and Science
Coimbatore
India

Tahir ul Gani Mir
Lovely Professional University
Phagwara
Punjab
India

Hriiziini Monica
North Eastern Hill University
Shillong, Meghalaya
India

Sagnik Nag
Vellore Institute of Technology
Tamil Nadu
India

Shaimaa H. Negm
Port Said University
Port Fouad City
Egypt

Jessica Pandohee
Telethon Kids Institute
Nedlands
Western Australia
Australia

Ajit Prakash
University of North Carolina
Chapel Hill
North Carolina
USA

Ridashisha Rymbai
North Eastern Hill University
Shillong, Meghalaya
India

Rohan Samir Kumar Sachan
Lovely Professional University
Phagwara
Punjab
India

Abu Saeid
NPI University of Bangladesh
Manikganj
Bangladesh

Ankita Saini
University of Delhi
New Delhi
India

Harshit Sajal
JSS Academy of Higher Education
and Research
Mysore
Karnataka
India

Bushra Shaida
Sharda University
Gr. Noida, U.P.
India

Rajani Sharma
Amity Institute of Biotechnology
Amity University Jharkhand
Ranchi
India

Vandana Singh
Sharda University
Gr. Noida, U.P.
India

Dwaipayan Sinha
Government General Degree College
Mohanpur
Paschim Medinipur
India

Yuvaraj Sivamani
Cauvery College of Pharmacy
Mysuru
Karnataka
India

Nimmy Srivastava
Amity Institute of Biotechnology
Amity University Jharkhand
India

Lisa F. M. Lee Nen That
RMIT University
Victoria
Australia

Ab Waheed Wani
Lovely Professional University
Punjab
India

Atif Khurshid Wani
Lovely Professional University
Phagwara
Punjab
India

Mulumebet Worku
North Carolina Agricultural and Technical
State University
Greensboro
North Carolina
USA

1

Structural and Dynamics of Healthy Adult's Microbiota

Mahdi Hussein Abdelrazig

Professor of Hematology, Omdurman Ahlia University, Sudan

1.1 Introduction

Microbiota are the range of microorganisms that may be commensal, symbiotic, or pathogenic found in and on all multicellular organisms, including plants. Microbiota include bacteria, archaea, protists, fungi, and viruses [1–3], and have been found to be crucial for immunologic, hormonal, and metabolic homeostasis of their host.

The term *microbiome* describes either the collective genomes of the microbes that reside in an ecological niche or within the microbes themselves [4–6]. The microbiome and host emerged during evolution as a synergistic unit from epigenetics and genetic characteristics, sometimes collectively referred to as a holobiont [7, 8]. The presence of microbiota in human and other metazoan guts has been critical for understanding the co-evolution between metazoans and bacteria [9, 10]. Microbiota play key roles in the intestinal immune and metabolic responses via their fermentation product (short-chain fatty acid), acetate [11]. All plants and animals, from simple life forms to humans, live in close association with microbial organisms [12]. Several advances have driven the perception of microbiomes, including:

- the ability to perform genomic and gene expression analyses of both single cells and entire microbial communities in the disciplines of metagenomics and metatranscriptomics [13];
- databases accessible to researchers across multiple disciplines [13]; and
- methods of mathematical analysis suitable for complex datasets [13].

Biologists have come to appreciate that microbes make up an important part of an organism's phenotype, far beyond the occasional symbiotic case study [13]. Commensalism, a concept developed by Pierre-Joseph van Beneden (1809–1894), a Belgian professor at the University of Louvain during the nineteenth century [14], is central to the microbiome, where microbiota colonize a host in a non-harmful coexistence. The relationship with their host is called mutualistic when organisms perform tasks that are known to be useful for the host [15, 16], and parasitic when disadvantageous to the host. Other authors define a situation as mutualistic where both benefit and commensal where the unaffected host benefits the symbiont [17]. A nutrient exchange may be bidirectional or unidirectional, may be context dependent, and may occur in diverse ways [17]. Microbiota that are expected to be

The Gut Microbiota in Health and Disease, First Edition. Edited by Nimmy Srivastava, Salam A. Ibrahim, Jayeeta Chattopadhyay, and Mohamed H. Arbab.
© 2023 John Wiley & Sons Ltd. Published 2023 by John Wiley & Sons Ltd.

present, and that under normal circumstances do not cause disease, are deemed normal flora or normal microbiota [15]; normal flora may not only be harmless, but may be protective of the host [18]. The human microbiota includes bacteria, fungi, archaea, and viruses. Micro-animals, which live on the human body, are excluded. The human microbiome refers to their collective genomes [15].

Humans are colonized by many microorganisms; the traditional estimate was that humans live with ten times more non-human cells than human cells; more recent estimates have lowered this to 3:1 and even to about 1:1 [19, 20]. In fact, these are so small that there are around 100 trillion microbiota on the human body [21]. The Human Microbiome Project sequenced the genome of the human microbiota, focusing particularly on the microbiota that normally inhabit the skin, mouth, nose, digestive tract, and vagina [15]. The Project reached a milestone in 2012 when it published initial results [22]. Organisms evolve within ecosystems so that the change of one organism affects the change of others. The hologenome theory of evolution proposes that an object of natural selection is not the individual organism, but the organism together with its associated organisms, including its microbial communities; coral reefs. The hologenome theory originated in studies on coral reefs [23]. Coral reefs are the largest structures created by living organisms, and contain abundant and highly complex microbial communities. Their innate immune systems do not produce antibodies, and they should seemingly not be able to respond to new challenges except over evolutionary time scales. The puzzle of how corals managed to acquire resistance to a specific pathogen led to a 2007 proposal that a dynamic relationship exists between corals and their symbiotic microbial communities. It is thought that by altering its composition, the holobiont can adapt to changing environmental conditions far more rapidly than by genetic mutation and selection alone. Extrapolating this hypothesis to other organisms, including higher plants and animals, led to the proposal of the hologenome theory of evolution [23]. As of 2007, the hologenome theory was still being debated [24]. A major criticism has been the claim that V. shiloi was misidentified as the causative agent of coral bleaching, and that its presence in bleached O. patagonica was simply that of opportunistic colonization [25]. If this were true, the basic observation leading to the theory would be invalid. The theory has gained significant popularity as a way of explaining rapid changes in adaptation that cannot otherwise be explained by traditional mechanisms of natural selection. Within the hologenome theory, the holobiont has not only become the principal unit of natural selection, but the result of other step of integration that it is also observed at the cell (symbiogenesis, endosymbiosis) and genomic levels [7].

Microbial therapeutics, including fecal microbiota transplants (FMTs), bacterial consortia, and probiotics are increasingly being tested in patients with Clostridium difficile (C. diff) infections and other gastrointestinal (GI) disorders [25] including inflammatory bowel disease (IBD), and more recently, non-GI indications such as autism [25, 26] and cancer. In parallel to microbial therapeutics, microbial signatures are being evaluated as a novel class of biomarkers, applied for stratification of efficacy and safety in clinical trials across multiple indications [28]. This rapid increase in microbial therapeutics and biomarkers notably demands a rigorous reevaluation of the factors influencing an individual's personal gut microbiome over time. Such understanding is essential for optimizing clinical trials with any microbial component. For example, without a complete understanding of the factors influencing the gut microbiome in health and disease, we cannot determine whether the optimal FMT should be sourced from a patient who previously responded to a therapy or a healthy donor who is matched for age and sex. In this text, we present a comprehensive assessment of the gut microbiome of 946 well-defined healthy French donors from the Milieu Interieur (MI) Consortium, with 1359 shotgun metagenomic samples. Designed to study the genetic and environmental factors underlying immunological variance between individuals, the MI Consortium comprises 500 women and 500 men evenly stratified across five decades of life, from 20 to 69 years of age, for whom extensive metadata, including demographic variables, serological measures, dietary information, and systemic immune profiles are available and easily accessible [28]. Integrating these data with those from cancer patients, we demonstrate clear evidence for altered microbial communities in cancer patients across multiple non-GI indications. To build on the findings of several landmark microbiome studies [29], many of which relied on an older reference library for taxonomic classification of microbial sequence reads [30], we leveraged an expanded set of reference genomes with a novel taxonomy that corrects many misclassifications in public databases to discover new biological insights, particularly around age and sex [31]. An independent dataset was used for replication of many of the findings [32]. Study of short-term longitudinal samplings from half the donors found that individuals are more similar to themselves over time compared with others [33]. However, the degree of stability between individuals was quite variable and was influenced by lifestyle factors as well as baseline composition. Overall, the aims of the study are threefold. First, we introduce a new microbiome analysis approach that uses an expanded set of reference genomes with a novel taxonomy to discover new, statistically robust insights into host/bacteria biology that will enable personalized medicine approaches for microbial therapeutics and biomarkers. Second, we provide the rich metadata and 1000-plus deep shotgun metagenomic samples described here as a resource on which future microbiome studies can test and build new computational tools, as well as be compared against disease cohorts. Finally, while demonstrating the utility of this resource as a control population, we define global shifts in the gut microbiomes of patients with non-GI tumors compared with healthy donors normalised based on relative evolutionary divergence [31]. The impact of this procedure was particularly prominent for species of the genus Clostridium, which were split into 121 unique genera spanning 29 families [31]. This could be especially meaningful for analysis of gut microbiome samples, as Clostridium species are prevalent community members and often emerge in association studies. The RefSeq sequences and taxonomic tree from the GTDB, including its naming conventions, were used to build a reference database for the k-mer-based program Kraken2 [33] and read-reassignment step [34]. This custom Kraken2/GTDB pipeline was applied to 1359 quality-controlled samples from 946 MI donors and compared using both the marker gene-based tool Metaphlan2 [35] and Kraken2, with the same 23 505 reference genomes using their original NCBI taxonomies. Consistently, more bacterial taxa were identified per sample with Kraken2 than Metaphlan2, a result of the updated reference database and higher sensitivity of this k-mer-based approach. Between the two Kraken databases (GTDB and NCBI), richness varied depending on how taxa were redistributed by GTDB. For example, GTDB split 2397 NCBI genera into 3205, while it collapsed 18 795 NCBI species into 13 446. Despite finer-level differences, the overall distribution of phyla across the three approaches was similar, indicating that Kraken2/GTDB pipeline results would be consistent with previous analyses. As such, a combination of k-mer-based read assignment and genome-based taxonomy allows higher resolution analysis of shotgun metagenomic samples. Using variable gut microbiomes in a restricted geographical region to complement our optimized taxa-based approach and further use of the resolution afforded by shotgun metagenomic sequencing, we applied HUMANn2 to identify the functional potential of microbial pathways present in the MI samples. Using both the Kraken2/GTDB and HUMANn2 pipelines, we identified a broad range of diversity across the 946 individuals in this geographically restricted cohort of healthy French adults. This diversity was observed in terms of metabolic pathway richness (282 ± 40, mean $\pm$ SD), species richness (248 ± 32), and Shannon diversity (3.7 ± 0.35), which account for both richness and evenness (Data S1, table 2). Across donors, our GTDB pipeline confirmed Firmicutes and Bacteroidota (formerly Bacteroidetes) as the most abundant phyla in the gut, but enabled distinction among the original Firmicutes phyla, which was further divided in the GTDB into 12 distinct categories; Firmicutes, Firmicutes_A, Firmicutes_B, ... Firmicutes_K (Data S1, table 1). Notably, throughout the GTDB, the group containing type material (if known) kept the original unsuffixed name. Of those, seven were present in this cohort, with Firmicutes_A the most abundant, followed by Firmicutes and Firmicutes, highlighting the finer granularity, even at the phylum level, provided by GTDB-based taxonomic calls. Subsequent application of the Bray–Curtis (BC) distance metric is a means to assess species presence/absence in addition to relative abundance.

References

1 Dastogeer, K.M., Tumpa, F.H., Sultana, A. et al. (2020). Plant microbiome–An account of the factors that shape community composition and diversity. *Cur. Plant Bio.* 23: 100161. https://doi.org/10.1016/j.cpb.2020.100161. Material was copied from this source, which is available under a Creative Commons Attribution 4.0 International License.

2 De Sordi, L., Lourenço, M., and Debarbieux, L. (2019). The battle within: interactions of bacteriophages and bacteria in the gastrointestinal tract. *Cell Host & Micro.* 25 (2): 210–218. https://doi.org/10.1016/j.chom.2019.01.018.

3 Peterson, J., Garges, S., Giovanni, M. et al. (2009). The NIH human microbiome project. *Genome Res. NIH HMP Work. Gr.* 19 (12): 2317–2323. https://doi.org/10.1101/gr.096651.109.

4 Backhed, F., Ley, R.E., Sonnenburg, J.L. et al. (2005). Host-bacterial mutualism in the human intestine. *Science* 307 (5717): 1915–1920. https://doi.org/10.1126/science.1104816.

5 Turnbaugh, P.J., Ley, R.E., Hamady, M. et al. (2007). The human microbiome project. *Nature* 449 (7164): 804–810. https://doi.org/10.1038/nature06244.

6 Ley, R.E., Peterson, D.A., and Gordon, J.I. (2006). Ecological and evolutionary forces shaping microbial diversity in the human intestine. *Cell* 124 (4): 837–848. https://doi.org/10.1016/j.cell.2006.02.017.

7 Salvucci, E. (2016). Microbiome, holobiont and the net of life. *Crit. Rev. Microbio.* 42 (3): 485–494. https://doi.org/10.3109/1040841X.2014.962478.

8 Guerrero, R., Margulis, L., and Berlanga, M. (2013). Symbiogenesis: the holobiont as a unit of evolution. *Int. Micro.* 16 (3): 133–143. https://doi.org/10.2436/20.1501.01.188.

9 Davenport, E.R., Sanders, J.G., Song, S.J. et al. (2017). The human microbiome in evolution. *BMC Bio.* 15: 127. https://doi.org/10.1186/s12915-017-0454-7.

10 Moeller, A.H., Li, Y., Ngole, E.M. et al. (2014). Evolution of the human gut flora. *Proc. Nat. Aca. Sci.* 111 (46): 16431–16435. https://doi.org/10.1073/pnas.1419136111.

11 Jugder, B.-E., Kamareddine, L., and Watnick, P.I. (2021). Microbiota-derived acetate activates intestinal innate immunity via the Tip60 histone acetyltransferase complex. *Immunity* 54 (8): 1683–1687.e3. https://doi.org/10.1016/j.immuni.2021.05.017.

12 Mendes, R. and Raaijmakers, J.M. (2015). Cross-kingdom similarities in microbiome functions. *ISME J.* 9 (9): 1905–1907. https://doi.org/10.1038/ismej.2015.7.

13 Bosch, T.C.G. and McFall-Ngai, M.J. (2011). Metaorganisms as the new frontier. *Zoology* 114 (4): 185–190. https://doi.org/10.1016/j.zool.2011.04.001.

14 Poreau B. (2014). Biologie et complexitéhistoire et modèles du commensalisme. *PhD Dissertation*, University of Lyon, France.

15 Sherwood, L., Willey, J., and Woolverton, C. (2013). *Prescott's Microbiology*, 9e, 713–721. New York: McGraw Hill.

16 Quigley, E.M. (2013). Gut bacteria in health and disease. *Gastroenterol. Hepatol. (NY)* 9 (9): 560–569.

17 Remy, W., Taylor, T.N., Hass, H. et al. (1994). Four hundred-million-year-old vesicular arbuscular mycorrhizae. *Pro. Nat. Acad. Sci. USA* 91 (25): 11841–11843. https://doi.org/10.1073/pnas.91.25.11841.

18 Copeland, C.S. (2017 September–October). The World within us. *Health. J. New Orleans*.

19 Compant, S., Duffy, B., Nowak, J. et al. (2005). Use of plant growth-promoting bacteria for biocontrol of plant diseases: principles, mechanisms of action, and future prospects. *App. Environ. Microbio.* 71 (9): 4951–4959. https://doi.org/10.1128/AEM.71.9.4951-4959.2005.

20 Tkacz, A., Cheema, J., Chandra, G. et al. (2015). Stability and succession of the rhizosphere microbiota depends upon plant type and soil composition. *ISME J.* 9 (11): 2349–2359. https://doi.org/10.1038/ismej.2015.41.

21 Copeland, C.S. (2019). What is Clostridium difficile? *Vital* 4.

22 (2014 January). *American academy of microbiology FAQ: human microbiome*. Archived 2016-12-31 at the Wayback Machine.

23 Judah L.. (2014). *Ten times more microbial cells than body cells in humans?* Rosner for Microbe Magazine.

24 Alison Abbott for Nature News. (2016 January 8). *Scientists bust myth that our bodies have more bacteria than human cells*.

25 Sender, R., Fuchs, S., and Milo, R. (2016). Are we really vastly outnumbered? Revisiting the ratio of bacterial to host cells in humans. *Cell* 164 (3): 337–340. https://doi.org/10.1016/j.cell.2016.01.013.

26 On and In You. *Micropia*. https://www.micropia.nl/en/discover/stories/on-and-in-you/#:~:text=They're%20on%20you%2C%20in,re%20known%20as%20human%20microbiota.

27 (2012 June 13). NIH Human Microbiome Project defines normal bacterial makeup of the body. *NIH News*.

28 Bataille, A., Lee-Cruz, L., Tripathi, B., et al. (2016). Microbiome variation across amphibian skin regions: implications for chytridiomycosis mitigation efforts. *Microb. Eco.* 71 (1): 221–232. https://doi.org/10.1007/s00248-015-0653-0.

29 Woodhams, D.C., Rollins-Smith, L.A., Alford, R.A. et al. (2007). Innate immune defenses of amphibian skin: antimicrobial peptides and more. *Anim. Conserv.* 10 (4): 425–428. https://doi.org/10.1111/j.1469-1795.2007.00150.x.

30 Brulc, J.M., Antonopoulos, D.A., Miller, M.E.B. et al. (2009). Gene-centric metagenomics of the fiber-adherent bovine rumen microbiome reveals forage specific glycoside hydrolases. *Proc. Natl. Acad. Sci. USA* 106 (6): 1948–1953. https://doi.org/10.1073/pnas.0806191105.

31 Russell, S.L., Gold, M.J., Hartmann, M. et al. (2012). Early life antibiotic-driven changes in microbiota enhance susceptibility to allergic asthma. *EMBO Rep.* 13 (5): 440–447. https://doi.org/10.1038/embor.2012.32.

32 Russell, S.L., Gold, M.J., Reynolds, L.A. et al. (2014). Perinatal antibiotic-induced shifts in gut microbiota have differential effects on inflammatory lung diseases. *J. All. Clin. Immu.* 135 (1): 100–109. https://doi.org/10.1016/j.jaci.2014.06.027.

33 Turnbaugh, P.J., Ley, R.E., Mahowald, M.A. et al. (2006). An obesity-associated gut microbiome with increased capacity for energy harvest. *Nature* 444 (7122): 1027–1031. https://doi.org/10.1038/nature05414.

34 Faith, J.J., Ahern, P.P., Ridaura, V.K. et al. (2014). Identifying gut microbe-host phenotype relationships using combinatorial communities in gnotobiotic mice. *Sci. Trans.Med.* 6 (220): 220. https://doi.org/10.1126/scitranslmed.3008051.

35 Barfod, K.K., Roggenbuck, M., Hansen, L.H. et al. (2013). The murine lung microbiome in relation to the intestinal and vaginal bacterial communities. *BMC Microbio.* 13: 303. https://doi.org/10.1186/1471-2180-13-303.

2

Composition and Diversity of Gut Microbiota

Lisa F.M. Lee Nen That[1] and Jessica Pandohee[2]

[1] School of Science, RMIT University, Bundoora, Victoria, Australia
[2] Telethon Kids Institute, Nedlands, Western Australia, Australia

2.1 Introduction

The human gastrointestinal tract, which has a surface of 250–400 m^2, is home to a rich, complex, and diverse microbial community which is evaluated at 100 trillion [1–3]. The community containing fungi, archaea, viruses, bacteria, and helminths constitute the gut microbiota [4]. Initially, the bacterial population was estimated to be 10^{14} bacterial cells, which is 10 times more than human cells and had 100 times more genes than the human genome [3, 5, 6]. However, an updated estimate indicated that the ratio of bacteria to human cells is 1:1 [7].

A co-dependent relationship has evolved leading to mutualistic interactions between the host and the microbial community as the microorganisms have provided many health benefits to the host [1]. Moreover, strong host selection and coevolution have shaped the diversity of the gut microbiota. Indeed, the relationship between mammals and the bacteria present in the gut is ancient and suggests coevolution due to the presence of several groups of similar and related bacteria in different mammals. This also highlights the beneficial impact on the host as both parties cooperate for a functionally stable ecosystem [1]. Humans have certainly benefited from interactions with the gut microbiota, as they prevent infections caused by pathogens [8, 9], allow synthesis and absorption of nutrients and metabolites [10, 11], and protect the gut barrier in behavioural disorders [12].

Previously, the study of the microbial community in the gastrointestinal tract relied on culture-based methods. However, advanced technology gave rise to new methods that allowed the amplification of conserved regions, such as the 16S rRNA gene using universal primers, and the amplified products may be compared to sequences in databases for identification [13]. Two large-scale projects, namely MetaHit and The Human Microbiome Project, have also contributed to our understanding and further characterised the microbial communities associated with humans [14, 15]. This chapter aims to provide an overview of the recent advances on the composition and diversity of the gut microbiota.

The Gut Microbiota in Health and Disease, First Edition. Edited by Nimmy Srivastava, Salam A. Ibrahim, Jayeeta Chattopadhyay, and Mohamed H. Arbab.
© 2023 John Wiley & Sons Ltd. Published 2023 by John Wiley & Sons Ltd.

2.2   Composition and Diversity of Gut Microbiota Throughout Lifespan

The bacterial community in the gastrointestinal tract undergoes several changes over a lifespan [3, 16]. From infant to adulthood, diversity in gut microbiota increases and becomes more complex [17]. At adulthood, the composition remains stable and as they age, interindividual variation is greater and there are shifts in the composition of the gut microbiota. Table 2.1 gives an overview of the bacterial composition at different life stages.

Table 2.1   Composition and diversity of gut microbiota throughout a lifespan.

Stages of lifespan		Composition and diversity of gut microbiota
Fetus		The gut microbiome starts developing before birth and is shaped by the mother's diet.
		Microorganisms detected in the placenta, amniotic fluid, fetal membranes, and cord blood.
		Community in placenta: Firmicutes, Tenericutes, Proteobacteria, Bacteroidetes, and Fusobacteria and resembles oral microbiome.
Baby	Preterm	Increase in pathogens, bacterial diversity is reduced compared to healthy term baby.
		Most abundant: facultative anaerobe; Enterobacteriaceae, Enterococcaceae, *Lactobacillus*.
		Less abundant: *Bifidobacterium, Bacteroides, Atopobium*.
	Delivery mode	Vaginal delivery: 72% similarity between infant and mother's fecal microbiota. High number of *Lactobacilli*. Early colonizers: facultative anaerobes (*Staphylococcus, Streptococcus, Enterococcus, Enterobacter*); obligate anaerobes (*Bifidobacterium, Bacteroides, Clostridium*).
		Caesarean birth (C-section): less bacterial diversity, bacterial community similar to skin and hospital environment. Increase in *Clostridium difficile*, absence of *Bifidobacterium* and *Bacteroides*.
		Difference in bacterial communities between elective and emergency C-section.
	At birth	Lower diversity and high interindividual variation. Dominant: Firmicutes, Proteobacteria, Actinobacteria. Less abundant: Bacteroidetes.
	Diet	Breast-fed babies: *Bifidobacteria* and *Lactobacillus* are dominant. Decrease in Firmicutes and Proteobacteria.
		Bottle-fed babies: Higher diversity. Increase in Bacteroidetes, *Clostridium coccoides, Staphylococcus*. Less abundant: *Bifidobacteria,*
Infant (first year)	Weaning	Microbiota becomes more complex, most abundant: *Bifidobacterium, Bacteroides*.
		Increase: *Clostridia* (*Clostridium coccoides*). Decrease: facultative anaerobes.

Table 2.1   (Continued)

Stages of lifespan	Composition and diversity of gut microbiota
Children	Main phyla: Bacteroidetes and Firmicutes, Interindividual variation in ratio of the 2 phyla, increase in diversity and similarity with adult microbiota increases.
	First four years: Enrichment in Proteobacteria and Actinobacteria.
	At 2.5 years, adult-like microbiota in terms of composition and diversity. Functional capabilities mostly involved in physical development.
	Preadolescent children: Increase in butyrate-producing bacteria (*Roseburia* spp., *Faecalibacterium* spp., *Ruminococcus* spp.), *Alistipes* spp., *Bacteroides vulgatus* and *Bacteroides xylanisolvens*.
Adolescents (11–18 years)	High level: *Bifidobacterium* and *Clostridium* spp.
Adults	Most abundant: Firmicutes, Bacteroidetes, and Actinobacteria. Less abundant: Proteobacteria, Verrucomicrobia. Stability is relatively unchanged in adulthood. Dominant: Lachnospiraceae and Ruminococcaceae (10–45% of total fecal bacteria), Bacteroidaceae and Prevotellaceae (remaining 12–60%).
Older adults	With age, both Firmicutes and *bifidobacteria* decline. Increase in Bacteroidetes and Proteobacteria. High interindividual variation. Diversity varies according to residence such as community, long-term care, hospital. Less diversity in adults in long-term care than those residing in community.
Centenarian	Increase: *Fusobacterium, Bacillus, Staphylococcus, Corynebacterium,* and Micrococcaceae family.
	Decrease: Butyrate-producing bacteria (*Faecalibacteriumprausnitzii, Eubacterium rectale, Eubacterium hallii, Eubacterium ventriosum*).

2.3   Composition of Bacterial Community in the Different Sections of the Gastrointestinal Tract

The composition and abundance of bacteria varies along the digestive tract due to the different environmental conditions within each section [18]. More than 90% of the bacteria found in the gastrointestinal tract belong to the phyla Firmicutes, Bacteroidetes, Actinobacteria, and Proteobacteria [3]. These microorganisms are usually found in the lumen, which is the gap in the digestive tract, and the mucosal layer of the digestive tract [16].

It has been estimated that saliva contains 10^9 cfu/ml [19, 20]. The cheeks, tongue, tooth surfaces, and saliva represent microenvironments in the oral cavity for a diverse community of bacteria which include *Streptococci, Clostridia*, fusobacteria, actinobacteria, proteobacteria, *Prevotella*, and *Bacteroides* [19]. In the esophagus, the most common microorganisms identified include *Streptococcus, Prevotella*, and *Veillonella* spp, and they only reside in the esophageal wall temporarily [16, 21]. Other bacteria such as *Veillonella, Clostridium*, and

Neisseria may also temporarily reside in the stomach [22]. *Helicobacter pylori* which is not acid-tolerant and has optimum growth conditions at pH 7 could be considered as an endemic gastric bacterium, as it has adapted to the harsh conditions inside the stomach, and resides mostly close to the antrum within the mucus layer where it has created its own suitable environment. There have been few studies carried out in the small intestine where the bacterial population is considered the lowest [16, 20]. Indeed, the duodenum had an estimated 10^3 cfu/ml of viable bacteria. Although it contains mostly acid-tolerant bacteria from incoming stomach content, other bacteria such as *Bacteroides*, *Bifidobacterium*, *Veillonella*, *Staphylococcus*, and Enterobacteria have also been identified in lesser numbers. The jejunum has similar microbial composition as the duodenum. The bacterial population in the ileum is more diverse and increases to 10^6–10^8 cfu/ml, as there is lesser movement and a neutral pH [20]. The bacteria present are mostly facultative anaerobes and aerobes [23]. The colon is home to one of the most populous and diverse microbial communities in nature with 300–1000 bacterial species present [16, 20]. Obligate anaerobes including *Bacteroides*, *Eubacterium*, and *Bifidobacterium* predominate the colon (90% of cultivable bacteria in the colon) followed by facultative anaerobes such as *Streptococcus* and enterobacteria [21].

The existence of community types in the gut microbiota has been demonstrated and are distinct in bacterial composition [24]. A study by Arumugam et al. has identified in individuals from 6 nationalities that the microbial can be grouped into three distinct enterotypes, namely *Bacteroides*, *Prevotella*, and *Ruminococcus* [25]. These enterotypes are distinguished by the different methods used for energy production from fermentable resources in the colon. *Bacteroides* break down carbohydrates and proteins to generate energy, while degradation of mucin glycoproteins is mainly caused by *Prevotella*. As for *Ruminococcus*, it is involved in mucin degradation and its uptake as the bacteria is involved in membrane transporters. It was argued that the term faecotypes would be more appropriate instead of enterotype, as enterotypes were identified by analysing fecal samples, and composition differs at different sections in the gastrointestinal tract [26].

There have been a few studies that questioned the existence of the three distinct enterotypes [27]. Wu et al. reported that in a long-term study looking at the effect of diet [28], there was a distinction between the two enterotype *Prevotella* and *Bacteroidetes* brought about by diet, and other genera responsible for the differences were *Alistipes*, *Parabacteroides*, *Paraprevotella*, and *Catenibacterium*. *Ruminococcus*, the third enterotype was not distinct and was associated with *Bacteroidetes*. Long-term diet strongly correlated with the enterotypes. The *Bacteroides* enterotype was characterised by animal protein and saturated fats, while *Prevotella* was mostly associated with a diet rich in carbohydrates and simple sugars.

Further research has also suggested that instead of three distinct enterotypes, bacterial communities may vary along a gradient and may be led by either *Prevotella* on one end or *Bacteroides* on the other [29, 30].

2.4 Stability, Resilience, and Functional Redundancy

Although diversity has been considered necessary for a stable ecosystem, many different and unrelated bacteria fulfil similar roles in the gut microbiota leading to functional redundancy, where taxonomic diversity varies among individuals while the functional stability is still maintained [1, 31]. Indeed, a study looking at obese and lean twins has revealed that a core functional group was present at the level of genes in bacteria that is crucial for several metabolic activities [32]. The existence of this functional group allows the resident bacteria to carry out a wide range of metabolic activities making the community functionally diverse [33]. Functional redundancy has also been considered a determinant in the stability and resilience of the gut microbiota, especially in response to perturbations. The stability of the gut microbiota depends on how the community can revert to its original state making it resilient [34]. Despite a change in taxonomic diversity, this is possible because more than one group of bacteria can carry out functions to restore to the state prior perturbation. Maintaining the core functional microbiota is important for health and any disruption may lead to diseases. The core microbiome is involved in various pathways including metabolism of amino-acid and carbohydrates [32]. Dysbiosis occurs when the gut microbiota fails to return to its original state and is usually dependent on how resilient and stable the gut microbiome is [32].

Specific functions may still be confined to certain groups of bacteria, which makes them keystone species. In the gut microbiota, keystone species play important roles in keeping the diversity and community structure by interacting with other resident bacteria [35, 36]. As they are usually relatively low in numbers, their loss would have a profound impact on the community. In a study looking at the amylolytic activity of four bacteria, namely *Eubacterium rectale*, *Bacteroides thetaiotaomicron*, *Bifidobacterium adolescentis*, and *Ruminococcusbromii*, the bacterium *R. bromii* had the most superior degradative ability when co-cultured with each of the four bacteria although it was inoculated in a medium that limited its growth [37]. This highlights the importance of *R. bromii* as a keystone species as many bacteria depend on it for provision of substrates. *Akkermansiamuciniphila* may be considered as another keystone species as it breaks down mucin to provide energy source, leading to increased growth of other bacteria in co-cultures [38].

2.5 Interactions in the Gut Microbiota

In the gut microbiota, no bacteria can survive on its own, and interactions between microbes and with the host are important to shape the community (Figure 2.1). Microbial interactions such as competition, predation, and cooperation in the gastrointestinal tract are constantly happening, and bacteria have had to adapt to tolerating surrounding bacteria while resisting invading pathogens, leading to a healthy state of the gut microbiota.

2.5.1 Microbe–microbe Interactions

Cooperation has been observed in bacteria such as congeners *Bacteroides ovatus* and *Bacteroides vulgatus* [39]. *B. ovatus* is a symbiont found in the gut that breaks down a large quantity of substrates such as inulin for *B. vulgatus* at its own expense. By doing so, the fitness of *B. ovatus* increases as it receives benefits from its congener, which may include generation of growth promoting factors.

Facilitation occurs because the presence of a closely related species, i.e., belonging to the same family in the gut microbiota, may also increase the chances of colonisation of a

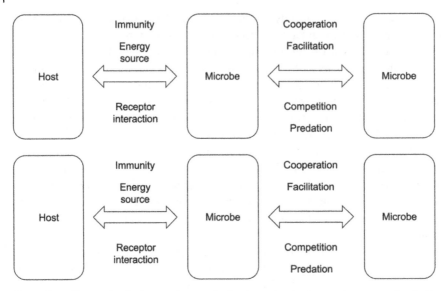

Figure 2.1   Host–microbe interactions and microbe–microbe interactions occurring in the gastrointestinal tract.

specific novel bacteria [2]. Factors that promote abundance of the related species may also encourage invasion of the bacterial species. A study by Stecher et al. showed that high levels of *E. coli* may have promoted the invasion of *Salmonella* as they require similar environmental conditions and are closely related [2]. Another example of facilitation occurred when rats with intestinal *Lactobacilli* were administered *Lactobacillus reuteri* and within 5 days, the population of *L. reuteri* was significantly increased and correlated with high levels of intestinal *Lactobacilli*.

Competition among bacteria has been reported when they occupy same ecological niche or require similar resources for survival [20]. When the gut microbiota is rich and diverse with the range of ecological niches filled, invading pathogens that compete for similar requirements may be less likely to invade. Resident bacteria such as *Bacteroides fragilis* have developed mechanisms such as toxin production or possess type IV secretion systems to combat other bacteria [40–42].

Bacteria in the gut are also subjected to predation by bacteriophages and other bacteria [43]. All these interactions indicate how complex and dynamic the microbial community in the gut is.

2.5.2   Host–microbe Interactions

Bacteria in the gastrointestinal tract has also developed a commensal and symbiotic relationship with the host whereby they coexist without harming each other and where one provides benefits to the other [44]. They also interact with each other to create a stable and healthy environment in the gastrointestinal tract, and resist any invasion from pathogens. Interaction with the host occurs through the modulation of the gut epithelium or when influencing the immune system [45].

Moreover, production of short chain fatty acids (SCFA) by resident bacteria from dietary fibres are energy sources for the intestinal epithelial cells and the gut microbiota. These SCFA play an important role in immunity and host physiology. A study by Maslowski et al. demonstrated that as the SCFA bind to a G-protein coupled receptor 43, it triggers an anti-inflammatory response that lead to modulation of apoptotic pathways [46].

The intestinal epithelium is covered by a layer of mucus made of glycoproteins to protect against pathogens such as *Salmonella*. It is also a food source for a select group of bacteria such as *Bacteroides fragilis*, *Akkermansiamuciniphila*, and *Bifidobacterium bifidum* as they produce enzymes that break down glycoproteins to release monosaccharides [47].

The mucus layer of the epithelium and the gut microbiota also work in concert to prevent pathogenic invasion [48]. Some bacteria also release toxins and antimicrobial peptides.

2.5.3 Colonisation of the Gut Microbiota

During the first years in a human lifespan, the process by which early colonisers settle and establish in the gut is termed *ecological succession* [20]. The community grows in complexity, diversity, and composition until it reaches a climax and remains stable throughout adulthood. Colonisation resistance occurs as residential bacteria protect the gut against pathogens.

Secondary succession is defined as the process by which the microbial community goes through a recovery phase after a perturbation such as antibiotic administration [49, 50]. The recovery stage is characterised by a complex process in multiple stages with interactions among bacterial species [51]. The presence of keystone taxa acts as a catalyst as it triggers a response that leads to restoration of the entire ecosystem. Moreover, 21 bacterial species have been linked to recovery and breakdown of complex polysaccharides and mucin is an important determinant for ecosystem recovery. Four ecological processes are also being considered to understand the microbial succession, namely dispersal potential, availability of resources, changes in environmental stresses, and predation by bacteriophages [52].

Chng et al. reported similar results from a meta-analysis of effect of antibiotic treatment on gut microbiota [51]. The initial step in the recovery phase includes the presence of rapid-growing facultative anaerobes that degrade complex substrates leading to biomass recovery, followed by aerotolerant bacteria that degrade fibre and mucin [50, 51]. At this stage, there is possibly functional redundancy in the community. Finally, the obligate anaerobes that break down fibre and other bacteria also return leading to stability and diversity in the ecosystem.

2.6   Conclusion

This chapter has highlighted the progress made in characterising the composition and diversity of the gut microbiota and demonstrated how the bacterial community has developed a close relationship with the host. Understanding the many processes that occur in the gut microbiota can allow us to translate the information into clinical practice and develop diagnostic strategies. As there are interindividual variations in the gut microbiota, and considering the important role of the microbiota in diseases, personalised medicine could become a new avenue and lead to development of next-generation tools [53, 54].

References

1 Bäckhed, F., Ley, R.E., Sonnenburg, J.L. et al. (2005). Host-bacterial mutualism in the human intestine. *Science* 307: 1915–1920.

2 Stecher, B., Chaffron, S., Käppeli, R. et al. (2010). Like will to like: abundances of closely related species can predict susceptibility to intestinal colonization by pathogenic and commensal bacteria. *PLoS Patho.* 6 (1): e1000711.

3 Thursby, E. and Juge, N. (2017). Introduction to the human gut microbiota. *Biochem. J.* 474: 1823–1836.

4 Vemuri, R., Shankar, E.M., Chieppa, M. et al. (2020). Beyond just bacteria: functional biomes in the gut ecosystem including virome, mycobiome, archaeome and helminths. *Microorganisms* 8: 483.

5 Savage, D.C. (1977). Microbial ecology of the gastrointestinal tract. *An. Rev. Microbio.* 31: 107–133.

6 Gill, S.R., Pop, M., DeBoy, R.T. et al. (2006). Metagenomic analysis of the human distal gut microbiome. *Science* 312 (5778): 1355–1359.

7 Sender, R., Fuchs, S., and Milo, R. (2016). Revised estimates for the number of human and bacteria cells in the body. *PLoS Bio.* 14 (8): e1002533.

8 Khosravi, A. and Mazmanian, S.K. (2013). Disruptions of the gut microbiome as a risk factor for microbial infections. *Cur. Opin. Microbio.* 16 (2): 221–227.

9 Chiu, L., Bazin, T., Truchetet, M. et al. (2017). Protective microbiota: from localized to long-reaching co-immunity. *Front. Immuno.* 8: 1678.

10 LeBlanc, J.G., Milani, C., de Giori, G.S. et al. (2013). Bacteria as vitamin suppliers to their host: A gut microbiota perspective. *Cur. Opin. Biotechno.* 24: 160–168.

11 Rinninella, E., Raoul, P., Cintoni, M. et al. (2019). What is the healthy gut microbiota composition? A changing ecosystem across age, environment, diet, and diseases. *Microorganisms* 7: 14.

12 Leclercq, S., Matamoros, S., Cani, P.D. et al. (2014). Intestinal permeability, gut-bacterial dysbiosis, and behavioral markers of alcohol-dependence severity. *Proceed. Nat. Acad. Sci.* 111 (42): E4485–E4493.

13 Zoetendal, E.G., Rajilić-Stojanović, M., and de Vos, W.M. (2008). High-throughput diversity and functionality analysis of the gastrointestinal tract microbiota. *Gut* 57: 1605–1615.

14 Qin, J., Li, R., Raes, J. et al. (2010). A human gut microbial gene catalogue established by metagenomic sequencing. *Nature* 464: 59–67.

15 The Human Microbiome Project Consortium. (2012). Structure, function and diversity of the healthy human microbiome. *Nature* 486 (7402): 207–214.

16 Ishiguro, E., Haskey, N. and Campbell, K. (2018). *Gut Microbiota: Interactive Effects of Nutrition and Health*. Elsevier.

17 Greenhalgh, K., Meyer, K.M., Aagaard, K.M. et al. (2016). The human gut microbiome in health: establishment and resilience of microbiota over a lifetime. *Environ. Microbio.* 18 (7): 2103–2116.

18 Zoetendal, E.G., Raes, J., van den Bogert, B. et al. (2012). The human small intestinal microbiota is driven by rapid uptake and conversion of simple carbohydrates. *ISME J.* 6: 1415–1426.

19 Maukonen, J., Mättö, J., Suihko, M. et al. (2008). Intra-individual diversity and similarity of salivary and faecal microbiota. *J.Med. Microbio.* 57: 1560–1568.

20 Lawley, T.D. and Walker, A.W. (2012). Intestinal colonization resistance. *Immunology* 138.

21 Wilson, M. (2005). *Microbial Inhabitants of Humans: Their Ecology and Role in Health and Disease*. New York: Cambridge University Press.

22 Nardone, G. and Compare, D. (2015). The human gastric microbiota: is it time to rethink the pathogenesis of stomach diseases? *United Euro. Gastroenter. J.* 3 (3): 255–260.

23 Hayashi, H., Takahashi, R., Nishi, T. et al. (2005). Molecular analysis of jejunal, ileal, caecal and recto-sigmoidal human colonic microbiota using 16S rRNA gene libraries and terminal restriction fragment length polymorphism. *J. Med. Microbio.* 54: 1093–1101.

24 Ding, T. and Schloss, P.D. (2014). Dynamics and associations of microbial community types across the human body. *Nature* 509: 357–360.

25 Arumugam, M., Raes, J., Pelletier, E. et al. (2011). Enterotypes of the human gut microbiome. *Nature* 473 (7346): 174–180.

26 Siezen, R.J. and Kleerebezem, M. (2011). The human gut microbiome: are we our enterotypes? *Microb. Biotechno.* 4 (5): 550–553.

27 Jeffery, I.B., Claesson, M.J., O'Toole, P.W. et al. (2012). Categorization of the gut microbiota: Enterotypes or gradients? *Nat. Rev. Microbio.* 10: 591–592.

28 Wu, G.D., Chen, J., Hoffmann, C. et al. (2011). Linking long-term dietary patterns with gut microbial enterotypes. *Science* 334 (6052): 105–108.

29 Huse, S.M., Ye, Y., Zhou, Y., and Fodor AA. (2012). A core human microbiome as viewed through 16S rRNA sequence clusters. *PLoS One* 7 (6): e34242.

30 Yong, E. (2012). Gut microbial 'enterotypes' become less clear-cut. *Nature*.

31 McCann, K.S. (2000). The diversity-stability debate. *Nature* 405: 228–233.

32 Turnbaugh, P., Hamady, M., Yatsunenko, T. et al. (2009). A core gut microbiome in obese and lean twins. *Nature* 457 (7228): 480–484.

33 Tian, L., Wang, X., Wu, A. et al. (2020). Deciphering functional redundancy in the human microbiome. *Nat. Comm.* 11: 6217.

34 Moya, A. and Ferrer, M. (2016). Functional redundancy induced stability of gut microbiota subjected to disturbance. *Trend. Microbio.* 24 (5): 402–413.

35 Trosvik, P. and de Muinck, E.J. (2015). Ecology of bacteria in the human gastrointestinal tract identification of keystone and foundation taxa. *Microbiome* 3: 44.

36 Pereira, F.C. and Berry, D. (2017). Microbial nutrient niches in the gut. *Environ. Microbio.* 19 (4): 1366–1378.

37 Ze, X., Duncan, S.H., Louis, P. et al. (2012). *Ruminococcus bromii* is a keystone species for the degradation of resistant starch in the human colon. *ISME J.* 6: 1535–1543.

38 Png, C.W., Lindén, S.K., Gilshenan, K.S. et al. (2010). Mucolytic bacteria with increased prevalence in IBD mucosa augment in vitro utilization of mucin by other bacteria. *Am. J. Gastroenter.* 105: 2420–2428.

39 Rakoff-Nahoum, S., Foster, K.R., and Comstock, L.E. (2016). The evolution of cooperation within the gut microbiota. *Nature* 533: 255–259.

40 Hecht, A.L., Casterline, B.W., Earley, Z.M. et al. (2016). Strain competition restricts colonization of an enteric pathogen and prevents colitis. *EMBO Rep.* 17: 1281–1291.

41 Roelofs, K.G., Coyne, M.J., Gentyala, R.R. et al. (2016). *Bacteroidales* secreted antimicrobial proteins target surface molecules necessary for gut colonization and mediate competition *in vivo*. *MBio* 7 (4): e01055–e01016.

42 Figueiredo, A.R.T. and Kramer, J. (2020). Cooperation and conflict within the microbiota and their effects on animal hosts. *Front. Eco. Evo.* 8: 132.

43 Gagliardi, A., Totino, V., Cacciotti, F. et al. (2018). Rebuilding the gut microbiota ecosystem. *Int. J. Environ. Res. Pub. Health* 15 (8): 1679.

44 Hooper, L.V. and Gordon, J.I. (2001). Commensal host-bacterial relationships in the gut. *Science* 292: 1115–1118.

45 Vivarelli, S., Salemi, R., Candido, S. et al. (2019). Gut microbiota and cancer: from pathogenesis to therapy. *Cancers* 11: 38.

46 Maslowski, K.M., Vieira, A.T., Ng, A. et al. (2009). Regulation of inflammatory responses by gut microbiota and chemoattractant receptor GPR43. *Nature* 461: 1282–1287.

47 Sicard, J., Le Bihan, G., Vogeleer, P. et al. (2017). Interactions of intestinal bacteria with components of the intestinal mucus. *Front. Cell. Inf. Microbio.* 7: 387.

48 Takiishi, T., Fenero, C.I.M., and Câmara, N.O.S. (2017). Intestinal barrier and gut microbiota: Shaping our immune responses throughout life. *Tiss. Bar.* 5 (4): e1373208.

49 Horn, H.S. (1974). The ecology of secondary succession. *An. Rev. Eco. Systemat.* 5: 25–37.

50 Gibbons, S.M. (2020). Keystone taxa indispensable for microbiome recovery. *Nat. Microbio.* 5: 1067–1068.

51 Chng, K.R., Ghosh, T.S., Tan, Y.H. et al. (2020). Metagenome-wide association analysis identifies microbial determinants of post-antibiotic ecological recovery in the gut. *Nat.Eco. Evol.* 4: 1256–1267.

52 David, L.A., Weil, A., Ryan, E.T. et al. (2015). Gut microbial succession follows acute secretory diarrhea in humans. *MBio* 6 (3): e00381–00415.

53 Hov, J.E. and Trøseid, M. (2015). Personalized medicine targeting the gut microbiota? *Tidsskr Nor Laegeforen* 135: 624.

54 Fassarella, M., Blaak, E.E., Penders, J. et al. (2021). Gut microbiome stability and resilience: elucidating the response to perturbations in order to modulate gut health. *Gut* 70: 595–605.

3

Factors Affecting Composition and Diversity of Gut Microbiota: A Disease Hallmark

Rohan Samir Kumar Sachan[1], Khushboo[1], Inderpal Devgon[1], Atif Khurshid Wani[1,], Nahid Akhtar[1], Tahir ul Gani Mir[1], Ab Waheed Wani[2], and Ajit Prakash[3]*

[1] *School of Bioengineering and Biosciences, Lovely Professional University, Punjab, India*
[2] *Department of Horticulture, Lovely Professional University, Punjab, India*
[3] *Department of Biochemistry and Biophysics, University of North Carolina, Chapel Hill, USA*
* *Corresponding author*

3.1 Introduction

Microbial communities modulate the influence of environmental factors on human health and diseases. They adapt to varying environments through series of molecular and cellular mechanisms [1]. These modulating communities are referred to as the human microbiota. The communities involve bacteria, archaea, eukaryotic viruses, bacteriophages, and fungi that coexist in human surface structures and body cavities, especially the gut. To coexist means to have a relationship status with humans that involves commensalism and mutualistic relationships [2]. The gut microbiota is of utmost importance due to its varied functions. Gut microbiota not only modulate and help in digestion or production of micronutrients, it also affects the hypothalamic–pituitary–adrenal axis (HPA), produces neurologically active substances like gamma-aminobutyric acid, short-chain fatty acids, and influences the immune system [3]. There is often an imbalance of gut microbiota due to environmental factors such as diet, xenobiotics, toxins, and pathogens, leading to dysregulation of physiological and metabolic microbiota processes. The term often used for such imbalance is dysbiosis. Approximately 100 genera and 1000 distinct bacterial species are identified from digestive tube niches. The common techniques used to identify are microbiological techniques involving pure culture isolation, limited to laboratory culturable microorganisms. Another is high-throughput DNA-based pyrosequencing depending upon conserved 16s RNA sequences to profile the complexity of microbial communities from human fecal samples. Nearly both culturable and non-culturable microorganisms are identified using the latter technique [4].

The scientific community proposes several therapies such as probiotics and prebiotics to maintain a balance between the microbial gut and its functions. The probiotic products are formed as the result of fermentation using probiotic microorganisms. In recent years, consumers worldwide have focused primarily on living a healthy life. Such a lifestyle has to change the paradigm of health and nutrients, and this has concerned the nutraceuticals sector who provide their services to share their health products with humans. The demand for probiotic food products has also increased due to the continuing research evidence regarding probiotics' beneficial role in creating a healthy lifestyle for humans. The products having probiotic microbial strains have GRAS (Generally Regarded as Safe) status, which can be used in different fermented food products for human consumption, where 10^6–10^7 CFU has been the standard probiotic dosage present per gram of probiotic products [5, 6]. Prebiotics also play a significant role in the positive modulation of gut microbiota. Prebiotics are regarded as the microbiome fertiliser as they nourish the desired or probiotic strains and outgrow the harmful microbial strains. Some of the active ingredients of prebiotics are arabinogalactan, pectin oligosaccharides, fructooligosaccharides, and many others [7]. Metagenomics, meta-omics [8, 9], and artificial intelligence strategies have opened new gateways in which to study the hidden microbial diversity through culture-independent techniques. This enables researches to predict the significance and implications of microorganisms thereby ensures human welfare.

This chapter provides insight into various microbial communities present in the gut and factors that affect such communities. The chapter also focuses on the role of probiotics and prebiotics in modulating gut microbiota and their effect on different microbial communities.

3.2 Composition of Gut Microbiota

The colonisation of microbes in the human gut has been estimated to be around 10^{11} to 10^{12} cells/mL, which is considered densely and diversely populated. These gut microbiota show symbiotic interaction with the human gut, and this interaction of a host with microorganisms is often called superorganisms. They function in immune and metabolic aspects of human body. Interestingly, the load of gut microbiota in humans differs with human development. At each development stage, from newborn to old age, the environment of gut microbiota varies to support specific microbes [10, 11].

3.2.1 Gut Microbiota of Infants and Newborns

The first-ever populating bacteria in an infant gut comes primarily from the mother via fecal–oral route. The gut microbiota offer three essential roles of protection, metabolism, and trophic during the infancy period. The infant gut microbiota also influences and takes a role during various immunological (infant acquired immunity and innate immunity), endocrine, and neural pathways. However, there is a transition of gut microbiota following development of infancy to maturity. During infant or birth phase, the gut is dominated by microbial genera of *Lactobacillus* and *Bifidobacterium*, and any change in concentration is related to non-communicable diseases. For instance, the change in the microbial load of *Bifidobacterium* in an infant gut may cause infant obesity and asthma [12, 13].

The infant gut microbiota is influenced by feeding mode (breast, formula, and mixed feeding) and later weaning. However, breast feeding highly shapes the gut microbiota of infants as breast milk is rich in biological factors which include immunological (antibodies, cytokines, and leukocytes), growth factors, and human milk oligosaccharides (HMOs) [14, 15]. Apart from shaping the gut, breast milk also provides healthy microbes to the infant gut, microbial genera such as *Bifidobacterium*, *Lactobacillus*, *Staphylococcus*, and *Streptococcus* to colonise the infant gut [16].

Other than providing protection, metabolising, or trophical functions towards newborns or infants, infant gut microbiota also provides an insight of future adult health by tracing plausible future colonisation of microbes in adult gut and their associated diseases [13].

3.2.2 Gut Microbiota of Adults

A healthy adult gut microbiota consists of 8 phyla, 18 families, 23 orders, 59 genera, and 109 species of bacteria, the majority belonging to Firmicutes, Actinobacteria, and Bacteroidetes [17]. These high taxa diversity with high gene richness and stable microbiome core functions defines a healthy gut microbiota [2]. The shaping of gut microbiota from infancy to adulthood is solely influenced by environmental factors.

3.3 Factors Affecting Gut Microbiota

Individuals' unhealthy habits deteriorate bodily functions leading to certain pathological diseases. The homeostatic maintenance of gut microbiome is a relationship between gut microbiome and health with multiple perspectives. Apart from the body's homeostasis mechanism, diversity of gut microbiome referring to a good gut microbiome also has a positive impact on individual's health. However, there are certain host–specific and non-specific factors that affect the diversity of gut microbiome, and such factors reform the gut microbiome having either positive or negative output. We will now focus on the factors responsible for changes in the gut microbiome over a period of infant–adult transition. Such factors altering gut microbiome leading to dysbiosis often result in risks to food allergy, asthma, diabetes, and obesity (Figure 3.1).

3.3.1 Age and Delivery Pattern

Aging is a predetermined factor of an individual; the changes that occur during aging are seen as dynamics that involves biological, environmental, social, and behavioral status. Similarly, with human aging, gut microbiota also changes, playing a role in longevity across species. As stated, microbiome is a critical factor that determines building of immune response against diseases, and dysbiosis leads to pro-inflammatory reactions [18].

The delivery of probiotics or microbiome to infants is significant in the first three months of their life and it changes after six months. After birth, infants are inhabited with microbiota via the mother's uterus. Looking for the dominancy of gut microbiome in infants, if an infant is delivered vaginally, *Lactobacillus* and *Bifidobacterium* [19] species are the primarily dominant strains. However, if delivered through caesarian, *Streptococcus*, *Corynebacterium*, and *Propionibacterium* colonise to dominance [20]. It has been documented that caesarian delivery showed decreased microbial evenness, richness, and phylogenetic diversity [21]. Apart from the type of infant delivery to colonise the gut

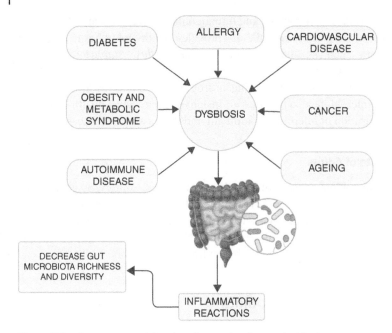

Figure 3.1 Consequences of various factors leading to dysbiosis.

microbiome, the mode of delivery of beneficial bacteria also affects the gut microbiome. During infancy, breast milk rich in certain oligosaccharides positively affects gut the microbiome [22]. After six months to a year, the associated dominant strains of microbiome become associated with the gut at later stage of infant development.

3.3.2   Diet

Diet is a variable factor in modulating or shaping gut microbiome. However, prolonged changes in diet may lead to permanent induced alteration in gut microbiome. The diet altering gut microbiome may be studied under two stages: infant diet and adult diet.

3.3.2.1   Infant diet on gut microbiome

A critical development chain is followed for the gut microbiota to be persistent in infants. The gut microbiome changes drastically after birth, during the lactation period, and at the introduction of solid food during the first three years of age. During these years, infants also tend to have lower bacterial diversity, but higher flux. Any disturbances in development chain, disease of autoimmune system, or metabolism at adulthood may occur [23].

Breast milk is a major source of HMOs and immunoglobulins (IgA). The predominant *Lactobacillus* and *Bifidobacterium* breaks down such oligosaccharides to short chain fatty acids. Such fatty acids tend to produce IgG as an immune response with stimulation of plasma cells, cytotoxic Th1 cells, NK cells, CD4+ cells, and CD8+ cells. These immune responses build up the immunity in infants [24, 25].

3.3.2.2 Adulthood diet on gut microbiome

The infancy gut microbiome develops in terms of shaping, modulating structure, and creating diversity with diet as a constant factor. HMOs help in maturation of gut microbiota, which is followed by higher bacterial richness. However, introduction of solid food reduces bacterial richness; one factor is age, and another is decreased food diversity. We know gut microbiota richness depends on constituents of food, interestingly, it responds differently towards the nutritional availability of food in both temporal and geographical contexts [26]. Not only the nature and geography of food affect the gut microbiota, but food additives have also shown to cause dysbiosis of gut microbiome through inflammatory responses of tissue injury [27].

The human diet normally consists of carbohydrates, proteins, and fats recommended in balance. The degradation of these complex structures to corresponding monomer relates to enhance body function and modulating gut microbiota. However, imbalance of any components may have severe effects on gut microbiota resulting in gastrointestinal diseases. For instance, increase in ammonia production from protein degradation may cause malignant growth, alteration of fat constituent in food, shown to decrease *Bacteroides* and increase *Firmicutes* and *Proteobacteria* species in the gut. The changes reduce microbial production of short chain fatty acid and thus, affect production of immunogenic molecules such as immunoglobulins. Such changes in the diet and lowering the "guard shield" (antibodies) lead to disease conditions such as various inflammatory diseases, diabetes, obesity, and cancer [28, 29].

3.3.3 Antibiotics

Antibiotics have also shown negative impact on growth of gut microbiota leading to antibiotic-associated diarrhea or recurrence of *Clostridioides difficile* infection. The following attributes are responsible for negative impact on gut microbiomes and their growth:

a) antibiotic mechanism;
b) antibiotic class;
c) resistant degree of antibiotic used;
d) treatment dosage;
e) administration route;
f) pharmacokinetic and pharmacodynamics properties;
g) antibiotic spectrum (broad or narrow).

All these attributes contribute towards loss of important gut microbiota taxa, reduction in species diversity, a shift in metabolism (metabolome), increase in gut susceptibility of non-beneficial microbes to colonise, and lastly, creation of bacterial antibiotic resistance [30, 31].

The human gut is a reservoir of many antimicrobial resistance genes (AGRs) belonging to the family *Enterobacteriaceae*. The use of short-term antibiotics alter the resistance gene composition of the AGRs, thus increasing the number above their average count in the gut [32]. Table 3.1 represents the effect of different classes of antibiotics on dysbiosis [33].

Table 3.1 Different classes of antibiotic creating dysbiosis.

Antibiotics used	Reason for dysbiosis
Amoxicillin Cephalosporins Macrolides Ketolides Clindamycin Tigecycline Quinolones Fosfomycin	Increased numbers of *Enterobacteriaceae* in the gut
Moxcillin Cephalosporins Macrolides Clindamycin Quinolones Sulphonamides	Decreases *Escherichia coli* growth
Clavulanate	Increases *Escherichia coli* growth
Amoxicillin Piperacillin Ticarcillin Cephalosporins Carbapenems Lipoglycopeptides	Increases *Enterococcus* growth
Macrolides Doxycycline	Decreases *Enterococcus* growth
Piperacillin Ticarcillin Carbapenems Macrolides Clindamycin Quinolones	Decreases abundance of anaerobic microbiome

3.3.4 Oxidative Stress

A healthy gut plays an important role in maintaining an antioxidative role due to the presence of a healthy microbiome. Dysbiosis leads to stress in an oxidative phase, which is interrelated to brain functioning. As the brain functions efficiently in the presence of oxygen, during oxidative stress oxygen levels in the brain are depleted resulting in neurological diseases [34]. The interaction between gut microbiota and oxidative stress has shown unwanted signaling leading to critical effects on gut–skin axis.

3.4 Modulation of Gut Microbiota

The gut microbiota in humans is a complicated ecology that plays a significant role in promoting gastrointestinal as well as systemic health. Microbiota dysbiosis is linked to a variety of disorders related to the gastrointestinal and digestive systems. The modulation of gut microbiota for human health is a hot topic in the medical world. The gut microbiota provides a basis of unique health-promoting bacteria, which are referred to as *next-generation probiotics* to differentiate them from conventional probiotics. The microbiome of the human intestine is a varied collection of microorganisms that includes bacteria, archaea, fungus, viruses, and protozoa and is thought to play an important role in maintaining the health of humans [2]. Changes in the composition, diversity, and temporal stability of the microbiota (microbiota dysbiosis) have been linked to a variety of gastrointestinal and systemic diseases. As a result, modulating the gut microbiota in order to preserve a positive ecological balance and promote the health of humans is of significant interest.

The term 'gut microbiota' was first introduced with established research by Joshua Lederberg. He referred to it as "the conservational local area of symbiotic, commensal, and pathogenic micro-organism that in a real sense share our body space and have been in essence unnoticed as determinants of health illnesses." The human body is comprised of trillions of microorganisms, for the most part inside the gastrointestinal tract, which consist of the small digestive system and colon. Utilising a 70 kg man as a type of perspective, 3.8×1013 organisms are accounted for to have a complete load of 0.2 kg [3]. The gut microbiota can ferment non-absorbable carbohydrates, which are notable as prebiotics, including galactose, inulin, xylose, oligofructose, and fructo-oligosaccharide, that contain oligosaccharides to satisfy the requirement of energy in the host body. The connections between these microorganisms and host cells were for quite some time accorded a pathogenic perspective, since toxin penetrates the stomach mucosa, and translocate, spread, and cause initial contaminations [4] In many cases, no consideration was paid to most of intestinal microorganisms, or their relationship with the health of the host. A few investigations have detailed useful partnerships between the commensal microbiota and the human body and have demonstrated that the microbiota serves as a genuine accomplice.

The microorganisms present in the body of the host affect the development of immunity and its functions, metabolism, and physiology. The symbiotic relationship functions through the synthesis of nutrients and protection from pathogenic colonisation. The protecting function of the relationship is a regulatory immune system that also modulates functional properties of gastrointestinal hormones [5, 13]. The enhancement of self-sufficient and atomic high output procedures provide the evidence regarding the distinguishing proof of unknown microscopic organisms, which would provide novel experiences in the practical and compositional variety of a portion of the fecal microbiota. What's more, a few examinations have recommended that problems such as oxidative pressure related sickness, inflammatory bowel disease (IBD), colorectal malignant growth, obesity, fatty liver infections, type 2 diabetes, and invulnerable immune related sicknesses are related with disease explicit dibiotic of changed compositions of microbiota [2, 12].

3.4.1 Probiotics and Prebiotics

Bacteria, fungi, archaea, protozoa, and viruses make up the gut microbiota, which interact with the host and each other to influence the host's physiology and health [18]. Gut bacteria serve important functions in human health, including vitamin B production, digestion enhancement, angiogenesis, and nerve stimulation [19]. Furthermore, when the gut ecology suffers significant aberrant changes, altering the gut microbiota might be hazardous. Actinobacteria Firmicutes (*Clostridium, Eubacteria,* and *Ruminococcus*), and Bacteroidetes (*Prevotella Porphyromonas*), are the most common phyla discovered in the human gut microbiome (Bifidobacterium) [18, 19], while small amounts of Escherichia coli Lactobacilli and Streptococci are detected in the stomach. Changes in the gut microbiota composition, on the other hand, have been linked to a variety of disorders in people and animals [22, 23].

According to current findings, the gut microbiota's activity and composition are linked to the health and illness of humans. Furthermore, the arrangement of the gut microbiota is anticipated to have an impact on a variety of organ systems, including the metabolic, cardiovascular, neurological, and immunological systems [16]. Many diseases affect the gut microbiota, including asthma, type 2 diabetes (T2D), cardiovascular disease, obesity, cancer, malignancy, colitis, mental disorders, gut–brain axis disorders, inflammatory disorders, and a variety of immunological illnesses [26]. The gut microbiota may help with a variety of health issues; in mice, probiotic feeding with a high-fat diet changed the gut microbiota composition resulting in a decrease in the gram-positive bacteria phyla Firmicutes and Actinobacteria [27].

3.4.1.1 Effect of probiotics on gut microbiota

The gut microbiome, which plays a crucial role in many illnesses, must be kept in balance. The gastrointestinal epithelium is the first line of defense against microorganisms. Infection and invasion of any pathogenic bacterium will alert the mucosa of the digestive tract, triggering an immune response [28]. Several gastrointestinal disorders including IBD, colon cancer, or irritable bowel syndrome (IBS), and few parenteral diseases like allergies, bronchial asthma, and cystic fibrosis are linked to changes in the composition and variety of microflora [29, 30].

Bifidobacterium spp. are the most *common* good bacteria found inside the human gut, and changes in the microbiota's quantity and composition are one of the most prevalent characteristics of disorders, including Crohn's disease [31], ulcerative colitis [32], respiratory infection disease [33], and autism [34]. Human gut flora might be modulated by probiotics, with toxic bacteria such as *Desulfovibrio* being inhibited, and helpful bacteria such as lactic acid bacteria being stimulated. In one study, pre-treatment with probiotic bacteria including *Bacillus cereus, Bifidobacterium infantis, Lactobacillus acidophilus,* and *Enterococcus faecalis* reduced the chance of colitis-linked cancer and tumor formation in mice by increasing the amount of *Lactobacillus acidophilus* and decreasing the amount of colitogenic bacteria such as *Odoribacter Mucispirillum* and *Desulfovibrio* [35].

According to this research, probiotics may help manage and reestablish intestinal microbiota balance by promoting the development and activity of helpful bacteria, while inhibiting the growth and activity of harmful bacteria. Although the exact mechanism of probiotics on gut microbiota modification is unknown, they may suppress pathogen development by producing short-chain fatty acids (SCFA) and some toxins [36, 37], as well as competing for colonisation sites with pathogens [35]. Furthermore, when new next-generation probiotic strains are discovered, their strain-specific effects and effective doses must be studied.

3.5 Gut Microbiota Hallmark in Disease Condition

The consequences of dysbiosis lead to development of a variety of pathologies ranging from bowel inflammation to cancerous and neurodegenerative conditions. Such consequences are due to overgrowth of pathogenic population within the commensal microbiota.

3.5.1 Cancer

The overgrowth of pathogens in the gut leading to dysbiosis compromises host's gut microbiota, metabolism, and immune system. These negative changes hallmark trigger tumorigenesis. According to Vivarelli et al. their surveys showed that 20% tumorigenesis was due to dysbiosis with rising population of pathogens [38]. Table 3.2 provides an insight of the ten pathogens most involved in cancer as per WHO report by International Agency for Research Centre (https://gco.iarc.fr/causes/infections/data-sources-methods)

However, antibiotic usage reduces gut microbiota population, which has been linked to defects in antitumor immune response. A study by Boursi et al. showed different antibiotic (antibacterial) treatment for the treatment of gastro-intestinal malignancies leads to risk of certain cancerous condition in Table 3.3 [39, 40].

3.5.2 COVID-19

COVID-19, caused by subacute respiratory syndrome virus (SARS-CoV-2) not only compromises the respiratory functions, but also the gut microbiome. If the coronavirus reaches the intestine, it is also linked to severe neurological diseases [41]. Studies have linked the severity of COVID-19 with depletion of symbiotic microbiota and bacteriophages [42, 43].

Table 3.2 WHO reporting ten pathogens most involved in different cancerous conditions.

Nature of microbe	Number as per WHO report	Examples included
Bacterium	01	*Helicobacter pylori*
Viruses	06	Hepatitis B virus, Hepatitis C virus, Human papilloma virus (type 16, 18, 6, 11, 31, 33, 45, 52, 58), Epstein-Barr virus, Human Herpes virus type 8 (Kaposi sarcoma virus), Human T-cell lymphotropic virus type 1 (HTLV-1)
Parasites	03	*Opisthorchis viverrine, Clonorchis sinensis, Schistosoma haematobium*

Table 3.3 Anti-GI drugs involved in different cancerous conditions.

Antibacterial drugs given to treat gastrointestinal malignancies	Type of cancer risk
Penicillin	Esophageal, gastric, and pancreatic cancer
Penicillin, cephalosporins, macrolides	Lung cancer
Penicillin, quinolones, sulphonamides, tetracyclines	Prostate cancer
Sulphonamides	Breast cancer
Quinolones, sulfonamides, trimethoprims	Colorectal cancer
Cephalosporins	Lymphoid and hematopoietic tissue cancer

The gut microbiota is mostly affected post-COVID-19-infection with higher tick of *Clostridium hathewayi*, *Actinomyces viscosus*, *Bacteroides nordii*, *Lactobacillus*, and *Streptococcus*, leading to secondary infection [44, 45]. The dysbiosis linked with COVID-19 can also be characterised by impaired gut-related metabolites such as acetyl-L-carnitine, betaine, choline, L-carnitine, and trimethylamine. Interestingly, a preliminary study showed impaired levels of betaine linked with severe dysbiosis, suggesting betaine as a marker to monitor gut microbiota health.

3.5.3 HIV

Human immunodeficiency virus (HIV) is grouped under genus Lentivirus of family Retroviridae, and is an immunodeficiency virus consisting of single-stranded RNA molecules enclosed in the core of the virus. It has also been linked to decreased gut microbiota richness and its diversity characterises it with systemic inflammation and immune activation, allowing HIV persistence through ART (anti-retroviral therapy) [46, 47]. The GI tract acts as an HIV reservoir, as the gut is a highly rich site of CD4+ T cells, and the site is necessary for early replication of HIV. As CD4+ T cells depletes, intestinal integrity is lost leading to epithelial dysfunction with loss of Th17 cells, which are vital for maintain gut homeostasis. The Th17 cells also prevent entrance of microbial antigens in systemic circulation [46].

People living with HIV (PLWH) have shown reduced abundance of Firmicutes and high abundance of Actinobacteria, and Proteobacteria. HIV also interferes with gut-intestinal metabolisms; for instance, altering tryptophan metabolism (amino acid metabolism), catabolism of tryptophan produced biologically activates metabolites necessary for neurotransmission, immune response, and intestinal homeostasis [48, 49].

3.6 Conclusion

A healthy gut is defined as having a healthy microbiome, and these microbiomes play a crucial role in maintaining the homeostasis of human body. The microbiome composition present in the gut functions diversely for the health of the gut, including protection, metabolism, and trophic aspects. However, various factors affect its composition, concerning host-specific or non-specificity. Apart from factors mentioned in the chapter, other factors such as geography, maternal diet, and lifestyle also affect the composition of gut microbiota in infants and adults.

The gut microbiota modulation with pro- or prebiotics seems to be therapeutically promising and many studies have proven to be effective. However, further studies are needed concerning loss or missing function of microbiota during dysbiosis. Depending upon the research and studies, specific probiotics and prebiotics as a medication regimen may be achieved to modulate dysbiosis.

References

1 Wani, A.K., Akhtar, N., Sher, F. et al. (2022). Microbial adaptation to different environmental conditions: molecular perspective of evolved genetic and cellular systems. *Arch. Microbiol.* 204 (2): 144.

2 Fan, Y. and Pedersen, O. (2021). Gut microbiota in human metabolic health and disease. *Nat. Rev. Microbiol.* 19 (1): 55–71.

3 Cheung, S.G., Goldenthal, A.R., Uhlemann, A.-C. et al. (2019). Systematic review of gut microbiota and major depression. *Front. Psychiatry*, 10.

4 Singh, R., Zogg, H., Wei, L. et al. (2021). Gut microbial dysbiosis in the pathogenesis of gastrointestinal dysmotility and metabolic disorders. *J. Neurogastro. Motil.* 27 (1): 19–34.

5 Gagliardi, A., Totino, V., Cacciotti, F. et al. (2018). Rebuilding the gut microbiota ecosystem. *Int. J. Environ. Res. Public. Health* 15 (8): E1679.

6 Tsai, Y.-L., Lin, T.-L., Chang, C.-J. et al. (2019). Probiotics, prebiotics and amelioration of diseases. *J. Biomed. Sci.* 26 (1): 3.

7 Appanna, V.D. (2018). Dysbiosis, Probiotics, and Prebiotics. In: diseases and health. *Hum. Microbes Power Within* 81–122.

8 Wani, A.K., Roy, P., Kumar, V. et al. (2022). Metagenomics and artificial intelligence in the context of human health. *Infect. Genet. Evol.* 10 (1): 105267.

9 Wani, A.K., Rahayu, F., Kadarwati, F.T. et al. (2022). Metagenomic screening strategies for bioprospecting enzymes from environmental samples. *IOP Conf. Ser. Earth Environ. Sci.* 974 (1): 012003.

10 Rodríguez, J.M., Murphy, K., Stanton, C. et al. (2015). The composition of the gut microbiota throughout life, with an emphasis on early life. *Microb. Ecol. Health Dis.* 26. https://doi.org/10.3402/mehd.v26.26050.

11 Rinninella, E., Raoul, P., Cintoni, M. et al. (2019). What is the healthy gut microbiota composition? A changing ecosystem across age, environment, diet, and diseases. *Microorganisms* 7 (1): 14.

12 Yang, I., Corwin, E.J., Brennan, P.A. et al. (2016). The Infant Microbiome: Implications for Infant Health and Neurocognitive Development. *Nurs. Res.* 65 (1): 76–88.

13 Yao, Y., Cai, X., Ye, Y. et al. (2021). The role of microbiota in infant health: from early life to adulthood. *Front. Immunol.* 12: 708472.

14 Brushett, S., Sinha, T., Reijneveld, S.A. et al. (2020). The Effects of urbanization on the infant gut microbiota and health outcomes. *Front. Pediatr.* 8: 408.

15 Jian, C., Carpén, N., Helve, O. et al. (2021). Early-life gut microbiota and its connection to metabolic health in children: perspective on ecological drivers and need for quantitative approach. *eBioMedicine* 69: 103475.

16 Moore, R.E. and Townsend, S.D. (2019). Temporal development of the infant gut microbiome. *Open Biol.* 9 (9): 190128.

17 King, C.H., Desai, H., Sylvetsky, A.C. et al. (2019). Baseline human gut microbiota profile in healthy people and standard reporting template. *PloS One* 14 (9): e0206484.

18 Badal, V.D., Vaccariello, E.D., Murray, E.R. et al. (2020). The gut microbiome, aging, and longevity: a systematic review. *Nutrients* 12 (12): E3759.

19 Rutayisire, E., Huang, K., Liu, Y. et al. (2016). The mode of delivery affects the diversity and colonization pattern of the gut microbiota during the first year of infants' life: a systematic review. *BMC Gastroenterol.* 16 (1): 86.

20 Hasan, N. and Yang, H. (2019). Factors affecting the composition of the gut microbiota, and its modulation. *Peer J.* 7: e7502.

21 Zhang, C., Li, L., Jin, B. et al. (2021). The effects of delivery mode on the gut microbiota and health: state of art. *Front. Microbiol.* 12: 724449.

22 Vandenplas, Y., Carnielli, V.P., Ksiazyk, J. et al. (2020). Factors affecting early-life intestinal microbiota development. *Nutr. Burbank Los Angel. Cty. CA* 78: 110812.

23 Leeming, E.R., Johnson, A.J., Spector, T.D. et al. (2019). Effect of diet on the gut microbiota: rethinking intervention duration. *Nutrients* 11 (12): E2862.

24 Riaz Rajoka, M.S., Shi, J., Mehwish, H.M. et al. (2017). Interaction between diet composition and gut microbiota and its impact on gastrointestinal tract health. *Food Sci. Hum. Well.* 6 (3): 121–130.

25 Singh, R.K., Chang, H.-W., Yan, D. et al. (2017). Influence of diet on the gut microbiome and implications for human health. *J. Transl. Med.* 15 (1): 73.

26 Zmora, N., Suez, J., and Elinav, E. (2019). You are what you eat: diet, health and the gut microbiota. *Nat. Rev. Gastroenterol. Hepatol.* 16 (1): 35–56.

27 Su, Q. and Liu, Q. (2021). Factors affecting gut microbiome in daily diet. *Front. Nutr.* 8: 644138.

28 Mansour, S.R., Moustafa, M.a.A., Saad, B.M. et al. (2021). Impact of diet on human gut microbiome and disease risk. *New Microb. New Infect.* 41: 100845.

29 Beam, A., Clinger, E., and Hao, L. (2021). Effect of diet and dietary components on the composition of the gut microbiota. *Nutrients* 13 (8): 2795.

30 Ramirez, J., Guarner, F., Bustos Fernandez, L. et al. (2020). Antibiotics as major disruptors of gut microbiota. *Front. Cell. Infect. Microbiol.* 10: 572912.

31 Yang, L., Bajinka, O., Jarju, P.O. et al. (2021). The varying effects of antibiotics on gut microbiota. *AMB Express* 11 (1): 116.

32 Ribeiro, C.F.A., de Oliveira Silva Silveira, G.G., de Souza Cândido, E., et al. (2020). Effects of antibiotic treatment on gut microbiota and how to overcome its negative impacts on human health. *ACS Infect. Dis.* 6 (10): 2544–2559.

33 Zimmermann, P. and Curtis, N. (2019). The effect of antibiotics on the composition of the intestinal microbiota a systematic review. *J. Infect.* 79 (6): 471–489.

34 Shandilya, S., Kumar, S., Kumar Jha, N. et al. (2022). Interplay of gut microbiota and oxidative stress: Perspective on neurodegeneration and neuroprotection. *J. Adv. Res.* 38: 223–244.

35 Prabhurajeshwar, C. and Chandrakanth, R.K. (2017). Probiotic potential of Lactobacilli with antagonistic activity against pathogenic strains: an in vitro validation for the production of inhibitory substances. *Biomed. J.* 40 (5): 270–283.

36 Sherman, P.M., Ossa, J.C., and Johnson-Henry, K. (2009). Unraveling mechanisms of action of probiotics. *Nutr. Clin. Pract. Off. Publ. Am. Soc. Parenter. Enter. Nutr.* 24 (1): 10–14.

37 Wani, A.K., Akhtar, N., Datta, B. et al. (2021). Ch. 14 – Volatiles and Metabolites of Microbes Cyanobacteria-derived small molecules. In: *A New Class of Drugs* (ed. A. Kumar, J. Singh, and J. Samuel), 283–303. Academic Press.

38 Vivarelli, S., Salemi, R., Candido, S. et al. (2019). Gut microbiota and cancer: from pathogenesis to therapy. *Cancers* 11 (1): E38.

39 Boursi, B., Mamtani, R., Haynes, K. et al. (2015). Recurrent antibiotic exposure may promote cancer formation: another step in understanding the role of the human microbiota? *Eur. J. Cancer Oxf. Engl. 1990* 51 (17): 2655–2664.

40 Roderburg, C., Loosen, S.H., Joerdens, M.S. et al. (2022). Antibiotic therapy is associated with an increased incidence of cancer. *J. Cancer Res. Clin. Oncol.* 149 (3): 1285–1293.

41 Chaves Andrade, M., Souza de Faria, R., and Avelino Mota Nobre, S. (2020). COVID-19: can the symptomatic SARS-CoV-2 infection affect the homeostasis of the gut-brain-microbiota axis? *Med. Hypoth.* 144: 110206.

42 Zuo, T., Liu, Q., Zhang, F. et al. (2021). Depicting SARS-CoV-2 faecal viral activity in association with gut microbiota composition in patients with COVID-19. *Gut* 70 (2): 276–284.

43 Yeoh, Y.K., Zuo, T., Lui, G.C.-Y. et al. (2021). Gut microbiota composition reflects disease severity and dysfunctional immune responses in patients with COVID-19. *Gut* 70 (4): 698–706.

44 Zuo, T., Wu, X., Wen, W. et al. (2021). Gut Microbiome Alterations in COVID-19. *Geno. Proteo. Bioinform.* 19 (5): 679–688.

45 Alharbi, K.S., Singh, Y., Hassan Almalki, W. et al. (2022). Gut Microbiota Disruption in COVID-19 or Post-COVID Illness Association with severity biomarkers: a possible role of Pre Pro-biotics in manipulating microflora. *Chem. Biol. Interact.* 358: 109898.

46 Koay, W.L.A., Siems, L.V., and Persaud, D. (2018). The microbiome and HIV persistence: implications for viral remission and cure. *Curr. Opin. HIV AIDS* 13 (1): 61–68.

47 Vujkovic-Cvijin, I. and Somsouk, M. (2019). HIV and the gut microbiota: composition, consequences, and avenues for amelioration. *Curr. HIV/AIDS Rep.* 16 (3): 204–213.

48 Chachage, M. (2021). The gut-microbiome contribution to HIV-associated cardiovascular disease and metabolic disorders. *Curr. Opin. Endocr. Metab. Res.* 21: 100287.

49 Ali, Z., Shahzadi, I., Majeed, A. et al. (2021). Comparative analysis of the serum microbiome of HIV infected individuals. *Genomics* 113 (6): 4015–4021.

4

Antibiotic-Induced Changes in the Composition of the Gut Microbiome

Gholamreza Abdi[1,], Abu Saeid[2], Ab Waheed Wani[3], and Vishal Johar[3]*

[1] Department of Biotechnology, Persian Gulf Research Institute, Persian Gulf University, Bushehr, Iran
[2] Department of Food Engineering, NPI University of Bangladesh, Manikganj, Bangladesh
[3] Lovely Professional University, Phagwara, Punjab, India
* Corresponding author

4.1   Introduction

Bacteria, fungi, archaea, viruses, and protozoans colonise the intestine and perform a variety of functions for the hosts, including food fermentation, vitamin and amino acid synthesis, immune system maturation and regulation, modulation of gastrointestinal hormone release, and brain-behavior regulation [1]. Two major phyla (Bacteroidetes and Firmicutes) and two minor phyla (Bacteroidetes and Firmicutes) make up the healthy gut microbiota (Actinobacteria and Proteobacteria). Bacteroidetes and Firmicutes dominated the phyla Bacteroidetes, and Firmicutes dominated the phyla Bacteroidetes and Firmicutes in the large intestine [2].

Humans are unaffected by the majority of intestinal microorganisms. Obesity, malnutrition, inflammatory bowel disease (IBD), neurological problems, and cancer are all caused by changes in the gut microbiota's composition, both qualitatively and quantitatively [3]. A variety of factors contributed to the change in gut microbiota, including food and nutritional changes, genetic and environmental factors, and antibiotic use [4].

Antibiotics have been used for decades to prevent infectious diseases, notably the creation of bacterial pathogens, as well as to treat bacterial infections that have already occurred [5]. Antibiotic use has a number of negative consequences for the gut microbiota, including reduced species diversity, altered metabolic activity, the selection of antibiotic-resistant organisms, and microbiome abnormalities, all of which may lead to antibiotic-induced diarrhea and C. diff. infections [6]. Dysbiosis, or imbalances in the microbiome, may cause autoimmune diseases, gastrointestinal problems, allergies, infections, arthritis, asthma, cancer, and obesity. Antibiotic use changes gut flora over time, which has been linked to the onset of neurological and mental diseases.

Antibiotics have been shown to affect the composition and functionality of the human microbiota, including the selection of resistant bacteria, pathogenic bacteria dominance of the microbial composition, bacterial diversity loss, decreased or loss of certain bacterial

The Gut Microbiota in Health and Disease, First Edition. Edited by Nimmy Srivastava, Salam A. Ibrahim, Jayeeta Chattopadhyay, and Mohamed H. Arbab.
© 2023 John Wiley & Sons Ltd. Published 2023 by John Wiley & Sons Ltd.

species, increased susceptibility to infections, and the risk of new infection and/or recurrence, according to numerous studies. This chapter focuses on the impact of antibiotics on the gut flora.

4.2 Gut Microbiota Composition

According to a recent large-scale study, the human gut microbiota contains approximately 35 000 different bacterial species. The gut microbiota contains 500–1000 different microorganisms [2], and the gastrointestinal tract is expected to contain more than 100 trillion germs. There are between 800 and 1000 different bacterial species and over 7000 diverse strains in the normal gut microbiota [7]. According to data from the Human Microbiome Project and the Human Microbiome Project and the Metagenome of the Human Intestinal Tract (MetaHIT), there are 2172 different species of human gut microbiota split into 12 different phyla [8]. The human microbiome may contain roughly 10 million non-redundant genes, according to research undertaken by MetaHIT [2].

Bacteroidetes and Firmicutes are the most common microbial phyla in the gut, followed by Actinobacteria, Proteobacteria, Fusobacteria, and Verrucomicrobia. Ninety percent of the gut microbiota is made up of Firmicutes and Bacteroidetes. Lactobacillus, Bacillus, Clostridium, Enterococcus, and Ruminicoccus are among the more than 200 genera that make up the Firmicutes phylum. The Clostridium genus makes up 95% of the Firmicutes phylum. Bacteroidetes is a phylum of bacteria that includes well-known taxa such as Bacteroides and Prevotella. The Actinobacteria phylum, which contains a lesser number of bacteria, is dominated by the Bifidobacterium genus. Figure 4.1 depicts the taxonomic composition of the gut microbiota. Bacteroides, Eubacterium, Bifidobacterium, Fusobacterium, Peptostreptococcus, and Atopobium are the most common stringent anaerobes in the gut microbiota, while facultative anaerobes such Enterococci, Lactobacilli, Enterobacteriaceae, and Streptococci make up a small percentage of the population. Three enterotypes of gut microbiota were discovered using multidimensional scaling and main coordinates analysis, each defined by a dominant genus; Bacteroides (enterotype 1), Prevotella (enterotype 2), or Ruminococcus (enterotype 3); despite the fact that clustering was unaffected by a host's age, gender, ethnicity, or BMI [9].

4.3 Antibiotic-induced Changes in the Composition of the Microbiota

In both short- and long-term, antibiotic treatment impacts the population structure of the indigenous microbiota, lowering bacterial diversity and rearranging member composition (see Figure 4.2). Changes in resource availability and species–species interactions result from changes in the highly co-evolved microbial community architecture, providing niches for pathogenic infiltration and contributing to the loss of colonisation resistance. Antibiotics also favour antibiotic-resistant members of the community, leading to a rise in the frequency of resistant genes in the microbiome. Antibiotic medication facilitates the transmission of genetic information between bacteria by boosting conjugation, phage transduction, and plasmid mobility, mostly through the activation of cellular stress responses [10].

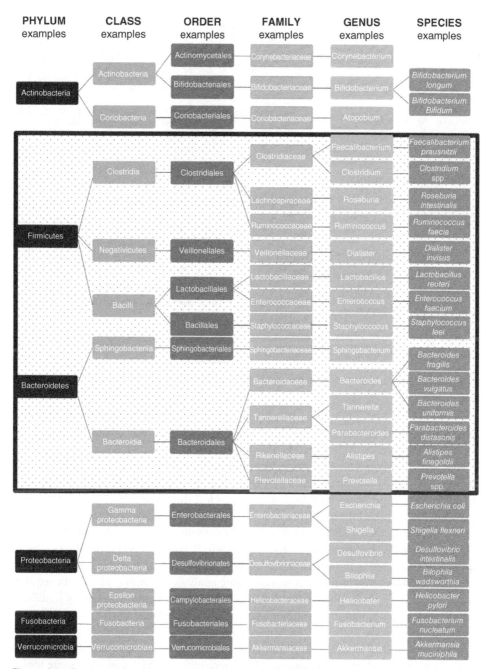

Figure 4.1 Taxonomic classification of gut microbiota composition.

The effects of antibiotics gut dysbiosis and the proposed role in disease even with short-term administration of antibiotics may shift the microbiota to long-term states of dysbiosis, which are characterised by changes in diversity, loss of important taxa, and consequent metabolic alterations leading to impaired colonisation resistance against intestinal pathogens. The interplay of gut immunity and microbiota is believed to contribute to the

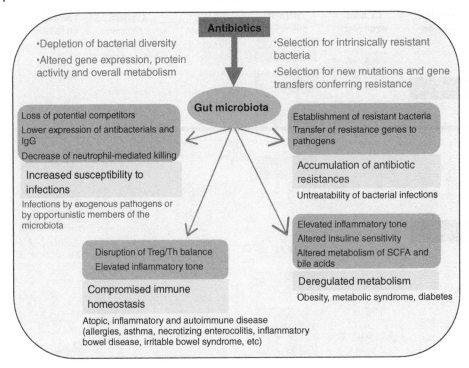

Figure 4.2 Overall consequences after administration of antibiotic in the host.

pathogenesis and severity of metabolic, (auto)-immune, infectious diseases, and cancer [11] (see Figure 4.3).

According to research, antibiotics encourage antibiotic-resistant members of the gut community, increasing the presence of resistance genes in the microbiome [10]. In clinical practice, fluoroquinolones have been shown to select fluoroquinolone-resistant microorganisms. Fluoroquinolone resistance acquired through nose Staphylococcus is prevalent in both community (42%) and hospitalised (94%) patients, and prevention in hospitals is nearly impossible. Resistance to fluoroquinolones in E. coli has also been linked to fluoroquinolone treatment in the stomach [12, 13]. Multidrug-resistant bacteria comprised about 20% of the total germs in a recent metagenomic analysis of the gut microbiota acquired from two healthy adults. Exogenous drugs, according to research, can have a significant impact on the accumulation of Antibiotic Resistance Genes (ARGs) [14]. Bacteria in animal body sites may evolve antibiotic resistance as a method to get past the host's defenses. For example, it was discovered that erythromycin resistance provided by a mutation in the 23s rRNA gene also conferred resistance to TLR13 recognition, which binds the same molecular target and is likely to exert selective pressure in vivo [15]. Antibiotics given exogenously to a host may cause ARGs to develop rapidly. Pigs were fed a meal laced with a growth-promoting antibiotic cocktail for two weeks in one experiment. As a result, their microbiome produced more ARGs, allowing them to tolerate medications that they had not been administered during the experiment [14].

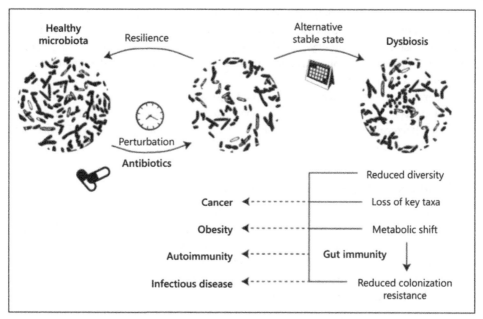

Figure 4.3 The interplay of gut immunity and microbiota is believed to contribute to the pathogenesis and severity of metabolic, (auto)-immune, and infectious diseases, and cancer [4]. *Source:* Lange et al., 2016 / Karger AG, Basel.

4.3.1 Loss of Bacterial Diversity and Domination of Pathogenic Bacteria

Broad-spectrum antibiotics limit bacterial diversity while increasing the number of micro-organisms available to opportunistic infections and reducing the number of helpful bacteria [10]. Antibiotics may also wreak havoc on the delicate balance of gut flora species. For example, antibiotics may contribute to pathobiont overgrowth by reducing species diversity, allowing pathobionts like toxigenic C. diff. to grow out of control [16]. Antibiotics may also reduce the quantity of bacteria in the gut microbiome by 30%, resulting in severe losses in taxonomic richness, variety, and evenness [16]. Antibiotic-induced dysbiosis may play a role in the onset and progression of inflammatory bowel disease (IBD). In truth, the number of potentially immunoprotective bacteria from the phylum Firmicutes, such as Faecalibacterium prausnitzii and Akkermansia muciniphila, is on the decline, while the number of adherent, invasive E. coli is on the rise [11].

Antibiotic exposure causes a rise in facultative anaerobic Proteobacteria such as E. coli in both animals and humans [17]. Oral supplementation with the subtherapeutic antibiotic ASP250 (a combination of chlortetracycline, sulfamethazine, and penicillin) increased E. coli populations and the number of functional genes associated with energy generation and antibiotic resistance genes in the feces of an 18-week-old pig model [5]. The quantity of Escherichia coli and Lachnobacterium in the cecum and colon digesta of adult pigs was increased by ASP250 [18]. Oral antibiotics (ampicillin, gentamycin, and metronidazole) were given to piglets for two weeks, and it was revealed that they reduced Bifidobacterium and Lactobacillus in the ileum digesta and feces while increasing Escherichia [19].

Antibiotic use has a variety of impacts on the gut microbiota, according to several research studies, but in most cases, it reduces the relative number of microbes in the gut while increasing the frequency of resistance genes. The use of macrolides, for example, results in a drop in Actinobacteria and an increase in Bacteroides and Proteobacteria in Finnish pre-school children [20].

Clindamycin treatment decreases the quantity of anaerobic bacteria such as Bacteroides while increasing the amount of Enterobacteriaceae in sick people [21]. Antibiotics decreased Bacteroidetes and increased Proteobacteria in teenage rats, as well as having a negative impact on anxiety and cognition [22].

4.3.2 Decrease or Loss of Certain Bacterial Species

Antibiotic-resistant bacteria are found in the Enterobacteriaceae, Lachnospiraceae, and Erysipelotrichaceae taxonomic groups [23]. Antibiotics produce a reduction in feces' secondary bile acids when they are taken orally. Members of the Firmicutes and Bacteroidetes phyla may be inhibited by this secondary bile acid [24]. Antibiotic treatment, according to research, lowers the microbiota composition, particularly Actinobacteria, Firmicutes, and Bifidobacterium (Table 4.1).

4.3.3 Increase in Susceptibility to Infections and Diseases

Over time, antibiotics alter the composition of the gut microbiota and decrease its density. As a result, signaling to the intestinal mucosa and peripheral organs is hampered, impairing immune system performance and causing illness in several host organs (Figure 4.4) [14]. Changes in the gut microbiota may play a role in the etiology and progression of non-communicable illnesses. Numerous studies have linked changes in the composition of the

Table 4.1 Microbiota variation by the impact of antibiotic treatments [25, 26].

| Antibiotic treatments | Gut microbiota abundance | | | | Bacterial diversity |
	Actinobacteria	Bacteroidetes	Firmicutes	Proteobacteria	
Macrolide	Actinobacteria* ↓	Bacteroides ↑	Firmicutes* ↓	Proteobacteria* ↑	↓
Clarithromycin	Actinobacteria* ↓	Bacteroides ↑	Firmicutes* ↓	Proteobacteria* ↑	↓
Vancomycin	—		Lactobacillus ↓ Clostridium ↓		↓
Ciprofloxacin	Bifidobacterium ↓	Alistipes ↓ Bacteroides ↑	Faecalibacterium ↓ Oscillospira ↓ Ruminococcus ↓ Dialister ↓		↓
Clindamycin	Bifidobacterium ↓ Lactobacillus ↓				↓

*Unknown genera
Source: Adapted from Fallani et al., 2011; Yatsunenko et al., 2012.

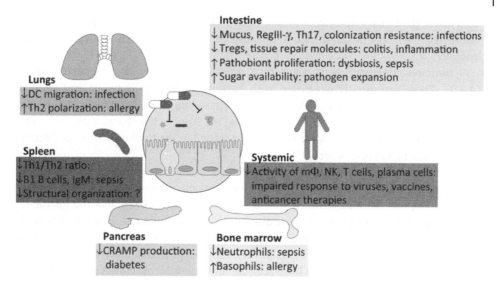

Figure 4.4 Diseases in multiple organs caused by antibiotic mediated microbiota depletion (mφ, macrophages; NK, natural killer cells).

gut microbiota to diseases such as advanced chronic liver disease, C. diff.-associated recurrent diarrhea, specific bowel disorders (including IBD), colorectal cancer, non-alcoholic steatohepatitis, type 2 diabetes (T2D), obesity, and certain bowel disorders [27].

Furthermore, regular use of macrolide antibiotics in the first two years of life has been associated to the later development of asthma and obesity, as well as the presence of these conditions [20]. Additionally, broad-spectrum antibiotics have a stronger relationship to asthma development, implying that bacterial diversity in the microbiota may play a role in antibiotics' effect on asthma development [28]. In patients with metabolic syndrome, oral vancomycin lowered fecal secondary bile acids while raising primary bile acids in plasma postprandially. Vancomycin affected the host's physiology by lowering peripheral insulin sensitivity [29]. Changes in bile acid metabolism caused by antibiotics may have an impact on the host's physiology and susceptibility to infection.

The early stages of life are critical for the development of the microbiota in both humans and animals, and its disruption increases the risk of disease later in childhood or adulthood, especially in cases of allergy and metabolic syndrome [14]. A number of research studies have looked into the link between dysbiosis and colorectal cancer (CRC). The interaction of dysbiotic microbiota with mucosal immune cells and epithelial cells, as well as the presence or absence of certain taxa following antibiotic therapy, could all have a role in the development of cancer. Chronic colonisation with single strains such as Bacteroides fragilis may induce epithelial proliferation, pulmonary endothelial stress, DNA damage, and facilitate a carcinogenic microbiome in mice when combined with other risk factors including genetic vulnerability [30].

Lowering butyrate after antibiotic therapy reduces epithelial oxygen use while increasing luminal oxygenation, leading to an increase in facultative anaerobic Proteobacteria [17]. Proteobacteria have been connected to gastrointestinal and extraintestinal disorders. In addition, studies suggest that it may play a role in lung illnesses such as asthma and chronic obstructive pulmonary disease, but there is little evidence to back this up. Rizzatti et al. conducted the same research about the asthma and chronic obstructive pulmonary disease [31].

A common consequence of nosocomial infections is antibiotic-associated diarrhea (AAD). These are usually associated with bacteria including Klebsiella pneumoniae, Staphylococcus aureus, and C. diff., which may cause long-term recurring infections and even potentially fatal pseudomembranous colitis [16]. Antibiotic-induced reductions of the variety of small and large intestine microbiota resulted in the formation of a persistent C. diff. infection in a mouse model [32].

Obesity and T2D are connected to gut microbiome dysbiosis, according to emerging data in animal models and people. Given that altered gut microbiota, inflammation, and gut barrier disruption are all associated with obesity and T2D, it's likely that the microbiota plays a role in the development of these diseases [33]. Antibiotics reduce the density of the gut microbiota, changing its composition over time. Decreasing signaling to the intestinal mucosa and peripheral organs, results in immune system dysfunction. The diagrams in Figure 4.4 represent diseases that have been found to develop or worsen due to antibiotic treatment in mouse models [14].

4.4 Conclusion

The gut microbiota is a natural part of the human body that performs metabolic, defense, and trophic activities. A healthy gut microbiota composition is characterised by the richness and diversity of gut microbiota that is produced early in life. An imbalanced diet, stress, antibiotic use, and infections, to name a few, have all had an impact on its composition, putting microbiota to the test. One of the primary causes of this occurrence is the use of antibiotic medication to treat infectious diseases, which has both acute and long-term consequences. The influence of antibiotic usage on gut microbiota composition was summarised in this chapter.

References

1 Pilmis, B., Le Monnier, A., and Zahar, J.R. (2020). Gut microbiota, antibiotic therapy and antimicrobial resistance: a narrative review. *Microorganisms* 8 (2): 1–17. https://doi. org/10.3390/microorganisms8020269.

2 Jandhyala, S.M., Talukdar, R., Subramanyam, C. et al. (2015). Role of the normal gut microbiota. *World J. Gastro.* 21 (29): 8836–8847. https://doi.org/10.3748/wjg.v21.i29.8787.

3 Leroy, N., Chirat, C., Lachenal, D. et al. (2004). Extended oxygen delignification. Part 2: multi-stage oxygen bleaching with intermediate hypochlorous acid stages. *Nature* 57 (3): 224–227.

4 Bibbò, S., Ianiro, G., Giorgio, V. et al. (2016). The role of diet on gut microbiota composition. *Euro. Rev. Med. Pharmaco. Sci.* 20 (22): 4742–4749.

5 Looft, T., Johnson, T.A., Allen, H.K. et al. (2012). In-feed antibiotic effects on the swine intestinal microbiome. *Proc. Natl. Acad. Sci. USA* 109: 1691–1696.

6 Yang, L., Bajinka, O., Jarju, P.O. et al. (2021). The varying effects of antibiotics on gut microbiota. *AMB Exp.* 11: 1. https://doi.org/10.1186/s13568-021-01274-w.

7 Huttenhower, C., Gevers, D., Knight, R. et al. (2012). Structure, function and diversity of the healthy human microbiome. *Nature* 486 (7402): 207–214. https://doi.org/10.1038/nature11234.

8 Zhang, X., Han, Y., Huang, W., et al. (2021). The influence of the gut microbiota on the bioavailability of oral drgs. *Acta Pharmac. Sinica B* 11 (7): 1789–1812. https://doi.org/10.1016/j.apsb.2020.09.013.

9 Arumugam M., Raes J., Pelletier E. et al. (2011). Enterotypes of the human gut microbiome. *Nature* 473: 174–180. https://doi.org/10.1038/nature09944.

10 Modi, S.R., Collins, J.J., and Relman, D.A. (2014). Antibiotics and the gut microbiota. *J. Clin. Invest.* 124: 4212–4218.

11 Lange, K., Buerger, M., Stallmach, A. et al. (2016). Effects of antibiotics on gut microbiota. *Dig. Dis.* 34 (3): 260–268. https://doi.org/10.1159/000443360.

12 Munier, A.-L., de Lastours, V., Barbier, F. et al. (2015). Comparative dynamics of the emergence of fluoroquinolone resistance in staphylococci from the nasal microbiota of patients treated with fluoroquinolones according to their environment. *Int. J. Antimicrob. Agen.* 46: 653–659. https://doi.org/10.1016/j.ijantimicag.2015.09.004.

13 de Lastours, V., Chau, F., Roy, C. et al. (2014). Emergence of quinolone resistance in the microbiota of hospitalized patients treated or not with a fluoroquinolone. *J. Antimicrob. Chemother.* 69: 3393–3400.

14 Becattini, S., Taur, Y., and Pamer, E.G. (2016). Antibiotic-induced changes in the intestinal microbiota and disease. *Trend. Molec. Med.* 22 (6): 458–478. https://doi.org/10.1016/j.molmed.2016.04.003.

15 Oldenburg, M., Kruger, A., Ferstl, R., et al. (2012). TLR13 Recognizes Bacterial 23S rRNA Devoid of Erythromycin Resistance-Forming Modification. *Science* 337 (6098): 1111–1115.

16 Francino, M.P. (2016). Antibiotics and the human gut microbiome: dysbioses and accumulation of resistances. *Front. Microbio.* 6 (1): 1–11. https://doi.org/10.3389/fmicb.2015.01543.

17 Litvak, Y., Byndloss, M.X., Tsolis, R.M. et al. (2017). Dysbiotic proteobacteria expansion: a microbial signature of epithelial dysfunction. *Curr. Opin. Microbiol.* 39: 1–6.

18 Looft, T., Allen, H.K., Cantarel, B.L. et al. (2014). Bacteria, phages and pigs: the effects of in-feed antibiotics on the microbiome at different gut locations. *ISME J.* 8: 1566.

19 Pi, Y., Gao, K., Peng, Y. et al. (2019). Antibiotic-induced alterations of the gut microbiota and microbial fermentation in protein parallel the changes in host nitrogen metabolism of growing pigs. *Animal* 13: 262–272.

20 Korpela, K., Salonen, A., Virta, L.J. et al. (2016). Intestinal microbiome is related to lifetime antibiotic use in Finnish pre-school children. *Nat. Commun.* 7: 10410. https://doi.org/10.1038/ncomms10410.

21 Pérez-Cobas, A.E., Artacho, A., Knecht, H. et al. (2013). Differential effects of antibiotic therapy on the structure and function of human gut microbiota. *PLoS One* 8: e80201. https://doi.org/10.1371/journal.pone.0080201.

22 Desbonnet, L., Clarke, G., Traplin, A. et al. (2015). Gut microbiota depletion from early adolescence in mice: implications for brain and behaviour. *Brain Behav. Immun.* 48: 165–173.

23 Bokulich, N.A., Chung, J., Battaglia, T. et al. (2016). Antibiotics, birth mode, and diet shape microbiome maturation during early life. *Sci. Transl. Med.* 8: 343ra82. https://doi.org/10.1126/scitranslmed.aad7121.

24 Caricilli, A.M. and Saad, M.J.A. (2014). Gut microbiota composition and its effects on obesity and insulin resistance. *Curr. Op. Clin. Nutri. Metab. Care* 17 (4): 312–318. https://doi.org/10.1097/MCO.0000000000000067.

25 Fallani, M., Amarri, S., Uusijarvi, A. et al. (2011). Determinants of the human infant intestinal microbiota after the introduction of first complementary foods in infant samples from five European centres. *Microbiology* 157: 1385–1392.

26 Yatsunenko, T., Rey, F.E., Manary, M.J. et al. (2012). Human gut microbiome viewed across age and geography. *Nature* 486: 222–227.

27 Duvallet, C., Gibbons, S.M., Gurry, T. et al. (2017). Meta-analysis of gut microbiome studies identifies disease-specific and shared responses. *Nat. Commun.* 8: 1784. https://doi.org/10.1038/s41467-017-01973-8.

28 Kozyrskyj, A.L., Ernst, P., and Becker, A.B. (2007). Increased risk of childhood asthma from antibiotic use in early life. *Chest* 131: 1753–1759. https://doi.org/10.1378/chest.06-3008.

29 Vrieze, A., Out, C., Fuentes, S. et al. (2014). Impact of oral vancomycin on gut microbiota, bile acid metabolism, and insulin sensitivity. *J. Hepatol.* 60: 824–831. https://doi.org/10.1016/j.jhep.2013.11.034.

30 Wu, S., Rhee, K.J., Albesiano, E. et al. (2009). A human colonic commensal promotes colon tumorigenesis via activation of T helper type 17 T cell responses. *Nat. Med.* 15: 1016–1022.

31 Rizzatti, G., Lopetuso, L.R., Gibiino, G. et al. (2017). Proteobacteria: a common factor in human diseases. *BioMed Res. Intl.* 9351507. DOI: 10.1155/2017/9351507.

32 Lawley, T.D., Clare, S., Walker, A.W. et al. (2009). Antibiotic treatment of *Clostridium difficile* carrier mice triggers a supershedder state, spore-mediated transmission, and severe disease in immunocompromised hosts. *Infect. Immun.* 77: 3661–3669. https://doi.org/10.1128/IAI.00558-09.

33 Wen, L. and Duffy, A. (2017). Factors influencing the gut microbiota, inflammation, and type 2 diabetes. *J. Nutr.* 147 (7): 1468S–1475S. https://doi.org/10.3945/jn.116.240754.

5

Dysbiosis and its Varied Impacts

Rajani Sharma and Kunal Kumar

Amity Institute of Biotechnology, Amity University, Jharkhand, Ranchi, India

5.1 Introduction

The omnipresence of microbes has intrigued researchers to implement its uses in different fields. Our bodies are invaded by microbes and commonly addressed as the microbiome; these microbes have a symbiotic relationship with our bodies. A healthy body has a calculated diversity of microbes (Table 5.1), and disturbance in their distribution causes the eruption of various diseases. Microbiome composition is affected by diet, physical environment, xenobiotics, and hygiene factors. Microbiomes are inherited from the mother during the time of vaginal delivery [1]. Even at early stages, there are certain fatty acids that are swallowed by the fetus that act as the supportive chemical for the microbiome. Further, microbes colonise during the lactation period, hence, the various studies support that babies born via Caesarean have weak immunity [2]. As life switches to a solid diet, the microbiome is further affected. Fat rich diet, use of preservatives, and consumption of less fibre lead to the rise in dysbiosis [3]. More specifically, immunocompromised hosts are more prone to develop dysbiosis. This chapter discusses the factors promoting dysbiosis and diseases related to this, a brief about these factors related to its treatment is also discussed.

5.2 Causes of Dysbiosis

The most prominent reasons for changes in the microbial diversity of the natural flora that lead to dysbiosis are changes in food habits, psychological stress, geographical location, history of unrestricted intake of antibiotics, and exposure to pesticides [12] (see Figure 5.1).

High fat and western diets such as saturated and trans-fat, simple sugar, refined flour, high-fructose corn syrup, and other processed foods contribute to changes in gut microbial populations and contribute to the imbalance of the microbiome [13]. It has also been found that infants feeding on breast milk have different dominant populations of microbes

The Gut Microbiota in Health and Disease, First Edition. Edited by Nimmy Srivastava, Salam A. Ibrahim, Jayeeta Chattopadhyay, and Mohamed H. Arbab.

Table 5.1   Some common microbiomes of the human body.

Organ	Natural Microbiome	Reference
Gut	Bacteroidetes, Firmicutes, and Actinobacteria comprised of *Bacteroides, Faecalibacterium, Clostridium, Ruminococcus, Eubacterium, Peptococcus, Bifidobacterium, Peptostreptococcus, Escherichia Lactobacillus*	[4, 5, 6]
	Fungal organisms such as *Aspergillus, Candida, Penicillium, Saccharomyces, Rhodotorula, Pleospora, Trametes, Sclerotinia, Bullera, Galactomyces*	
Urogenital	*Lactobacillus, Gardnerella, Actinobaculum, Coriobacterium, Rhodococcus, Fusobacterium, Azospira, Corynebacterium, Pseudomona, Prevotella, Streptococcus*	[7, 8]
Skin	*Propionibacterium, Staphylococcus, Corynebacterium, Micrococcus Malassezia* spp., *Aspergillus* spp., *Cryptococcus* spp., *Rhodotorula* spp., *Epicoccum* spp.	[9,10]
Oral cavity	*Peptostreptococcus, Abiotrophia, Stomatococcus Streptococcus, Corynebacterium, Bifidobacterium, Pseudoramibacter, Propionibacterium, Neisseria, Moraxella, Veillonella, Treponema, Desulfovibrio*	[11]
	Fungal genera include *Candida, Fusarium, Aspergillus*	

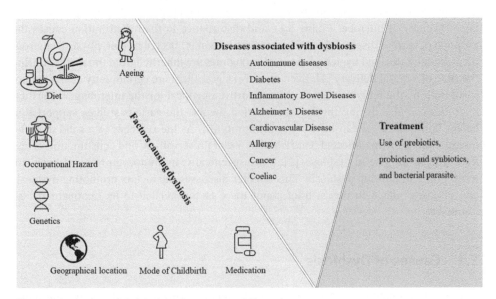

Figure 5.1   Impact of dysbiosis and treatments followed.

in comparison to infants fed on formula [14]. More recent studies have highlighted the presence of *Bifidobacteria* spp. in breast-fed infants, while *Bacteroides* spp., *Clostridium coccoides*, and *Lactobacillus* spp. were seen in higher numbers in formula-fed infants [15]. The work carried out by Zhang et al. [16] revealed that mice fed on diets high in fat lost gut protecting *Bifidobacteria* spp. The study also demonstrated that a complete dietary change could cause more than 50% structural variation in gut microbiota. Human fecal microbiota could maintain a balanced population upon transplantation in a germ free (GF) mouse model under low fat, high plant polysaccharide-rich diet. However, on sudden shift in western diet, overgrowth of *Eubacterium dolichum*, *Clostridium innocuum*, *Catenibacteriummitsuokai*, and *Enterococcus* spp. belonging to Firmicutes was accounted for, with substantial decline in numerous *Bacteroides* spp. [17]. Diets with high complex carbohydrate content do not promote pathogenic species such as *Mycobacterium avium* and Enterobacteriaceae [18]. Beneficial *Bifidobacteria* spp. including *B. longum* and *B. thetaiotaomicron* were seen in high numbers in subjects consuming complex carbohydrates, while refined sugar consumption led to overgrowth of opportunistic strains of *C. difficile and C. perfringens* [19].

Antibiotics are consumed by patients to overcome the deleterious effect of pathogens; however, overdose and unrestricted use contribute to factors of dysbiosis. Broad-spectrum activities of antibiotics indiscriminately kill and inhibit commensal microbes of the human gut. Different sets of antibiotics have specific detrimental effects on specific species. Microbes of the Firmicutes group are prone to destruction by vancomycin antibiotics. On the contrary, the amoxicillin group of antibiotics does not cause significant inhibitory effects on microbial diversity of natural flora. However, cocktails of gentamicin, ampicillin, metronidazole, vancomycin, and neomycin have significantly inhibited the proliferation of natural flora and shifted the structure and composition of gut microbiota [20]. Many synthetic and semi-synthetic antibiotics, specifically penicillin, cephalosporin, and vancomycin significantly affect colonisation of microbiota, probably because they inhibit the gram-positive nonsporulating, lactic acid-producing Bacillus species [21].

Symbiosis and co-dependency are common traits among different groups of gut microbiota. The secondary metabolites produced by one set of gut microbes may be a substrate for another set of microbes. Such a trend has been seen in case of *Bifidobacterium adolescentis* and butyrate producing anaerobes. *B. adolescentis* could produce lactate and acetate utilising fructooligosaccharides and starch. Lactate and acetate are growth factors for butyrate-producing anaerobes as these strains have shown inability to utilise starch and fructooligosaccharides [22]. Butyrate has anti-inflammatory and immunomodulatory effect, and is a vital metabolite of the human colon; this is an excellent example of cross-feeding, and any member of symbionts affected by unrestricted use of antibiotics may directly affect the growth of other symbiont. Similar cross-feeding association has been established between Escherichia coli and Rhodopseudomonas palustris, Bacteroides, and Methanobrevibactersmithii [23]. The population sub-set of dominant Bifidobacteria, accounting for 90% of the total colon natural flora in breast-fed infants, could fall drastically to less than 5% of the total microbial count in adults associated with antibiotic associated diarrhea [20]. One unfavourable impact of antibiotics is development of antibiotic resistance genes in organisms. These antibiotic resistant organisms may eliminate sensitive strains through competitive habitation. Moreover, antibiotic-resistance genes may be transmitted through conjugation, transduction, and transformation across other microbial species leading to a rapid propagation of antibiotic resistance in other members of the gut microbiota [24].

Another prominent cause of dysbiosis is exposure to pesticides and insecticides; the changes in the population are dependent on exposure duration and chemical composition of pesticides [25]. Studies on mice suggested that in general, the amounts of *Bacteroidetes*,

Firmicutes, Actinobacteria, Proteobacteria, and *Verrucomicrobia,* and were seriously diminished on exposure and bioaccumulation of benzimidazolecarbendazim (CBZ) [25]. The mice subjected to penconazole exhibited a decreased amount of *Proteobacteria,* while *Cyanobacteria Bacteroidetes* and *Actinobacteria* considerably improved. Similar results were obtained in cases on exposure to the fungicide azoxystrobin. The direct outcome of change in microbial load may lead to impairment of intestinal barrier function, affecting glucolipid metabolism and normal liver function and promoting liver damage [26].

5.3 Dysbiosis, Immune System, and Associated Diseases

A key attribute of the microbiome is conferring protection from pathogenic organisms, and promoting the growth of other symbionts involved in short chain fatty acid synthesis responsible for anti-inflammatory and immunomodulatory properties. Furthermore, vitamins, essential amino acids synthesised by microbes, regulate fat metabolism indirectly modulating the synthesis of molecules of immune system [27].

Studies conducted recently on germ-free animal models have proved that the natural microbiome of the human body have profound effects in the growth of bone marrow, thymus, spleen, and lymph nodes, and play a pivotal role in generation of CD4+ and CD8+ intestinal T cell subsets [28]. Development of T-cell effector subsets is linked to specific bacterial communities. T helper 17 cells, potent sources of interleukin-17 (IL-17), play a critical role in the development of a pathogen-free gut and maintain the integrity of mucosal barrier [28]. A unique interaction between the mucosal immune system and gut microbiota revealed that the human body causes no negative immune response on non-pathogenic microbes suppressing the harmful microbes with the downregulation of interleukin 8 secretion, macrophage-attracting chemokine production, and NF-kB dependent gene expression [29]. Bifidobacterium and lactic acid bacteria of the gut, among many other microbes, upregulate anti-inflammation. Short chain fatty acids of colon-inhabiting microbes modulate the immune response via methylation, demethylation activity within the promoter region of certain genes, and by involvement of G-Protein coupled receptors. G-Protein coupled receptors also promote anti-inflammatory function by the suppression of histone deacetylases activity in regulatory T cells (T_{regs}) [30]. Onset of dysbiosis with imbalance in gut microbiome causes inappropriate mucosal inflammation leading to various immune mediated conditions of inflammatory bowel disease, rheumatoid arthritis, multiple sclerosis, and systemic lupus erythematosus diseases [12].

5.3.1 Dysbiosis in the Immune-Compromised Host

Our bodies have two defense mechanisms; innate and adaptive immunity to fight against infection [31], but certain environmental and host-related factors alter the ecosystem favouring the survival of pathogens. Microbes adopt a sensing mechanism to colonise by coordinating with Pattern Recognition Receptors (PRRs), so the invasion of pathogens is possible only in the immune-compromised host [32]. In general, microbiota of the intestine prevents the growth of pathogens; however, induction of inflammation along with genetic deficiency of interleukin-10 favours the growth of enteric pathogens. As in the case of T1D, an autoimmune disease that is developed due to the destruction of β-cells (producing insulin by T-cell) changes the healthy ecosystem of intestinal microbiomes leading to dysbiosis. This seems to be directly associated with the deficient function of Myeloid differentiation primary response protein 88 (MyD88), an adaptor for TLR (Toll-like receptor) [33]. Susceptibility of pathogens is due to downregulation of IgA transporter or class switching to IgE, intestinal mucosal protein such as mucin-2, antimicrobial peptide including RegIIIγ, and Defa-res1. *Klebsiella pneumonia* is one of the pathogens associated with malfunctioning of MyD88. In response to MyD88 class switching is seen with asthma [34].

Inflammation, a component of innate immunity, is a mechanism to check the growth of pathogens. In diseases such as IBD, there is increase in pathogenesis and a decrease in the richness of beneficial microbes. Under such conditions, there is switching of obligatory to facultative microbes. Moreover, there is decrease in the frequency of butyrate-producing bacteria causing increase in permeability of the epithelial layer by increasing sulphate reduction. Celiac disease is also a result of inflammatory response activated by Th1 and Th17 [35]. In the case of a celiac patient there is a significant increase in *Shigella, Klebsiella, Bacteroids,* and *Staphylococcus,* and decreased species of *Lactobacillus, Bifidobacter,* and *Enterococcus* were noticed [36, 37]. An increase in pathogens elevated the metabolism of ethyl-acetate, short-chain fatty acid, free amino acids, and glutamine. Likewise in rheumatoid arthritis, there is alteration in the metabolism of sulfur, zinc, iron, and arginine along with transportation system and redox environment [38]. There is depletion of the *Haemophilus* spp. colony, and overgrowth of *Prevotellacopri* and *Lactobacillus salivarius* were observed in cases of rheumatoid arthritis [39].

Dysbiosis may directly influence immune-mediated diseases, and autoimmune diseases are believed to be a cause of dysbiosis, which will be discussed and summarised next.

5.3.2 Intestinal Bowel Disease (IBD)

IBD is a disorder characterised by the acute inflammation of the intestinal mucosal wall and associated organs of the intestine. The changes in microbial diversity of the gut play a leading role in the pathogenesis of IBD. Several studies have failed to find a bacterium for a single associated cause of the disease. It has been proposed that in addition to changes in microbial diversity as one of leading causes of IBD, diminishing production of metabolites like butyrate and increasing sulphate reduction also contribute to IBD [40, 41].

5.3.3 Rheumatoid Arthritis

Rheumatoid arthritis is an autoimmune disease represented by joint destruction. Studies on GF mice suggest that intestinal commensal bacteria play a fundamental role in the development and progression of rheumatoid arthritis. Increased susceptibility to this autoimmune disease has been credited to *Prevotellacopri*, and metagenomic analysis indicated natural flora, *Lactobacillus salivarius*, as a marker of rheumatoid arthritis. Patients with rheumatoid arthritis harbour commensal bacteria exhibiting deviation in several metabolic pathways and metagenomic functions. These set of microbes in patients with rheumatoid arthritis have different mechanism of metal ion and arginine metabolism [42, 43].

5.3.4 Type 1 Diabetes

T1D is T cell-mediated damage of insulin-producing cells of the pancreas, and therefore characterised as an autoimmune disease, destroying the normal mechanism of glucose metabolism. Genetic factors such as the presence of Human Leukocyte Antigen (HLA), risk alleles along with non-genetic factors contribute to T1D [44]. Dysbiosis in humans cause T1D through alteration of multiple metabolites mediated signalling, as suggested by several works [45]. More recently, studies have demonstrated that autoimmune risk of T1D in children with high-risk of insulin dependent diabetes mellitus (IDDM) is linked with special major histocompatibility complex (MHC) gene products, designated as antigens HLA-DR3 and DR genotype reduced to 60% on administration of probiotics. These works suggest that changes in microbiota causally contributes to the instigation of autoimmunity [33].

5.3.5 Dysbiosis of Skin Microbiome in Carcinogenesis

Human skin harbours a multitude of diverse communities of microbes. The skin provides a range of environments with diverse pH, salinity, moisture, temperature, sebum content, and associated internal factors to promote specific and selective microbes [46]. For example, *Staphylococcus epidermidis* remain in commensal association with other microbes and does not allow the growth of pathogenic *Staphylococcus aureus* by secretion of serine protease. However, a balanced microbial community of skin changes during injury, and the region is inhabited by pathogenic microbes causing numerous complications. In-vivo studies in mice have revealed that flagellated microorganisms such as *Escherichia coli* and *Pseuodomonas aeruginosa* supported carcinogenesis through an intrinsic signalling mechanism in the host at the site of tissue injury. Flagellin and similar microbial molecules provoke inflammation and activate toll-like receptor 5 (TLR-5) for tumour growth [10, 47].

5.3.6 Dysbiosis of Oral Microbiota Impacts Carcinogenesis

Oral cavities have many ecological niches harbouring sets of microbiomes in lips, gingivae, teeth, hard palate, buccal mucosa, tongue, and floor of the mouth. Every region of the oral cavity represents an ecological niche, and each of these niches have a different microbial diversity [48]. Several physical and chemical factors released by the commensal microorganisms protect the oral cavity from invading pathogens; however, physical factors and tobacco consumption alter the microbiome of the mouth. It is a well-known fact that tobacco leads to oral cancers, and an overabundance of a few commensal microbial species such as *Streptococcusanginosus* or *Fusobacterium nucleatum* have been noted in a few oral cancers. These sets of microorganisms overproduce nitric oxide, damaging the DNA of cells and cause carcinogenesis. Studies have found *F. nucleatum* and *Porphyromonas Gingivalis* activate immunocytes leading to tumour progression with the release of reactive oxygen species. *P. gingivalis* induces expression of prostaglandin–endoperoxide synthase with the aid of expression of cyclooxygenase-2 gene [49]. These phenomenon initiate symptoms of inflammation by bringing pro-inflammatory mediators at the site of pathogenesis, thereby indirectly inducing inflammation mediated carcinogenesis and tumour progression [47].

5.3.7 Dysbiosis of Urobiome

Urobiome is the microbial community of the urinary tract and are dominated by *Lactobacillus, Gardnerella, Streptococcus, Staphylococcus, Klebsiella*, and *Enterococcus*. The variations in the human urinary microbiome aggravate the concern of globally prevalent diseases influencing kidney function, such as diabetes mellitus, chronic kidney disease, hypertension, and urinary tract infection [8].

5.3.8 Pigmented Gallstone

Gallstone, or cholelithiasis, is considered a metabolic disease, but many of the researchers had evidence of the association of microbes in the mechanism of the formation of gallstone. The bacterial isolates had urease, β-glucuronidase, and slime producing activity. Under normal conditions, bile solubilises the cholesterol released from the liver to the gallbladder by the formation of micelles. When the cholesterol to phospholipid ratio is disturbed, there is the precipitation of cholesterol forming nidus [50].

The composition of gallstone is largely determined by epidemiological factors and dietary habits, but chemical analysis of gallstone states the presence of some common elements and compounds in all types of gallstones, such as $CaCO_3$ and its precipitated product (vaterite). Further, the microbial isolates from the cholesterol gallstone had urease activity [51]. The urease activity was supposed to generate $CaCO_3$ by degrading urea. This increase concentration of $CaCO_3$ precipitate, with further deposition, led to the formation of gallstone. Major research has supported the association of $CaCO_3$ with cholesterol gallstone. The microbial role was also seen to be associated with pigmented gallstone; bilirubin is the major content of pigmented gallstone [52]. This is formed by the precipitation of unconjugated bile salts. Bacteria with β-glucuronidase activity were directly responsible for pigmented gallstone. Bile salts remain soluble in their conjugated form. β-glucuronidase activity of bacteria is responsible for deconjugation of bile salts causing their precipitation [53, 54], hence, it initiates the mechanism for pigmented gallstone formation. The common isolates from gallstone are *Escherichia, Vibrio, Helicobacter, Salmonella, Streptococcus, Klebsiella, Enterococcus*, and *Salmonella*. Another remarkable property of the bacteria isolated from gallstone has slime producing activity, which is supposed to bind the precipitated particles together; this process further challenges the dissolution process of gallstone. In an in-vitro study it was analysed that the presence of bacteria enhances the rate of solidification of precipitates [54]. The increase in the solidification process decreases the chances of dissolution by oral treatment.

5.3.9 Cholangitis

Cholangitis is a condition of obstruction of bile in hepatobiliary system, and may lead to mild to life threatening septic shock intestinal disease. Under normal circumstances there is the flawless movement of sterile bile with antimicrobial activity [55]. In the case of a pathogenic invasion, the bile drains to the duodenum and the rest are checked by bile salt. Infection is further checked by the secretion of IgA by the epithelial lining of biliary tract. The obstruction of bile causes increased duct pressure to more than 25 cm H2O; under high pressure, the defense system fails, leading to dysbiosis [56]. Under such pressure, the tight junction widened and decreases the production of IgA and the Kuffer cells malfunction. The dysbiosis condition is usually associated with acute or secondary cholangitis, and less common in primary sclerosis and IgG4 associated cholangitis [57]. Under such a malfunctioning immune system, there is an increase in the pathogenesis of *E.coli*, *Pseudomonas*, *Klebsiella*, *Candida*, etc.

5.4   Intestinal Colonisation in Neonates and Dysbiosis

The timing of intestinal colonisation in neonates is a concluding factor to determine their immune system and microbial colonisation. Neonates are inoculated with the microbes at the time of vaginal birth while passing through the birth canal. This can be evidenced from the similarity of microbiota of a newborn's intestine with the colonisation of mother vaginal microbes. So, if the mother has dysbiosis condition, there is the chance of the passage of this stage to neonates [1]. Such a condition is not associated with caesarean births but those newborns are at greater risk of celiac disease, asthma, obesity, and other dysbiotic diseases such as IBD, as there is delay in the microbial colonisation. Delayed colonisation also decreases the microbial diversity and challenges the immune system. A study on germ-free mice stated that there is hypermethylation of Cxc116 gene, which results in the accumulation of invariant natural killer T cells in the lungs and colon; this causes morbidity in IBD mice and asthma [58]. Initially, the neonates have aerobic colonies of both gram-positive and negative bacteria, these earliest colonising bacteria inside the gut of neonates eventually establish an anaerobic environment, which leads to the establishment of bacterial population belonging to obligate anaerobes, including Firmicutes. The diversity of bacterial colonies is largely influenced by the diet during pregnancy, maternal genetics, and environmental exposures. After this first inoculation the compounds present in the gut of neonates and further act as prebiotics, which promotes further commensals. Vernix caseosa is one of them, these are short chain fatty acids (SCFAs) that form a waxy coating around the fetus [59], and have been swallowed by the fetus in-utero. Its presence in the intestine of the fetus upregulates the Interleukin 10, and hence maintain the intestinal microbial ecology. Like SCFAs, breast milk is also rich in oligosaccharides, which promotes the growth of *Bifidobaterium* spp. During pregnancy, there is an increase in intestinal permeability, which leads to the translocation of gut bacteria to the mammary glands through enteromammary pathway. The presence of such prebiotics and catabolite products of SCFAs and lactate check the growth of pathogens such as *E. coli* and *Enterococcus* [60]. Further, breast milk is rich in lysozyme and lactoferrin, which have antibacterial properties, and the glycan content of milk misguides the attachment of pathogens as it mimics cell surface adhesion molecules [61].

In the later stage of development of childhood, the challenge to maintain the microbiomes lies with the diet. Children with shorter periods of breast feeding, and consumption of more calories, animal proteins, fats, and less fibre have less diverse microbes.

5.5   Treatment or Therapeutics

Dysbiosis resembles the state of dominance of pathogens over favourable microbes, so, a major step to overcome the condition of dysbiosis is to provide the environment to favour the growth of prebiotics, probiotics, and synbiotics [62]. This methodology has proven efficient even under immunocompromised conditions, mental stress, and prolonged antibiotic therapies. Under immune stress, prebiotics activate the innate immunity and stimulate the modulation of cytokines. The modulation of cytokines further targets the production of immunoglobulin and activate macrophages and inflammation [63].

Sedentary lifestyle is also responsible for dysbiosis and studies have proved that physical activity enhances the number of beneficial microorganisms, reducing the risk of dysbiosis-related disorders in the human body [64]. Regular workouts lead to greater abundance of *Faecalibacterium prausnizii*, *Roseburia hominis*, and *A. muciniphilia* compared with sedentary routines [12]. Some of the probiotic's role in dysbiosis treatment is mentioned in Table 5.2. The probiotics could regulate the pH of the surrounding by secreting certain chemicals such as acetic acid and lactic acid, which check the growth of pathogens. Secretion of certain extracellular enzymes such as α-amylase, DNase, and β-glucanacase are some other well-proved chemicals that could check the growth of pathogens which are responsible for diarrhea [65]. There are certain predators, which seem to balance the microbial ecology; *Bdellovibrio bacteriovorus* in one such bacterial species which is predominant in the duodenum and checks the growth of gram-negative bacteria [66]. Another option is to use a predator for phage therapy; here the virus specific for pathogenic bacteria were used.

Fecal transplantation is another preferable technique and has been in use since the 1950s [67]. In this technique, a healthy stool is transplanted, which is considered as a rich source of gut microflora. This has been proven effective in pseudomembranous colitis and

Table 5.2 Role of the probiotic for the treatment of dysbiosis.

Bacterial Species	Target characteristics for treatment	Treatment process
Lactobacilli	Modulate innate immune system	Effective against inflammation, diarrhea, enteric pathogens, and prevention of infant colic
Bifidobacteria	Source for enzymes, vitamins, acetic, and lactic acids. Inhibit pathogens by regulating pH of the colon	Effective against allergic IgE
Bacillus subtilis	Secrete many extracellular enzymes (α-amylase, arabinase, cellulose, β-glucanacase, and DNase	Anti-diarrheal
Escherichia coli strain Nissle *1917*	Modulate immune system	Microbial homeostasis and reduction of pathogen invasion to intestinal epithelial cells
Streptococcus thermophilus	Anti-inflammatory properties	Fight against pathogenic bacteria
Enterococcus faecium	Lactic and butyric acid producer	Regulate immune function and prevent enteric pathogens
Saccharomyces boulardii	Produces lactic acid and group B vitamins	Effective against diarrhea

inflammation [68]. Initially, it was administered as an enema, but now colonoscopy and nasogastric are preferred. A major advantage of fecal transplantation is that its glycerol can be stored at –80°C.

5.6 Conclusion

Several studies have revealed that natural flora present in the human body play a pivotal role in maintaining health. A slight variation in our food habits, lifestyle, exposure to occupational hazards, and non-discriminate use of antibiotics alter the diversity and structure of the microbiome, leading to dysbiosis. Dysbiosis is one of the leading causes of many life-threatening conditions such as IBD, T1D, autoimmune diseases, and cancers. Treatment strategies should incorporate steps for providing the environment to favour the growth of prebiotics, probiotics, and synbiotics, along with the adoption of healthy food habits and lifestyles, and precautionary measures to overcome exposure of occupational hazards.

References

1 Dunn, A.B., Jordan, S., Baker, B.J. et al. (2017). The maternal infant microbiome: considerations for labor and birth. *MCN Am. J. Matern. Nurs.* 42 (6): 318–325. https://doi. org/10.1097%2FNMC.0000000000000373.

2 Kalbermatter, C., Fernandez Trigo, N., Christensen, S. et al. (2021). Maternal microbiota, early life colonization and breast milk drive immune development in the newborn. *Front. Immunol.* 12. https://doi.org/10.3389/fimmu.2021.683022.

3 Hrncirova, L., Machova, V., Trckova, E. et al. (2019). Food preservatives induce proteobacteria dysbiosis in human-microbiota associated Nod2-deficient mice. *Microorganisms* 7 (10): 383. https://doi.org/10.3390%2Fmicroorganisms7100383.

4 Guarner, F., Malagelada, J.-R. (2003). Gut flora in health and disease. *Lancet* 361 (9356): 512–519.

5 Beaugerie, L., Petit, J.-C. (2004). Antibiotic-associated diarrhoea. *Best Pract. Res. Clin. Gastroenterol.* 18 (2): 337–352.

6 Cui, L., Morris, A., and Ghedin, E. (2013). The human mycobiome in health and disease. *Genome Med.* 5 (7): 63.

7 Perez-Carrasco, V., Soriano-Lerma, A., Soriano, M. et al. (2021). Urinary microbiome: yin and yang of the urinary tract. *Front Cell Infect. Microbiol.* 11.

8 Wolfe, A.J., Brubaker, L. (2019). Urobiome updates: Advances in urinary microbiome research. *Nat. Rev. Urol.* 16 (2): 73–74.

9 Byrd, A.L., Belkaid, Y., Segre, J.A. (2018). The human skin microbiome. *Nat. Rev. Microbiol.* 16 (3): 143–155.

10 Grice, E.A. and Segre, J.A. (2011). The skin microbiome. *Nat. Rev. Microbiol.* 9 (4): 244–253.

11 Deo, P.N. and Deshmukh, R. (2019). Oral microbiome: unveiling the fundamentals. *J. Oral Maxillofac. Pathol.* 23 (1): 122–128.

12 Martinez, J.E., Kahana, D.D., Ghuman, S. et al. (2021). Unhealthy lifestyle and gut dysbiosis: a better understanding of the effects of poor diet and nicotine on the intestinal microbiome. *Front Endocrinol.* 12: 667066.

13 Sonnenburg, E.D. and Sonnenburg, J.L. (2014). Starving our microbial self: the deleterious consequences of a diet deficient in microbiota-accessible carbohydrates. *Cell Metab.* 20 (5): 779–786.

14 Ma, J., Li, Z., Zhang, W. et al. (2020). Comparison of gut microbiota in exclusively breast-fed and formula-fed babies: a study of 91 term infants. *Sci. Rep.* 10 (1): 1–11.

15 Zhang, Y.J., Li, S., Gan, R.Y. et al. (2015). Impacts of gut bacteria on human health and diseases. *Int. J. Mol. Sci.* 16 (4): 7493.

16 Zhang, C., Zhang, M., Wang, S. et al. (2009). Interactions between gut microbiota, host genetics and diet relevant to development of metabolic syndromes in mice. *ISME J.* 4 (2): 232–41.

17 Turnbaugh, P.J., Ridaura, V.K., Faith, J.J. et al. (2009). The effect of diet on the human gut microbiome: a metagenomic analysis in humanized gnotobiotic mice. *Sci. Transl. Med.* 1 (6): 6ra14.

18 Walker, A.W., Sanderson, J.D., Churcher, C. et al. (2011). High-throughput clone library analysis of the mucosa-associated microbiota reveals dysbiosis and differences between inflamed and non-inflamed regions of the intestine in inflammatory bowel disease. *BMC Microbiol.* 11.

19 Brown, K., DeCoffe, D., Molcan, E. et al. (2012). Diet-induced dysbiosis of the intestinal microbiota and the effects on immunity and disease. *Nutrients* 4 (8): 1095.

20 Zhang, S., Chen, D.C., and Chen, L.M. (2019). Facing a new challenge: the adverse effects of antibiotics on gut microbiota and host immunity. *Chin. Med. J.* 132 (10): 1135.

21 Rafii, F., Sutherland, J.B., and Cerniglia, C.E. (2008). Effects of treatment with antimicrobial agents on the human colonic microflora. *Ther. Clin. Risk Manag.* 4 (6): 1343–1358.

22 Rivière, A., Selak, M., Lantin, D. et al. (2016). Bifidobacteria and butyrate-producing colon bacteria: Importance and strategies for their stimulation in the human gut. *Front. Microbiol.* 7: 979.

23 Heinken, A. and Thiele, I. (2015). Anoxic conditions promote species-specific mutualism between gut microbes in silico. *Appl. Environ. Microbiol.* 81 (12): 4049–4061.

24 Willing, B.P., Russell, S.L., and Finlay, B.B. (2011). Shifting the balance: Antibiotic effects on host-microbiota mutualism. *Nat. Rev. Microbiol.* 9 (4): 233–243.

25 Giambò, F., Teodoro, M., Costa, C. et al. (2021). Toxicology and microbiota: how do pesticides influence gut microbiota? A review. *Int. J. Environ. Res. Public Heal.* 18 (11): 5510.

26 Meng, Z., Liu, L., Jia, M. et al. (2019). Impacts of penconazole and its enantiomers exposure on gut microbiota and metabolic profiles in mice. *J. Agric. Food Chem.* 67 (30): 8303–8311.

27 Berer, K. and Krishnamoorthy, G. (2014). Microbial view of central nervous system autoimmunity. *FEBS Lett.* 588 (22): 4207–4213.

28 Gensollen, T., Iyer, S.S., Kasper, D.L. et al. (2016). How colonization by microbiota in early life shapes the immune system. *Science* 352 (6285): 539–544.

29 Delcenserie, V., Martel, D., Lamoureux, M. et al. (2008). Immunomodulatory effects of probiotics in the intestinal tract. *Curr. Issues Mol. Biol.* 10 (1–2): 37–54.

30 Andrade, M.E.R., Araújo, R.S., de Barros, P.A.V. et al. (2015). The role of immunomodulators on intestinal barrier homeostasis in experimental models. *Clin. Nutr.* 34 (6): 1080–1087.

31 Pandey, V.K., Sharma, R., Prajapati, G.K. et al. (2022). N-glycosylation, a leading role in viral infection and immunity development. *Mol. Biol. Rep.* https://doi.org/10.1007/s11033-022-07359-4.

32 Chu, H. and Mazmanian, S.K. (2013). Innate immune recognition of the microbiota promotes host-microbial symbiosis. *Nat. Immunol.* 14 (7): 668–675. https://doi.org/10.1038/ni.2635.

33 Durazzo, M., Ferro, A., and Gruden, G. (2019). Gastrointestinal microbiota and type 1 diabetes mellitus: the state of art. *J. Clin. Med.* 8 (11): 1843. https://doi.org/10.3390/jcm8111843.

34 Li, Y., Chen, Q., Ji, W. et al. (2021). TLR2 deficiency promotes IgE and inhibits IgG1 class-switching following ovalbumin sensitization. *Ital. J. Pediatr.* 47 (1): 162. https://doi.org/10.1186%2Fs13052-021-01088-3.

35 Mazzarella, G. (2015). Effector and suppressor T cells in celiac disease. *World J. Gastroenterol.* 21 (24): 7349. https://doi.org/10.3748%2Fwjg.v21.i24.7349.

36 Abdukhakimova, D., Dossybayeva, K., and Poddighe, D. (2021). Fecal and duodenal microbiota in pediatric celiac disease. *Front Pediatr.* 9: 652208. https://doi.org/10.3389/fped.2021.652208.

37 Arrieta, M.-C., Stiemsma, L.T., Amenyogbe, N. et al. (2014). The intestinal microbiome in early life: health and disease. *Front. Immunol.* 5. https://doi.org/10.3389/fimmu.2014.00427.

38 Horta-Baas, G., Romero-Figueroa, M.del S, Montiel-Jarquín, A.J. et al. (2017). Intestinal dysbiosis and rheumatoid arthritis: a link between gut microbiota and the pathogenesis of rheumatoid arthritis. *J. Immunol. Res.* 1–13. https://doi.org/10.1155/2017/4835189.

39 De Luca, F. and Shoenfeld, Y.. (2018). The microbiome in autoimmune diseases. *Clin. Exp. Immunol.* 195 (1): 74–85. https://doi.org/10.1111/cei.13158.

40 Strauss, J., Kaplan, G.G., Beck, P.L. et al. (2011). Invasive potential of gut mucosa-derived fusobacterium nucleatum positively correlates with IBD status of the host. *Inflamm. Bowel. Dis.* 17 (9): 1971–1978.

41 Li, J., Butcher, J., Mack, D. et al. (2015). Functional impacts of the intestinal microbiome in the pathogenesis of inflammatory bowel disease. *Inflamm. Bowel. Dis.* 21 (1): 139–153.

42 Zhang, X., Zhang, D., Jia, H. et al. (2015). The oral and gut microbiomes are perturbed in rheumatoid arthritis and partly normalized after treatment. *Nat. Med.* 21 (8): 895–905.

43 Scher, J.U., Sczesnak, A., Longman, R.S. et al. (2013). Expansion of intestinal Prevotella copri correlates with enhanced susceptibility to arthritis. *Elife* 2: e01202.

44 Achenbach, P., Bonifacio, E., Koczwara, K. et al. (2005). Natural history of type 1 diabetes. *Diabetes* 2: S25–31.

45 Wen, L., Ley, R.E., Volchkov, P.Y. et al. (2008). Innate immunity and intestinal microbiota in the development of type 1 diabetes. *Nature* 455 (7216): 1109–1113.

46 Somerville, D.A. (1969). The normal flora of the skin in different age groups. *Br. J. Dermatol.* 81 (4): 248–58.

47 Vimal, J., Himal, I., and Kannan, S. (2020). Role of microbial dysbiosis in carcinogenesis & cancer therapies. *Indian J. Med. Res.* 152 (6): 553–561.

48 Dewhirst, F.E., Chen, T., Izard, J. et al. (2010). The human oral microbiome. *J. Bacteriol.* 192 (19): 5002–5017.

49 Castellarin, M., Warren, R.L., Freeman, J.D. et al. (2012). Fusobacterium nucleatum infection is prevalent in human colorectal carcinoma. *Genome Res.* 22 (2): 299–306.

50 Sharma, R., Kumar, A., Jha, N.K. et al. (2012). Probing into the prevalence and factors of gallstones formation in Jharkhand region in India. *IJABPT* 3 (3): 36–41.

51 Sharma, R., Soy, S., Kumar, C. et al. (2015). Analysis of gallstone composition and structure in Jharkhand region. *Indian J. Gastroenterol.* 34 (1).

52 Soloway, R.D. and Malet, P.F. (1984). Classification and pathogenesis of pigment gallstones. In: *Epidemiology and Prevention of Gallstone Disease* (ed. L. Capocaccia, G. Ricci, F. Angelico et al.), 58–63. Dordrecht: Springer Netherlands. https://doi.org/10.1007/978-94-009-5606-3_10.

53 Sharma, R., Sachan, S.G., and Sharma, S.R. (2013). Urease positive and slime producing bacterial activity: results in gallstone precipitation and solidification. *Arch. Clin. Infect. Dis.* 8 (4).

54 Sharma, R., Sachan, S.G., and Sharma, S.R. (2020). In vitro analysis of gallstone formation in the presence of bacteria. *Indian J. Gastroenterol.* 39 (5).

55 Ahmed, M. (2018). Acute cholangitis an update. *World J. Gastrointest. Pathophysiol.* 9 (1): 1–7. https://doi.org/10.4291/wjgp.v9.i1.1.

56 Furukawa, M., Moriya, K., Nakayama, J. et al. (2020). Gut dysbiosis associated with clinical prognosis of patients with primary biliary cholangitis. *Hepatol. Res.* 50 (7): 840–852. https://doi.org/10.1111/hepr.13509.

57 Goodchild, G., Pereira, S.P., and Webster, G. (2018). Immunoglobulin G4-related sclerosing cholangitis. *Korean J. Intern. Med.* 33 (5): 841–850. https://doi.org/10.3904/kjim.2018.018.

58 Olszak, T., An, D., Zeissig, S. et al. (2012). Microbial exposure during early life has persistent effects on natural killer T cell function. *Science* 336 (6080): 489–493. https://doi.org/10.1126/science.1219328.

59 Park, D.H., Kim, J.W., Park, H.-J. et al. (2021). Comparative analysis of the microbiome across the gut–skin axis in atopic dermatitis. *Int. J. Mol. Sci.* 22 (8): 4228. https://doi.org/10.3390/ijms22084228.

60 Sun, Y. and O'Riordan, M.X.D. (2013). Regulation of bacterial pathogenesis by intestinal short-chain fatty acids. *Adv. Appl. Microbiol.* 84: 93–118. https://doi.org/10.1016/B978-0-12-407672-3.00003-4.

61 Hennart, P.F., Brasseur, D.J., Delogne-Desnoeck, J.B. et al. (1991). Lysozyme, lactoferrin, and secretory immunoglobulin A content in breast milk: influence of duration of lactation, nutrition status, prolactin status, and parity of mother. *Am. J. Clin. Nutr.* 53 (1): 32–39. https://doi.org/10.1093/ajcn/53.1.32.

62 Gagliardi, A., Totino, V., Cacciotti, F. et al. (2018). Rebuilding the gut microbiota ecosystem. *Int. J. Environ. Res. Public Health* 15 (8): 1679. https://doi.org/10.3390%2Fijerph15081679.

63 Zhang, J.-M. and An, J. (2007). Cytokines, inflammation, and pain. *Int. Anesthesiol. Clin.* 45 (2): 27–37. https://doi.org/10.1097/aia.0b013e318034194e.

64 Monda, V., Villano, I., Messina, A. et al. (2017). Exercise modifies the gut microbiota with positive health effects. *Oxid. Med. Cell Longev.* 3831972. https://doi.org/10.1155%2F2017%2F3831972.

65 Zhang, H.-L., Li, W.-S., Xu, D.-N. et al. (2016). Mucosa-reparing and microbiota-balancing therapeutic effect of Bacillus subtilis alleviates dextrate sulfate sodium-induced ulcerative colitis in mice. *Exp. Ther. Med.* 12 (4): 2554–2562. https://doi.org/10.3892%2Fetm.2016.3686.

66 Cavallo, F.M., Jordana, L., Friedrich, A.W. et al. (2021). Bdellovibrio bacteriovorus: a potential 'living antibiotic' to control bacterial pathogens. *Crit. Rev. Microbiol.* 47 (5): 630–646. https://doi.org/10.1080/1040841X.2021.1908956.

67 Eiseman, B., Silen, W., Bascom, G.S. et al. (1958). Fecal enema as an adjunct in the treatment of pseudomembranous enterocolitis. *Surgery* 44 (5): 854–859. https://pubmed.ncbi.nlm.nih.gov/13592638/.

68 Sharma, S.R., Sharma, R., and Kar, D. (2020). Novel Microbial Compounds as a Boon in Health Management. In: *Biotechnological Advances for Microbiology, Molecular Biology, and Nanotechnology, An Interdisciplinary Approach to the Life Sciences. I.* (ed. J.R. Rout, G.K. Rout, and A. Dutta), 77–118. Apple Academic Press.

6

Connection between Dysbiosis and Diet

Sagnik Nag[1], Nimmy Srivastava[2], Rohan Dutta[1], Aparajita Bagchi[1], Israrahmed Adur[1], and Shuvam Chakraborty[1]

[1] *Department of Biotechnology, School of Biosciences & Technology, Vellore Institute of Technology (VIT), Tamil Nadu, India*
[2] *Assistant Professor, Amity Institute of Biotechnology, Amity University, Jharkhand, India*

6.1 Introduction

6.1.1 Gut Microbiota and Dysbiosis

The gastrointestinal tract, which includes the oesophagus, stomach, small intestine, and large intestine, extends from the mouth to the anus [1]. Along the gastrointestinal tract, the associated host microbe symbiotic relationship plays a key role in digestion and influences host health. Gut microbiota is a dynamic composition with trillions of microorganisms, 35 000 species of bacteria, archaea and yeasts [2]. It constitutes the genus *Bacteroidetes, Fermicutes, Prevotella, Bifidobacterium, Lactobacillus, Eubacterium, Propionibacterium, Escherichia, Enterococcus, Peptostreptococcus, Fusobacteria,* and *Ruminococcin* [3, 4]. The composition of human gut microbiota gradually changes from birth to adult stage and remains unaltered until there is a bacterial infection, antibiotic treatment, lifestyle, or long-term change in diet plan [5]. Maternal microbiota acts as an inoculum from birth, resembling bacteria from the mother's vagina or skin, depending on whether the route of delivery is vaginal birth or assisted delivery of the newborn (C-section) [6]. At infancy, family environment, breast feeding, lactation period, genetics, and the environment define the gut microbiome. The diet lifestyle, medication during adulthood, and elderly age effectively influence the gut microbiota [5]. The gut microbiota is also responsible for the regulation of adaptive immunity, inflammatory signalling, physiology, and regulation [7].

Dysbiosis is the imbalance of gut microflora that interferes with the digestive system and causes various pathological ailments. There are several factors that contribute to dysbiosis of the gut microbiota and can have an influence on host health, the most important of which is diet or nutrition [8]. According to Kashtanova et al., increasing food intake in kcal per day with 24% protein, 16% fat, and 60% carbs for three days can increase firmicutes while decreasing Bacteroidetes [3]. Studies reveal the protein content in diet from plant and animal sources, 30% of fat with stable proportions of short chain fatty acid, Mono-unsaturated Fatty acids (MUFA), Poly-unsaturated Fatty acids (PUFA), and type of oligosaccharides have a significant impact on gut microbes [9]. Dysbiosis of the beneficial microbes in the gut may lead to an imbalance between the metabolic activity and by-product, and the bacterial toxins [10]. Dysbiosis is related to many diseases such as IBD, Crohn's disease (CD), and ulcerative colitis (UC), gastrointestinal disorders, IBS, celiac disease, CRC, and Central nervous system (CNS) related disorders [8]. Although diet plays a key role in dysbiosis, 60–70% of mothers diet during pregnancy, and breast feeding, genetics and, epigenetics crucially defines one's gut microbial diversity [3]. Therefore, the World Health Organisation (WHO) recommends six months of breastfeeding for an infant, as it plays a key role in the infant's metabolic and immunological programming, influencing the gut microbiota [9].

Recent studies suggest the association of gut microbiota with human appetite, where leptin plays a crucial role in microbiota regulation, may be used to detect dysbiosis based on bacterial composition in the gut [3]. However, as a part of diet one may consume probiotics and prebiotics or use therapeutic manipulation to improve the gut symbiotic relationship [7]. Therefore, this chapter emphasises how various dietary components are a major factor in shaping gut microbiota and its role in dysbiosis.

6.1.2 Importance of Diet in regulation of Gut Microbiota

The term microbiome denotes the microorganism's collective genomes in a specific environment and microbiota remains the microorganism's community itself. In the gastrointestinal tract of humans, nearly 100 trillion microorganisms are present, with bacteria being the largest proportion; however, viruses, fungi, and protozoa are also found [11], therefore, the microbiome is now considered to be the body's virtual organ. The human genome comprises nearly 23 000 genes, while nearly 3 million genes are encoded by the microbiome that produce thousands of metabolites, replacing varied host functions and consequently impacting the health, phenotype, and fitness of the host [11].

Gut microbes play an important role in many areas of human health, including immunological [12], metabolic [13], and neurobehavioral characteristics [14, 15]. Even though there is a heritable element to gut microbiota, twin studies have revealed that environmental factors such as nutrition, medicines, and anthropometric measurements are more important predictors of microbiota composition [13, 16]. The importance of gut microbiota in human health has been supported by several levels of evidence, including animal models [17] and human research [16, 18–20].

The host benefits greatly from the homeostatic equilibrium of the intestinal microflora; nevertheless, if the microbial composition changes causing a severe imbalance amongst helpful and possibly pathogenic bacteria, the gut becomes sensitive to pathogenic assault with gut microbial modifications. Dysbiosis is a disruption to gut microbiota homeostasis caused by a disparity in the flora themselves, alterations in their functional makeup as well as in the metabolic functions, or alterations in their distribution infrastructure [21, 22]. Many chronic diseases have become more prevalent in recent decades, for example, dysbiosis caused by environmental variables such as use of antibiotics has been hypothesised to modify the microbiome in ways that enhance inflammation and the emergence of chronic disease. Dysbiosis is characterised accordingly as the gain or loss of microorganisms that promote or cause disease [23].

Particular foods and dietary habits may all have an impact on the quantity of different bacterial types in the gut, which may have a negative impact on health (see Figure 6.1 and Table 6.1). High-intensity sweeteners, which are several times sweeter than sugar yet have fewer calories, are often employed as sugar substitutes. Despite the fact that these sugar substitutes are 'generally regarded as safe' by regulatory bodies, animal research has indicated that they may have deleterious effects on the gut microbiome. Sucralose, saccharin, and aspartame have all been demonstrated to affect the gut microbiota's balance and diversity [24]. Sucralose-fed rats showed significantly greater proportions of total aerobic bacteria, clostridia, and Bacteroides in their stomachs, as well as a substantially higher fecal pH, than sucralose-free rats [25]. Sucralose increased the expression of pro-inflammatory bacterial genes in the gut and disturbed fecal metabolites in mice that were administered sucralose for six months [26].

Animals' gut microbiome has been demonstrated to be affected by dietary additives such as emulsifiers, which are widespread in processed diets [27]. Mice given low doses of two frequently used emulsifiers—polysorbate and carboxymethylcellulose-80—had less microbial diversity than mice that were not given emulsifiers. Inflammation-promoting *Proteobacteria* linked with mucus were abundant, while *Verrucomicrobia* and *Bacteroidales* were reduced [27].

The consequences of trendy restricted diets on gut health are another source of concern. Some stringent vegan diets, raw food diets, gluten-free diets, and low FODMAP (fermentable oligosaccharides, disaccharides, monosaccharides, and polyols) diets for IBS are among these [17, 28].

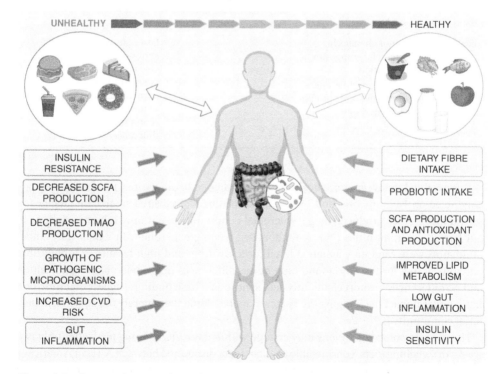

Figure 6.1 Comparative analysis on the impact of dietary intake on gut health.

Table 6.1 Role of different dietary elements and patterns affecting constituent microbial species, and its subsequent effect on human health.

Dietary element	Status	Constituent microbial species	Impact on gut microbiome mediated health outcomes	References
FODMAP diet	Low-FODMAP diet	Elevated *Actinobacteria*	Lessened IBS symptoms	[17, 28]
	High-FODMAP Diet	Reduced gas-producing bacteria		
Cheese	Bacteria providing good health advantages to their hosts	Increased *Bifidobacteria*	Increased SCFA production, Decreased TMAO output	[30–32]
	Some strains linked with intestinal illnesses	Decreased *Bacteroides* and *Clostridia*		
Prebiotics and fibre	SCFA production	Increased microbial diversity	Reduced risk of T2D and cardiovascular disease	[33–35]
Polyphenols	Increased butyrate-producing bacteria and decreased Lipopolysaccharide producers	*Lactobacillus, Bifidobacterium, Roseburia, Faecalibacterium prausnitzii, Akkermansia muciniphila, Bacteroides vulgatus, E. coli,* and *Enterobacter cloacae*	Decline in metabolic syndrome and cardiovascular risk indicators	[36–38]
Vegan	Minor changes in microbial composition and variety. Significant differences in metabolomic profile compared to omnivorous diet.	—	Some studies showed that a vegetarian diet is superior to an omnivorous one, while others report no difference.	[29, 39, 40]

It is assumed that vegans are healthy when compared to omnivores; however, in a study conducted on 16 omnivores and 15 vegans, researchers discovered significant changes in serum metabolites produced by gut microbial communities, but only minor variations in gut bacterial communities [29]. A randomised feeding experiment in which ten human omnivores were randomly assigned to either a low-fibre and high-fat diet or a high-fibre and low-fat diet for ten days found only minor differences in gut microbiota composition and no differences in short chain fatty acid synthesis. These findings suggest that nutrition has a larger impact in changing the bacterial metabolome than merely the short-term bacterial community [29].

The gut microbiota alterations may emerge within days after altering food; after only two weeks of switching diets, considerable changes were discovered between African Americans and rural Africans [41]. Butyrate production swelled 2.5 times and secondary bile acid synthesis was inhibited in African Americans eating a rural African diet, due to a rise in the frequency of known butyrate-generating bacteria [41]. Another study that compared dramatic swings between animal and plant protein-based diets found that these alterations occurred only after five days [42]. Healthy microbiota, on the other hand, are resistant to temporal alterations caused by dietary treatments, indicating that homeostatic reactions re-establish the original community makeup, as demonstrated recently in the case of bread [15].

6.2 Different Dietary Patterns Resulting in Dysbiosis

6.2.1 Breastfeeding

To promote ideal health, growth, and development, the WHO recommends that women completely breastfeed newborns for the first six months. Following that, they should be fed nutritional complementary foods and breastfed until they are two years old or older. A systematic assessment of the evidence on this topic was published, and the review's findings, which encompassed two randomised controlled trials with 18 other studies from both developing and developed nations, backed up existing WHO recommendations. The findings of the systematic review revealed that exclusively breastfeeding infants for six months with no other foods or drinks had various advantages over exclusively breastfeeding for three to four months preceded by combined breastfeeding. These benefits encompass a low risk of gastrointestinal infections for the newborn, faster maternal weight loss following delivery, and a longer duration between menstrual periods [43].

Abnormalities in the infant gut microbiota, upon immune system maturation and the colonisation of gut with bacteria, have been associated with disease risk in later age, as revealed by animal and epidemiological studies [44]. This demonstrates that there is a clear opportunity for prevention of illness, inclusive of atopic disease, that coincides with breast-feeding. Since B lymphocytes undertake greater isotype class switching to IgE in Peyer's patches and mesenteric lymph nodes in germ-free mice, serum immunoglobulin (Ig)E levels are higher. If a varied microbiome is used, microbial colonisation of germ-free canine progenies between birth and one week after weaning totally prevents IgE induction. This implies that a certain degree of microbial diversity is required after birth to inhibit induction of IgE [45]. Colonisation early in development of germ-free mice with gut microbiota, but not as adults, is also enough to protect them from lung mucosal invariant natural killer T cell (iNKT) accumulation and allergic inflammation of airways [46]. Only when antibiotic treatment began early in childhood did it worsen inflammation of allergic airways, diminish FoxP3+ regulatory T cells (Treg) in the colon, and raise serum IgE [47]. In humans, a relationship was shown between dysbiosis of gut microbiota and a heightened incidence of asthma in the first 100 days of life [48]. Other research has also discovered a link between the early gut microbiome and the development of allergy sensitisation [49–51]. All show a relationship amongst dysbiosis of early gut microbiota and a heightened incidence of allergies (see Figure 6.2).

Aside from the direct impact of gut microorganisms on the immune response, metabolites produced by the dietary fibre fermentation and other complex macronutrients that, in the small intestine, evade digestion, play an essential role. Molecules synthesised or acquired from bacterial metabolism control cellular host processes, including the

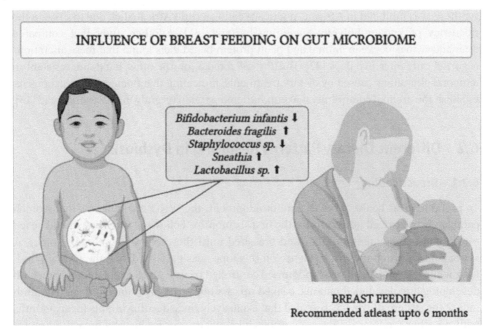

Figure 6.2 Breast feeding and its impact on the gut microbiota.

immunological, epithelial, vascular, and neurological systems in the intestine [52]. Bacterial metabolites may cause epigenetic modifications such as chromatin alterations, allowing the microbiota to have a long-term impact on immunity [53]. Choline metabolites, phenolic derivatives, and vitamins are examples of microbial metabolites [52]. Bacterial metabolism may convert primary bile acids into secondary bile acids, which may stimulate the bile acid receptors farnesoid X receptor (FXR) and G protein-coupled bile acid receptor (TGR5) in distinct ways [54]. The essential amino acid tryptophan is metabolised by commensal bacteria, particularly *Lactobacilli*, creating derivatives of indole that may attach to aryl hydrocarbon receptors (AHR) exhibited by immunological and epithelial cells. ILC3 stimulation and function of intestinal barrier are both dependent on AHR signalling [55]. To date, the AHR ligand's role in immune development during the newborn period is mainly unknown. Bacterial amino acid metabolism produces branched-chain fatty acids such as isovalerate, isobutyrate, and valerate. When dietary fibre is broken down, SCFAs such as propionate, acetate, and butyrate are generated. Succinate and lactate are intermediary metabolites in the formation of SCFA, but they may also influence the immune system [56, 57]. SCFA's are a vital source of energy for intestinal epithelial cells; furthermore, SCFA signalling via G protein coupled receptors found on immune and epithelial cells, including GPR41, GPR43, and GPR109A, inhibits histone deacetylases [55, 58]. SCFA has been shown to improve intestinal barrier integrity, produce tolerogenic DC, and boost anti-inflammatory Treg in the colon in adult mice, all of which contribute to immunological tolerance [55]. SCFA reduces innate lymphoid type 2 cell (ILC2) multiplication and function in the lungs by impairing dendritic cell's (DCs) ability to stimulate T helper 2 responses [59, 60]. There is currently a scarcity of information on the impact of SCFA on the gastrointestinal and immune system maturation in the neonate; however, there is some evidence that increased acetate levels in infants may help protect them from hypersensitivity reactions [48].

Breastmilk's ability to influence the early gut microbiome of children is a promising strategy for immunological education and allergy management, as seen in Table 6.2. This necessitates determining what constitutes a favourable microbiota for allergy management in today's world, what factors in breastmilk are required to assist the creation of such a

Table 6.2 Breastfeeding and gut microbiota.

Breast milk constituents	Related Microbiota	Effects	References
Human Milk Oligosaccharides (HMO)	*Bifidobacterium*	Prebiotics, helps beneficial bacteria to grow or activate.	[56, 61–64]
		Anti-adhesives; inhibiting pathogen attachment to mucosal surfaces and preventing colonisation.	
		Promote the proliferation of Bifidobacterium and are their favoured substrates.	
Tryptophan metabolites	Gut microbiota	Tryptophan and its metabolites have a significant impact on the infant's gut bacteria makeup, metabolism, and function.	[65–67]
		Antimicrobial activities of kynurenines can have a direct impact on the gut microbiota.	
		AHR signalling pathway can potentially affect the microbiome composition.	
Lipids	*Clostridium, Streptococcus, Veillonella, Enterobacteriaceae,* and *Bacteroides*	Lipids impact gut ecology microbiota by fuelling bacteria or by causing the host to release bile acids and hormones.	[54, 68, 69]
		Bile acids are bacterial detergents, which cause low bacterial count in the duodenum.	
		The relative abundance of five taxa in the gut microbiota of breastfed neonates was linked to human milk fatty acid profiles.	
Antimicrobial proteins and peptides	*Bifidobacteria* and *lactobacilli, S. aureus* and group B *streptococci*	Lactoferrin from breastmilk defends infants from bacterial infection.	[70–72]
		The fecal bifidobacteria and lactobacilli number in infants was linked to fecal lactoferrin that encourages specific microbial compositions.	
		The growth of manganese-sensitive bacteria inhibited as calprotectin levels in human milk are high shortly after birth.	

beneficial microbiota, and in what way to enhance breast milk with the necessary elements (see Figure 6.2). In recent years, significant progress has been made in identifying a beneficial microbiome for the prevention of allergy illness. The importance of a diversified gut microbiota and the role of microbial metabolism have been highlighted in particular. The importance of the microbiota of breastmilk and HMOs in the development of the neonatal gut microbiota has lately become increasingly apparent. Nevertheless, there is still a lack of understanding on how to manipulate breastfeeding elements that shape the microbiota. Administration of probiotics to nursing mothers has yielded mixed results in terms of changing the milk microbiota [73,74], and currently there is no indication that HMO's content in breastmilk may be altered. There is a requirement for randomised intervention trials to investigate the allergy-prevention effects of supplementing nursing mothers with milk-modulating substances such as pre- and probiotics in order to change the infant's microbiome and, as a result, programme the immune response [75].

6.2.2 Carbohydrate-rich Diet

Carbohydrates are one of the most essential bio-molecules that constitute the living organism and are mainly obtained from sources such as fruits, legumes, vegetables, and cereals. These in turn provide energy to the host and help in constituting the gut microbiota. There are three main carbohydrates types; resistant starches, non-starch polysaccharides, and oligosaccharides. These three types of carbohydrates are difficult to digest and are therefore fermented in the gut by the gut microbiota, which contributes to the major source of energy production [76]. Recent studies show that incorporating milk into the diet leads to an increase in *Bifidobacterium longum* and other *Bacteroides* species, as milk consists of fucosylated oligosaccharides which act as nutrients for these microorganisms, and as a result they tend to outcompete other organisms such as *Escherichia coli* and *Clostridium perfringens* [2]. Another provision of carbohydrates for the gut microbiota is the intestinal mucus which lines the entire gastrointestinal tract [77]. The glycans in the mucin responsible for the mucus formation consist of N-acetylglucosamine, N-acetylgalactosamine, and galactose, which elongate and are terminated by fucose and sialic acid residues [78].

With an increase in the demand for carbohydrate-rich food, there has been a surge in metabolic disorders; this is seen in both the glycemic index (GI) and the glycemic load (GL). The higher the value of GI and GL, the higher the risk of contracting metabolic disorders such as Type-II diabetes and cardiovascular diseases. Higher carbohydrate-containing foods such as factory processed grains tend to increase triglycerides, decrease high-density lipoprotein cholesterol, and aggravate dyslipidemia. When foods with higher content of GI are consumed, they lead to decreased beta-oxidation of fatty acids and higher adipogenesis; whereas when foods with higher GL content are consumed, they increase energy storage and inflammatory markers such as C-reactive proteins. These factors indicate that a high carbohydrate diet may be correlated to diabetes and obesity [79].

Recent studies also show that the intake of a starchy diet is associated with high metabolic disorders and hyperlipidemia. It was observed that there was an increase in visceral fats and serum triglyceride levels and decrease in High Density Lipoprotein (HDL) [80]. Moreover, with the consumption of refined grains and tubers with a higher glycemic index and glycemic load, there was an increase in the incidence of glycemia and insulin resistance; but consumption of whole grains reduced the risk of diabetes by a rate of 21% [81].

Sugar-sweetened beverages have a higher glycemic load, and thus consumption of them leads to an increase in blood sugar and insulin levels. This, in turn, leads to the exhaustion of the β cells of the pancreas [79]. Diets rich in monosaccharides and disaccharides are associated with Crohn's disease and ulcerative colitis, and disaccharides metabolised in the liver lead to lipogenesis, dyslipidemia, and insulin resistance [82]. One of the well-known monosaccharides, i.e., fructose, is a key dietary component in the induction of gut dysbiosis [83], and it has an impact on the lipoprotein profile, which leads to various cardiovascular diseases and increased risk of T2D [84, 85].

Some recent studies suggest that consumption of non-digestible carbohydrates may decrease the risks of ulcerative colitis and Crohn's disease [86]. Dietary fibres such as cellulose are beneficial to bowel health as it increases the digesta mass and is hydrophilic. This gives a positive edge to health by toxin dilution, intracolonic pressure reduction, and by increasing desecration frequency. Furthermore, it induces fermentation which induces bacterial procreation and acts as an energy source for the bacterial population [87]. One major end-product of carbohydrate fermentation is the production of short-chain fatty acids which also contribute to bowel health [88].

Table 6.3 gives a detailed description of all the metabolic disorders and alterations of gut microbiota intertwined with carbohydrates.

Prebiotics play a vital role in constituting the gut microbiota and act as a means of treating dysbiosis, as prebiotic carbohydrates induce the growth of microorganisms such as *Bifidobacteria*, *F. prausnitzii*, *Akkermansia muciniphila*, and *Roseburia* [96]. The growth of these microorganisms enhances the fermentation process of the carbohydrates and lowers the risk of developing any metabolic disorders or cardiovascular diseases. The technical studies suggest that the induction of prebiotic imbibed bacterial strains results in improved functioning of the gut concerning host energy homeostasis. As a result, the bioactive metabolites such as SCFA's, conjugated linoleic acid (CLA), and bile acids improve the host health in terms of overfeeding and obesity [97]; thus, the introduction of such types of food in the diet is not only essential in improving gut health but also in preventing various diseases.

Given the symbiotic relationship between the gut and the indigenous microbiota, there is a likely probability that it may become impacted by the plethora of disease states, but detailed studies have paved a path through which gut health may be maintained. Recent studies on metabolomics have correlated gut health and diet and have given a clear understanding of the health and disease phenotypes [2]. Moreover, dual therapeutic strategies such as combining immunotherapy and microbiota-targeted approaches may be applied to restore the gut environment. The introduction of non-digestible carbohydrates in the diet such as dietary fibres and resistant starch have also proved to be extremely effective against various metabolic diseases, dysbiosis, and cardiovascular diseases [79]. Thus, more mechanistic studies on diet and gut health will pave new paths to successfully overcome the problems of dysbiosis, obesity, cardiovascular diseases, and many more metabolic disorders.

6.2.3 Protein-rich Diet

Proteins and amino acids play an essential role in constituting the human diet; the composition of these dietary proteins has an impact on the gut microbiota and microbial metabolites. Recent studies have suggested that higher levels of undigested proteins accentuate the growth of pathogenic microorganisms, facilitating various diseases [98]. A series of studies

Table 6.3 Metabolic disorders and gut alterations associated with carbohydrate.

Class	Possible Sources	Principle Components	Effects on Gut Microbiota	–/+	Effect on Human Health	References
Long term agrarian diets	High starch and fibres	Carbohydrates from starchy foods	*Prevotella* and *Xylanibacter*	+	Risk of metabolic disorders and hyperlipidemia	[79, 80, 89, 90]
		Total carbohydrate, starch, and refined sugar	*Bacteroides*	–	Increased visceral fat and serum TG level	
		Refined grains and tubers			Low HDL-C level	
					Risk of Crohn's disease and ulcerative colitis	
					Risk of glycemia and insulin resistance	
Monosaccharides and Disaccharides	Sugar-sweetened beverages (SSB) Daily fruits	Lactose	*Bifidobacteria*	+	Risk of type-II diabetes	[79, 85, 91, 92]
		Fructose	*Bacteroides*	–	Risk of cardiovascular disease	
		Sugar	*Clostridia*	–	Increased Lipogenesis, dyslipidemia, and visceral adiposity	
		Total sugars sucrose	*Lactobacilli*	+	Insulin resistance	
					Risk of Crohn's disease	
					Risk of ulcerative colitis	
					Risk of pancreatic cancer	

Category	Food source	Microbe	+/−	Health effect	References
Artificial Sweeteners	Diet soda	Bifidobacteria	−	High adipogenesis and low lipolysis	[79, 92, 93]
	Artificially sweetened beverages	Bacteroides	+	Insulin resistance	
	Sucralose	Clostridia	+	Risk of dysbiosis and metabolic abnormalities	
	Aspartame	Lactobacilli	−	Risk of type-II diabetes and cardiovascular disease	
				Risk of hypertension	
				Risk of urinary tract tumor and laryngeal cancer, breast and ovarian cancer	
				Risk of stroke and dementia	
Non-digestible carbohydrates	Cereal fibres	Bifidobacteria	+	Decreased risk of cardiovascular disease	[79, 94, 95]
	Wheat bran cereals	Actinobacteria	+	Decreased risk of T2D	
	Fruits and vegetable fibres	Bacteroides	+	Decreased risk of colorectal cancer	
	Oligosaccharides mixture,	Firmicutes	+	Decreased risk of Crohn's disease	
	Polysaccharide peptides	Ruminococcus	−	Decreased risk of gastric cancer	
	Polydextrose	Eubacteria	+		
	Fructo-oligosaccharide	Parabacteroides	+		
	Galactooligosaccharides	Lactobacilli	+		
	FODMAP	Clostridia	+		
		Enterococcus	−		

have revealed that plant proteins such as soybean and peanut have less digestibility, as they contain glycinin and β-conglycinin, whereas animal proteins are easier to digest as they are easily fermented by aerobic microorganisms and produce different metabolites such as ammonia, hydrogen sulfide, phenol, indole, polyamine, and short-chain fatty acids [99].

A diet with higher content of peanut proteins has been shown to increase the *Bifidobacterium* species and decrease *Enterobacteria* and *Clostridium perfringens* [100], as a result, *Bifidobacterium* produces more lactic acids and acetic acids that inhibit toxic metabolites. On the other hand, adding soybean to the diet increases *Escherichia* and *Propionibacterium* [101]. Another important source of protein is casein, as it not only increases *Lactobacilli* and *Bifidobacterium* species but also decreases *Staphylococci*, *Coliforms*, and *Streptococci* species [102], and recent studies have shown that casein also decreases the *Eubacterium rectale* and *Marvinbryantia formatexigens* population [103]. Supplementation of dried skimmed milk has been shown to increase the growth of aerobes and anaerobes, while the introduction of animal proteins leads to a decrease in the short chain fatty acid levels, and an increase in gut pH and ammonia concentration [104].

Soybean plays an important role in the diet as it contains proteins such as conglycinin and glycinin, which have the properties of immunogenicity and thermal stability [105]. Soybean has also been seen to stimulate the overgrowth of pathogens and so has been associated with both advantages and disadvantages. Studies have shown that dietary proteins and peptides are broken down after digestion, but some of the anti-nutritional proteins tend to pass through the intestinal epithelial and trigger the immune response of the host. Such a response is mediated by the soybean as the T lymphocytes are triggered with the secretion of IgE, which is harmful for the gut microbiota as it impairs the villi and proliferates the cryptic cells [99, 105]. The hypersensitivity to soybean protein triggers the overgrowth of pathogenic microorganisms as well as enteropathogens such as Escherichia coli. As a result, when the pathogens colonise in the lumen, dysbiosis of the gut microbiota takes place [98]. Recent studies have also shown that soybean consists of pepsin hydrolysate conglycinin (PHC), which plays a significant role in lowering hypertension, has antioxidant properties, and acts as immunogens [106].

Another protein that plays an important role is casein as it induces the transcription of amino acid transporters in the gut. Lysine and arginine are transported with the help of Cationic amino acid transporters (CAT1) and their levels increase on the supplementation of casein [107]. Casein also upregulates the levels of Excitatory amino acid carrier 1 (EAAC1) which transport aspartate and glutamate and levels of Peptide transporter 1 (PePT1). Thus, incorporating casein in diet accentuates the expression of amino acids and peptide transporters, as a result of which there is increased transportation of all these amino acids in the intestinal environment [98]. These changes play an important role in constituting the microbiota by synthesising various bacterial proteins.

Dietary proteins are closely associated with gut microbiota and foods such as milk, cheese, curd, and other dairy products should be incorporated in meals, as they induce the growth of many probiotics such as *Lactobacillus bulgaricus* and *Lactobacillus gasseri*, which help in the reinstitution of the microecology of the intestine. Supplementation of fermented milk is beneficial as it has been seen that the consumption of 200 grams of fermented milk consisting of *Lactobacillus gasseri* over 12 weeks help reduce obesity by a high margin by affecting the visceral, abdominal, and subcutaneous fat [107]. Furthermore, various metadata analyses should be conducted using metabolomics, proteomics, microbiomics, and bioinformatics to get a better understanding of the interpersonal relationship of dietary proteins and gut microbiota [98].

6.2.4 Fats and Oil-rich Diet

Lipids and an oil rich diet encompass fatty acids, including saturated (SFA), monounsaturated (MUFA), and polyunsaturated (PUFA) fatty acids, their derivatives, including monoglycerides, diglycerides, triglycerides, and phospholipids, as well as sterols such as cholesterol [108]. Fatty acids offer a wide range of antibacterial properties, including the lysis and solubilisation of bacterial cell membranes, as well as the suppression of adenosine triphosphate (ATP) synthesis. Carbon chain length, saturation, and double bond location all influence fatty acid antibacterial activity, which in turn causes dysbiosis [109]. A number of studies have been investigated between dyslipidemia (high cholesterol level or fats in the blood) and the gut flora. The unabsorbed starch and non-starch polysaccharide or fibres are broken down by the gut microbes into short chain fatty acids (SCFA) that are again categorised into three main acids; acetate, propionate, and butyrate [110]. These play a crucial role in mucosal energy metabolism, absorption of sodium, mucosal blood flow and mucous release, cellular differentiation, mucosal cell proliferation, and prevention of colitis [111].

In addition, fatty propanoic acid produced by bacteria during breakdown of carbohydrates and amino acids inhibits carnitine transport across the gut and may trigger autism spectrum disorders (ASDs) [112]. Studies also reveal the treatment of distal ulcerative colitis of the gut is possible with SCFA. SCFA also facilitates contraction and limits ileal emptying, thus protecting the ileal mucosa from the potentially damaging effects of colonic content reflux [113]. The effect of medium-chain fatty acids (MCFAs) such as caprylic, capric, and lauric acids in coconut, palm kernel, and human milk, respectively, are studied on animal models, growth of certain microbial genus was observed; namely, *Bacteroidetes* and *Firmicutes* [114]. On the other hand, almond oil was found to regulate gut microbiota related to glucose metabolism and increase the abundance level of the genus *Lactobacillus*, *Bacteroides*, and *Lachnospiraceae* [115]. Walnut oil was similarly investigated for its preventive and protective effects on the intestinal mucosa, including anti-oxidant, anti-inflammatory, immunity, and gut microbiota modulation [116].

The MUFAs include palmitoleic, oleic, and eicosenoic acids obtained from safflower, sesame, pumpkin seed, rice bran, human milk, rapeseed, olive, peanut, wheat germ, and hemp [117]. A recent study using healthy and unhealthy animal models, including humans under risk of metabolic syndrome, found that a high-fat MUFAs-rich diet, including extra-virgin olive oil, increased the gut microbiota diversity with a decrease in metabolic disorders such as obesity and hypertension [118]. The MUFA-rich diet showed lower *Escherichia coli* and *Candida albicans* abundance, and higher *Bifidobacteria* to *Eschericia coli* ratio, suggesting a negative effect on the gut.

The polyunsaturated fatty acids (PUFAs) are essential fatty acids in the unsaturated group containing two or up to six double bonds in their structures, such as α-linolenic acid (ALA) from the n-3 PUFA family and linoleic acid (LA) from the n-6 PUFA family. The n-3 long-chain polyunsaturated fatty acid (PUFA), dietary sources of ω-3 PUFAs, are mainly fish oil (FO) and algae oil (AO), having positive impacts on the host. According to a study conducted by Mujico et al., mice model fed with a diet rich in ω-6 PUFAs, the abundance of *Enterobacteriaceae* and *Clostridia* supplemented with fish oil, showed reduced inflammation. These bacteria species are known to cause inflammation and other ill effects [119].

Another study supports the claim that the combination of n-6 and n-3 PUFA, like DHA/EPA, leads to increased oxidative stress and exacerbate gastrointestinal dysbiosis in the elderly, which can be reversed by supplementing fish oil on an n-6 PUFA [120]. Studies also suggest perilla oil-derived ω-3 PUFA supplementation on gut microbiota improves glucolipid metabolism and thereby modulates gut microbiota in diabetic KK Ay mice [121]. Martinez et al. proposed the influence of obesity and Western-style diets rich in a complex mixture of fats. The dysbiosis of gut microbiome is evident within 24–48 hours and sustained if a high density fat (HFD) diet habit persists, led to changes in *Firmicutes* to *Bacteroidetes* ratio [122], and may not be recoverable without change in diet, reintroduction of affected microbial strains, or dietary supplementation such as prebiotics and probiotics [117]. Finally, gut microbial composition and an imbalanced dietary lipid pattern, such as HFD, may contribute to gut dysbiosis, which may lead to gut inflammatory disorders. However, consumption of the PUFA rich diet, oils from sources such as fish and algae, may have significant improvement in intestinal disorders and maintain the gut microbiota homeostasis. Furthermore, it is important to understand additional clinical evidence and molecular mechanisms regarding how these fats and oils interact causing microbiota homeostasis.

6.3 Future Prospects in Establishing a Healthy Connection between Diet and Gut Microbiota

Despite being one of the most studied communities, only around 1% of bacteria may be cultured from various environments, yet some may be cultivated from the gut microbiome [123]. The gut microbiome is vital for health, showing strong insights on digestion and benefits to one's immune system. An imbalance of harmful and good microbes in the intestines can promote weight gain, high blood sugar, high cholesterol, and other disorders [124].

Nutrition education has a bright future, and the gut microbiota plays a crucial role. Consumption of helpful bacteria and fibrous foods is a viable solution to a healthy gut microbiome. Dietary fibre is defined as a component of food obtained from plant cells that is resistant to hydrolysis and digestion by the human enzyme system [124]. It is made up of hemicellulose, cellulose, and pectins among other things. Dietary fibres play a critical role in the prevention of diabetes, colon cancer, coronary heart disease, and weight loss. Both Type 1 and Type 2 diabetics will benefit from dietary fibre and complex carbohydrates, as such diets reduce insulin needs while increasing insulin sensitivity in peripheral tissues [81]. High-carbohydrate, high-fibre diets boost glucose metabolism while lowering insulin secretion. They reduce fasting serum and peripheral insulin concentrations in diabetic and non-diabetic people in response to oral glucose treatment [124]. Several theories have been proposed to explain how dietary fibre prevents colon cancer and helps people lose weight. It dilutes or binds to bile acids in colon cancer, reducing their role in mutation or cell proliferation. Fermentation of dietary fibres produces short-chain fatty acids, which lowers the

PH of the intestine and prevents the conversion of main bile acids to secondary acids, which is thought to promote gastrointestinal mutation [113]. High fibre diets aid weight loss by increasing satiety and delaying stomach emptying through the release of specific gut hormones. Fatty acids from starch and nitrogen from high-fibre meals may be poorly absorbed [125]. Beneficial bacteria, opportunistic bacteria, and bad bacteria are the three categories of bacteria found in the gut. Beneficial bacteria promote digestion, absorption, and immunity while also helping to maintain weight, health, and anti-aging effects; *Bifidobacterium* and *Lactobacillus* bacteria are two examples [126]. Beneficial bacteria, such as *Bifidobacterium*, may help reduce intestinal inflammation and improve gut health. The Human Microbiome Project (HMP) arose as a result of all of these circumstances [126], the HMP is a method for better understanding the microbial components of the human genetic and metabolic landscape, as well as how they contribute to normal physiology and disease predisposition. The initiative primarily focused on extracting otherwise inaccessible nutrients or sources of energy from the diet, vitamin synthesis, xenobiotic and other metabolic phenotype metabolism, gut epithelial cell renewal, and immune system growth and function [127].

There has been a growing interest in understanding the microbiome in order to capitalise on the therapeutic potential of manipulating it, which has led to the development of fecal microbiota transplantation as a new practice [128]. Fecal microbiota transplantation (FMT) is the process of introducing a solution of feces from a donor into the digestive system of a recipient in order to directly influence the recipient's microbial makeup and provide a health benefit [129]. The first stage is usually to choose a donor who does not have a family history of autoimmune, metabolic, or malignant illnesses, as well as to check for any potential infections. A filtration step is conducted after mixing the feces with water or normal saline to remove any particle components [129]. The mixture may be given using a nasogastric tube, a nasojejunal tube, an esophagogastroduodenoscopy, a colonoscopy, or a retention enema. The majority of FMT's clinical experience has come from treating *Clostridium difficile* infections (CDI) that are recurring or resistant [130]. The therapeutic potential of FMT in treating CDI, (IBD), and other disorders are discussed in this chapter [131]. Vitamin A deficiency causes offspring to be born with low vitamin A levels in their livers, resulting in poor intestinal absorption and excessive excretion. Vitamin D deficiency is common in many parts of India, resulting in toneless and flabby muscles from childhood, leading to weak abdominal muscles, atony of intestinal musculature, and intestinal fermentation, as well as gastrointestinal upsets and diarrhea, which may be caused by a high-carbohydrate diet [132]. Zinc deficiency may alter the gut microbiome by causing excessive phytates and phosphates in the diet, as well as excessive copper and malabsorption. Folic acid deficiency produces inadequate nutritional intake, which results from a lack of milk, fresh fruits, and vegetables [133]. This deficiency also leads to low absorption of diet because folic acid cannot be converted to its active form in the absence of certain vitamins [133].

To stay healthy and fit, one's gut, food, and gut flora must all be in good working order. As a result, metabolic profiling, which is the measurement in biological systems of the complement of low molecular weight metabolites and their intermediates that reflects the dynamic response to genetic modification, as well as physiological, pathophysiological, and developmental stimuli, is a viable option [134]. Nuclear magnetic resonance (NMR) and mass spectrometry are the most prevalent technologies; the magnetic resonance shift or mass/charge ratio of individual analytes in the sample is used to separate the metabolites, resulting in a separation spectral profile [66]. Using Metabolomics to unravel compounds affecting human health, we see the gut microbiota is made up of a wide diversity of bacteria that produce a wide range of compounds that are vital for microbe selection and the formation of a metabolic signalling network [135].

The gut microbiota's future is bright, and there are still many improvements to be made in terms of healthy solutions. Probiotics, prebiotics, and eubiotics are currently recent terms, therefore they are getting quite a bit of attention [136]. Probiotics are living bacteria found in certain food supplements that give a variety of health benefits; whereas prebiotics are carbohydrate-derived compounds that are consumed by the good bacteria in your intestines. Eating a balanced diet of probiotics and prebiotics can help maintain your gut microbiota health by ensuring that you have the proper balance of bacteria [63]. Eubiotics are a type of feed additive that includes prebiotics, probiotics, essential oils, and organic acids. However, according to databases, as additional compounds are evaluated, the number of categories will surely increase [5].

Vitamin K and SCFAs are also produced by microorganisms in one's stomach, and the cells that line the colon get their sustenance primarily from SCFAs [34]. They aid in the maintenance of a healthy gut barrier, which keeps harmful chemicals, viruses, and bacteria at bay. This also helps to reduce inflammation and may help to reduce the risk of cancer. One's diet has a significant impact on the balance of good and bad bacteria in one's gut; for example, a high-sugar, high-fat diet harms gut bacteria and may contribute to insulin resistance and other disorders [88]. As there aren't as many beneficial bacteria to block the bad bacteria, when we feed on the wrong bacteria on a daily basis, they may grow faster and colonise more easily [137]. A greater body mass index has also been linked to the presence of dangerous bacteria and a less healthy gut flora. Additionally, organic food has been seen to play a major positive role on the gut microbiome [138].

The escalating trends in the domains of gut microbiota, diet, and dysbiosis have paved the way towards novel research leading to establishing a connection between a person's overall well-being and gut health. Moreover, additional scientific expedition is being performed in this domain to learn more about the gut microbiota and it's intervention on healthy physiological functioning of the human body [1, 139].

6.4 Conclusion

Human gut microbiota is a manifold of a dynamic population of microbes, which obtain their nutritional requirements and energy for sustenance from metabolism of complex food in the human gut. The production of a variety of enzymes by the microbial diversity present in the human gut plays an imperative role in catabolic processes such as digestion, contributing to the maintenance of good physiological health of an individual. Robust occurrence and growth of microbial population in humans is essential for maintenance of the immune system. The role of proper food intake and dietary measures and other factors influence the composition of gut microbiota. Macronutrients such as carbohydrates, proteins, and fats play a significant role in building up the composition and controlling functioning of the gut microbiota. The presence of diverse types of good bacterial population competes with harmful bacteria in terms of utilisation of essential nutrients and location of colony formation. Routine implementation of a carbohydrate, protein, and fat rich dietary regime adversely affects the normal physiological functioning of the body and affects the various metabolic pathways leading to chronic dysbiosis and disorders such as obesity and cardio-vascular ailments. The impact of carbohydrate rich diet on gut microbiome has been a dimension of research in recent years; whereas the effect of fat and protein rich diet on gut microbiome remains as a huge area to be explored. Incessant smoking, lack of physical movements, and unhealthy lifestyle affects the stable human gut microbiota adversely, leading to dysbiosis. Chronic stress also has an indirect impact on colonic microbial profiles. Diet involving fibres helps to control and maintain a healthy gut microbiota and as a result it can resist the pathogenic bacteria from causing harm. Infant oligosaccharides present in colostrum leads to the formation of bacteria such as *Lactobacillus* which aids in development of the immune system of their body. Change in dietary habits with growing age lead to changes in bacterial population in the gut. With age, maturation of microbial population in the human gut happens, leading to the production of vitamins and other essential components in the human body. Further research shows evidence that an imbalanced diet may lead to the onset of various clinical complications such as IBD. The sedentary and stressed lifestyle of an individual leads to imbalance of proper dietary requirements and also fluctuates the gut microbial population, which in many cases brings adverse effects. A balanced diet plays a substantial role in keeping good health and obviating severe chronic diseases. Change of diet for either a transient time or long term affects the gut microbiota and has consequences over one's immune system. It is very important to have nutrient-dense food in our diet in order to maintain a healthy lifestyle. Additionally, it is important to understand and find out which component of diet provides substrate for the stabilisation of the microbial community present in the gut to use it for the adjustment of microbial population in the body and maintaining healthy outcomes. Remedial measures for rebuilding the gut microbiota involve cost effective methods such as usage of prebiotic, probiotics, etc. Early analysis and understanding of growth of the gut microbial profile would aid in preventing clinically unwanted microbial profile formation in the gut and strengthen the immune system. Medically complex and expensive methods such as fecal transplantation are used at times. In this retrospective, various researches are being conducted in this domain, which are accentuating the better understanding of gut health and its impact on healthy physiological functioning of the human body, and thus this heralds a promising future.

References

1 Sommer, F. and Bäckhed, F. (2013). The gut microbiota: masters of host development and physiology. *Nature Rev. Microbiol.* 11 (4): 227–238.
2 Thursby, E. and Juge, N. (2017). Introduction to the human gut microbiota. *Biochem. J.* 474 (11): 1823–1836.
3 Kashtanova, D.A., Popenko, A.S., Tkacheva, O.N. et al. (2016). Association between the gut microbiota and diet: fetal life, early childhood, and further life. *Nutrition* 32 (6): 620–627.
4 Umu, Ö.C.O., Rudi, K., and Diep, D.B. (2017). Modulation of the gut microbiota by prebiotic fibres and bacteriocins. *Microb. Ecol. Health Dis.* 28 (1): 1348886.

5 Rodríguez, J.M., Murphy, K., Stanton, C. et al. (2015). The composition of the gut microbiota throughout life, with an emphasis on early life. *Microb. Ecol. Health Dis.* 26: 0.

6 Hill, C.J., Lynch, D.B., Murphy, K. et al. (2017). Evolution of gut microbiota composition from birth to 24 weeks in the INFANTMET Cohort. *Microbiome* 5 (1).

7 Neish, A.S. (2009). Microbes in gastrointestinal health and disease. *Gastroenterology* 136 (1): 65–80.

8 Carding, S., Verbeke, K., Vipond, D.T. et al. (2015). Dysbiosis of the gut microbiota in disease. *Microb. Eco. Health Dis.* 26: 0.

9 Moszak, M., Szulińska, M., and Bogdański, P. (2020). You are what you eat—the relationship between diet, microbiota, and metabolic disorders—a review. *Nutrients* 12 (4).

10 Bamola, V.D., Ghosh, A., Kapardar, R.K. et al. (2017). Gut microbial diversity in health and disease: experience of healthy Indian subjects, and colon carcinoma and inflammatory bowel disease patients. *Microb. Eco.Health Dis.* 28 (1): 1322447.

11 Rath, C.M. and Dorrestein, P.C. (2012). The bacterial chemical repertoire mediates metabolic exchange within gut microbiomes. *Cur. Opin.Microbio.* 15 (2): 147–154.

12 Zhang, H., Sparks, J.B., Karyala, S.V. et al. (2015). Host adaptive immunity alters gut microbiota. *ISME J.* 9 (3): 770–781.

13 Rothschild, D., Weissbrod, O., Barkan, E. et al. (2018). Environment dominates over host genetics in shaping human gut microbiota. *Nature* 555 (7695): 210–215.

14 Hakansson, A. and Molin, G. (2011). Gut microbiota and inflammation. *Nutrients* 3 (6): 637–687.

15 Korem, T., Zeevi, D., Zmora, N. et al. (2017). Bread affects clinical parameters and induces gut microbiome-associated personal glycemic responses. *Cell Metabo.* 25 (6): 1243–1253.e5.

16 Goodrich, J.K., Waters, J.L., Poole, A.C. et al. (2014). Human genetics shape the gut microbiome. *Cell* 159 (4): 789–799.

17 McIntosh, K., Reed, D.E., Schneider, T. et al. (2017). FODMAPs alter symptoms and the metabolome of patients with IBS: a randomised controlled trial. *Gut* 66 (7): 1241–1251.

18 Beaumont, M., Goodrich, J.K., Jackson, M.A. et al. (2016). Heritable components of the human fecal microbiome are associated with visceral fat. *Geno. Bio.* 17 (1).

19 Falony, G., Joossens, M., Vieira-Silva, S. et al. (2016). Population-level analysis of gut microbiome variation. *Science* 352 (6285): 560–564.

20 Sonnenburg, E.D. and Sonnenburg, J.L. (2014). Starving our microbial self: The deleterious consequences of a diet deficient in microbiota-accessible carbohydrates. *Cell Metab.* 20 (5): 779–786.

21 Bien, J., Palagani, V., and Bozko, P. (2013). The intestinal microbiota dysbiosis and Clostridium difficile infection: Ii there a relationship with inflammatory bowel disease? *Ther. Adv. Gastro.* 6 (1): 53–68.

22 Knights, D., Lassen, K.G., and Xavier, R.J. (2013). Advances in inflammatory bowel disease pathogenesis: linking host genetics and the microbiome. *Gut* 62 (10): 1505–1510.

23 Wilkins, L.J., Monga, M., and Miller, A.W. (2019). Defining dysbiosis for a cluster of chronic diseases. *Sci. Rep.* 9 (1).

24 Nettleton, J.E., Reimer, R.A., and Shearer, J. (2016). Reshaping the gut microbiota: impact of low calorie sweeteners and the link to insulin resistance? *Phys.Behav.* 164: 488–493.

25 Abou-Donia, M.B., El-Masry, E.M., Abdel-Rahman, A.A. et al. (2008). Splenda alters gut microflora and increases intestinal P-glycoprotein and cytochrome P-450 in male rats. *J. Toxi. Environ. Health Part A: Curr. Iss.* 71 (21): 1415–1429.

26 Bian, X., Chi, L., Gao, B. et al. (2017 July). Gut microbiome response to sucralose and its potential role in inducing liver inflammation in mice. *Front. Phys.* 8.

27 Chassaing, B., Koren, O., Goodrich, J.K. et al. (2015). Dietary emulsifiers impact the mouse gut microbiota promoting colitis and metabolic syndrome. *Nature* 519 (7541): 92–96.

28 Gibson, P.R. (2017). The evidence base for efficacy of the low FODMAP diet in irritable bowel syndrome: is it ready for prime time as a first-line therapy? *J. Gastro. Hepa. (Australia)* 32: 32–35.

29 Wu, G.D., Compher, C., Chen, E.Z. et al. (2016). Comparative metabolomics in vegans and omnivores reveal constraints on diet-dependent gut microbiota metabolite production. *Gut* 65 (1): 63–72.

30 Montel, M.C., Buchin, S., Mallet, A. et al. (2014). Traditional cheeses: rich and diverse microbiota with associated benefits. *Int. J. Food Micro.* 177: 136–154.

31 Uchida, M., Mogami, O., and Matsueda, K. (2007). Characteristic of milk whey culture with Propionibacterium freudenreichii ET-3 and its application to the inflammatory bowel disease therapy. *Inflammopharmacology* 15 (3): 105–108.

32 Zheng, H., Yde, C.C., Clausen, M.R. et al. (2015). Metabolomics investigation to shed light on cheese as a possible piece in the French paradox puzzle. *J. Agri. Food Chem.* 63 (10): 2830–2839.

33 Cheng, W., Lu, J., Li, B. et al. (2017 September). Effect of functional oligosaccharides and ordinary dietary fiber on intestinal microbiota diversity. *Front. Micro.* 8.

34 Sasaki, D., Sasaki, K., Ikuta, N. et al. (2018). Low amounts of dietary fibre increase in vitro production of short-chain fatty acids without changing human colonic microbiota structure. *Sci. Rep.* 8 (1).

35 Zhao, L., Zhang, F., Ding, X. et al. Gut bacteria selectively promoted by dietary fibers alleviate type 2 diabetes. *Science* 359 (6380): 1151–1156. https://pubmed.ncbi.nlm.nih.gov/29590046/.

36 Etxeberria, U., Arias, N., Boqué, N. et al. (2015). Reshaping faecal gut microbiota composition by the intake of trans-resveratrol and quercetin in high-fat sucrose diet-fed rats. *J. Nutri. Biochem.* 26 (6): 651–660.

37 Moreno-Indias, I., Sánchez-Alcoholado, L., Pérez-Martínez, P. et al. (2016). Red wine polyphenols modulate fecal microbiota and reduce markers of the metabolic syndrome in obese patients. *Food Fun.* 7 (4): 1775–1787.

38 Ozdal, T., Sela, D.A., Xiao, J. et al. (2016). The reciprocal interactions between polyphenols and gut microbiota and effects on bioaccessibility. *Nutrients* 8 (2).

39 Mihrshahi, S., Ding, D., Gale, J. et al. (2017). Vegetarian diet and all-cause mortality: evidence from a large population-based Australian cohort the 45 and up Study. *Prev. Med.* 97: 1–7.

40 Orlich, M.J., Singh, P.N., Sabaté, J. et al. (2013). Vegetarian dietary patterns and mortality in adventist health study 2. *JAMA Int. Med.* 173 (13): 1230–1238.

41 O'Keefe, S.J.D., Li, J.V., Lahti, L. et al. (2015). Fat, fibre and cancer risk in African Americans and rural Africans. *Nat. Comm.* 6.

42 David, L.A., Maurice, C.F., Carmody, R.N. et al. (2014). Diet rapidly and reproducibly alters the human gut microbiome. *Nature* 505 (7484): 559–563.

43 Renz, H., Adkins, B.D., Bartfeld, S. et al. (2018). The neonatal window of opportunity— early priming for life. *J. All. Clin. Imm.* 141 (4): 1212–1214.

44 Tamburini, S., Shen, N., Wu, H.C. et al. (2016). The microbiome in early life: implications for health outcomes. *Nat. Med.* 22 (7): 713–722.

45 Cahenzli, J., Köller, Y., Wyss, M. et al. (2013). Intestinal microbial diversity during early-life colonization shapes long-term IgE levels. *Cell H. Mi.* 14 (5): 559–570.

46 Olszak, T., An, D., Zeissig, S. et al. (2012). Microbial exposure during early life has persistent effects on natural killer T cell function. *Science (1979)* 336 (6080): 489–493.

47 Russell, S.L., Gold, M.J., Hartmann, M. et al. (2012). Early life antibiotic-driven changes in microbiota enhance susceptibility to allergic asthma. *EMBO Rep.* 13 (5): 440–447.

48 Arrieta, M.-C., Stiemsma, L.T., Dimitriu, P.A. et al. (2015). Early infancy microbial and metabolic alterations affect risk of childhood asthma. *Sci. Trans. Med.* 7 (307): 307ra152. https://pubmed.ncbi.nlm.nih.gov/26424567/.

49 Azad, M.B., Konya, T., Guttman, D.S. et al. (2015). Infant gut microbiota and food sensitization: associations in the first year of life. *Clin. Ex. All.* 45 (3): 632–643.

50 Bisgaard, H., Li, N., Bonnelykke, K. et al. (2011). Reduced diversity of the intestinal microbiota during infancy is associated with increased risk of allergic disease at school age. *J. All. Clin. Imm.* 128 (3).

51 Johansson, M.A., Sjögren, Y.M., Persson, J.O. et al. (2011). Early colonization with a group of Lactobacilli decreases the risk for allergy at five years of age despite allergic heredity. *PLoS ONE* 6 (8).

52 Nicholson, J.K., Holmes, E., Kinross, J. et al. (2012). Host-gut microbiota metabolic interactions. *Science (1979)* 336 (6086): 1262–1267.

53 Amenyogbe, N., Kollmann, T.R., and Ben-Othman, R. (2017). Early-life host-microbiome interphase: the key frontier for immune development. *Front. Ped.* 5.

54 Baars, A., Oosting, A., Knol, J. et al. (2015). The gut microbiota as a therapeutic target in ibd and metabolic disease: a role for the bile acid receptors fxr and tgr5. *Microorganisms* 3 (4): 641–666.

55 Rooks, M.G. and Garrett, W.S. (2016). Gut microbiota, metabolites and host immunity. *Nat. Rev. Imm.* 16 (6): 341–352.

56 Bridgman, S.L., Azad, M.B., Field, C.J. et al. (2017). Fecal short-chain fatty acid variations by breastfeeding status in infants at 4 months: differences in relative versus absolute concentrations. *Front. Nutr.* 4.

57 Iraporda, C., Errea, A., Romanin, D.E. et al. (2015). Lactate and short chain fatty acids produced by microbial fermentation downregulate proinflammatory responses in intestinal epithelial cells and myeloid cells. *Immunobiology* 220 (10): 1161–1169.

58 van den Elsen, L.W.J., Poyntz, H.C., Weyrich, L.S. et al. (2017). Embracing the gut microbiota: the new frontier for inflammatory and infectious diseases. *Clin. Trans. Immunol.* 6 (1).

59 Trompette, A., Gollwitzer, E.S., Yadava, K. et al. (2014). Gut microbiota metabolism of dietary fiber influences allergic airway disease and hematopoiesis. *Nat. Med.* 20 (2): 159–166.

60 Thio, C.L.P., Chi, P.Y., Lai, A.C.Y. et al. (2018). Regulation of type 2 innate lymphoid cell–dependent airway hyperreactivity by butyrate. *J. All. Clin. Immu.* 142 (6): 1867–1883.e12.

61 Ayechu-Muruzabal, V., van Stigt, A.H., Mank, M. et al. (2018). Diversity of human milk oligosaccharides and effects on early life immune development. *Front. Ped.* 6.

62 Bode, L. (2012). Human milk oligosaccharides: every baby needs a sugar mama. *Glycobiology* 22 (9): 1147–1162.

63 Roberfroid, M. (2007). Prebiotics: the concept revisited. *J. Nutri.* 137 (3 Suppl 2): 830S–7S. https://pubmed.ncbi.nlm.nih.gov/17311983/.

64 Zivkovic, A.M., German, J.B., Lebrilla, C.B. et al. (2011). Human milk glycobiome and its impact on the infant gastrointestinal microbiota. *Proc. Natl. Acad. Sci. USA* 108 (Supp. 1): 4653–4658.

65 Gao, J., Xu, K., Liu, H. et al. (2018 February). Impact of the gut microbiota on intestinal immunity mediated by tryptophan metabolism. *Front. Cell. Inf. Micro.* 8.

66 Gómez-Gallego, C., Morales, J.M., Monleón, D. et al. (2018). Human breast milk NMR metabolomic profile across specific geographical locations and its association with the milk microbiota. *Nutrients* 10 (10).

67 Korecka, A., Dona, A., Lahiri, S. et al. (2016). Bidirectional communication between the Aryl hydrocarbon Receptor (AhR) and the microbiome tunes host metabolism. *NPJ Biof. Micro.* 2.

68 Jiang, T., Liu, B., Li, J. et al. (2018). Association between sn-2 fatty acid profiles of breast milk and development of the infant intestinal microbiome. *Food Func.* 9 (2): 1028–1037.

69 Ojeda, P., Bobe, A., Dolan, K. et al. (2016). Nutritional modulation of gut microbiota the impact on metabolic disease pathophysiology. *J. Nutri. Biochem.* 28: 191–200.

70 Demmelmair, H., Prell, C., Timby, N. et al. (2017). Benefits of lactoferrin, osteopontin and milk fat globule membranes for infants. *Nutrients* 9 (8).

71 Mastromarino, P., Capobianco, D., Campagna, G. et al. (2014). Correlation between lactoferrin and beneficial microbiota in breast milk and infant's feces. *Bio. Met.* 27 (5): 1077–1086.

72 Pirr, S., Richter, M., Fehlhaber, B. et al. (2017 December). High amounts of S100-alarmins confer antimicrobial activity on human breast milk: targeting pathogens relevant in neonatal sepsis. *Front. Imm.* 8.

73 Wickens, K., Barthow, C., Mitchell, E.A. et al. (2018). Maternal supplementation alone with Lactobacillus rhamnosus HN001 during pregnancy and breastfeeding does not reduce infant eczema. *Ped. All. Immu.* 29 (3): 296–302.

74 Jiménez, E., Fernández, L., Maldonado, A. et al. (2008). Oral administration of Lactobacillus strains isolated from breast milk as an alternative for the treatment of infectious mastitis during lactation. *Appl. Environ. Micro.* 74 (15): 4650–4655.

75 van den Elsen, L.W.J., Garssen, J., Burcelin, R. et al. (2019 February). Shaping the gut microbiota by breastfeeding: the gateway to allergy prevention? *Front. Ped.* 7.

76 Senghor, B., Sokhna, C., Ruimy, R. et al. (2018). Gut microbiota diversity according to dietary habits and geographical provenance. *Hu. Micro. J.* 7–8: 1–9.

77 Tailford, L.E., Owen, C.D., Walshaw, J. et al. (2015). Discovery of intramolecular trans-sialidases in human gut microbiota suggests novel mechanisms of mucosal adaptation. *Nat. Comm.* 6.

78 Arike, L. and Hansson, G.C. (2016). The densely O-glycosylated MUC2 mucin protects the intestine and provides food for the commensal bacteria. *J. Mol. Bio.* 428 (16): 3221–3229.

79 Seo, Y.S., Lee, H.-B., Kim, Y. et al. (2020). Dietary carbohydrate constituents related to gut dysbiosis and health. *Microorganisms* 8 (3).

80 Feng, R., Du, S., Chen, Y. et al. (2015). High carbohydrate intake from starchy foods is positively associated with metabolic disorders: a cohort study from a Chinese population. *Sci. Rep.* 5.

81 Hu, F.B. (2011). Globalization of diabetes: the role of diet, lifestyle, and genes. *Diab. Care* 34 (6): 1249–1257.

82 Hou, J.K., Abraham, B., and El-Serag, H. (2011). Dietary intake and risk of developing inflammatory bowel disease: a systematic review of the literature. *Am. J. Gastro.* 106 (4): 563–573.

83 Tang, W.H.W., Kitai, T., and Hazen, S.L. (2017). Gut microbiota in cardiovascular health and disease. *Circ. Res.* 120 (7): 1183–1196.

84 Stanhope, K.L. and Havel, P.J. (2010). Fructose consumption: recent results and their potential implications. *Ann. NY Acad. Sci.* 1190: 15–24.

85 Sonestedt, E., Wirfält, E., Wallström, P. et al. (2012). High disaccharide intake associates with atherogenic lipoprotein profile. *Br. J. Nutr.* 107 (7): 1062–1069.

86 Knight-Sepulveda, K., Kais, S., Santaolalla, R. et al. (2015). Diet and inflammatory bowel disease. *Gastro. Hepa.* 11.

87 den Besten, G., van Eunen, K., Groen, A.K. et al. (2013). The role of short-chain fatty acids in the interplay between diet, gut microbiota, and host energy metabolism. *J. Lip. Res.* 54 (9): 2325–2340.

88 Conlon, M.A. and Bird, A.R. (2015). The impact of diet and lifestyle on gut microbiota and human health. *Nutrients* 7 (1): 17–44.

89 de Filippo, C., di Paola, M., Ramazzotti, M. et al. (2017 October). Diet, environments, and gut microbiota. A preliminary investigation in children living in rural and Urban Burkina Faso and Italy. *Front. Micro.* 8.

90 Kau, A.L., Planer, J.D., Liu, J. et al. (2015). Functional characterization of IgA-targeted bacterial taxa from undernourished Malawian children that produce diet-dependent enteropathy. *Sci. Transl. Med.* 7 (276): 276ra24. https://pubmed.ncbi.nlm.nih.gov/25717097/.

91 Ruiz-Ojeda, F.J., Plaza-Díaz, J., Sáez-Lara, M.J. et al. (2019). Effects of sweeteners on the gut microbiota: a review of experimental studies and clinical trials. *Adv. Nut.* 10: S31–S48.

92 Suez, J., Korem, T., Zeevi, D. et al. (2014). Artificial sweeteners induce glucose intolerance by altering the gut microbiota. *Nature* 514 (7521): 181–186.

93 Pase, M.P., Himali, J.J., Beiser, A.S. et al. (2017). Sugar- and artificially sweetened beverages and the risks of incident stroke and dementia: a prospective cohort study. *Stroke* 48 (5): 1139–1146.

94 Halmos, E.P., Christophersen, C.T., Bird, A.R. et al. (2015). Diets that differ in their FODMAP content alter the colonic luminal microenvironment. *Gut* 64 (1): 93–100.

95 Yu, Z.T., Liu, B., Mukherjee, P. et al. (2013). Trametes versicolor extract modifies human fecal microbiota composition in vitro. *Plant Foods Hu. Nut.* 68 (2): 107–112.

96 Zhang, X., Shen, D., Fang, Z. et al. (2013). Human gut microbiota changes reveal the progression of glucose intolerance. *PLoS ONE* 8 (8).

97 Hennessy, A.A., Barrett, E., Paul Ross, R. et al. (2012). The production of conjugated α-linolenic, γ-linolenic and stearidonic acids by strains of bifidobacteria and propionibacteria. *Lipids* 47 (3): 313–327.

98 Zhao, J., Zhang, X., Liu, H. et al. (2018). Dietary Protein and Gut Microbiota Composition and Function. *Cur. Pro. Pep. Sci.* 20 (2): 145–154.

99 He, L., Han, M., Qiao, S. et al. (2015). Soybean antigen proteins and their intestinal sensitization activities. *Cur. Pro. Pep. Sci.* 16 (7): 613–621.

100 Peng, M., Bitsko, E., and Biswas, D. (2015). Functional properties of peanut fractions on the growth of probiotics and foodborne bacterial pathogens. *J. Food Sci.* 80 (3): M635–M641.

101 Lozupone, C.A., Stombaugh, J.I., Gordon, J.I. et al. (2012). Diversity, stability and resilience of the human gut microbiota. *Nature* 489 (7415): 220–230.

102 Hooper, L.V., Littman, D.R., and Macpherson, A.J. (2012). Interactions between the microbiota and the immune system. *Science (1979)* 336 (6086): 1268–1273.

103 Faith, J.J., McNulty, N.P., Rey, F.E. et al. (2011). Predicting a human gut microbiota's response to diet in gnotobiotic mice. *Science (1979)* 333 (6038): 101–104.

104 Windey, K., de Preter, V., and Verbeke, K. (2012). Relevance of protein fermentation to gut health. *Mole. Nut. Food Res.* 56 (1): 184–196.

105 Ma, X., He, P., Sun, P. et al. (2010). Lipoic acid: an immunomodulator that attenuates glycinin-induced anaphylactic reactions in a rat model. *J. Agri. Food Chem.* 58 (8): 5086–5092.

106 Song, P., Zhang, R., Wang, X. et al. (2011 June). Dietary grape-seed procyanidins decreased post-weaning diarrhea by modulating intestinal permeability and suppressing oxidative stress in rats. *J. Agri. Food Chem.* 59 (11): 6227–6632.

107 Woyengo, T.A., Weihrauch, D., and Nyachoti, C.M. (2012). Effect of dietary phytic acid on performance and nutrient uptake in the small intestine of piglets. *J. An. Sci.* 90 (2): 543–549.

108 Butteiger, D.N., Hibberd, A.A., McGraw, N.J. et al. (2016). Soy protein compared with milk protein in a western diet increases gut microbial diversity and reduces serum lipids in Golden Syrian hamsters. *J. Nutr.* 146 (4): 697–705.

109 Schoeler, M. and Caesar, R. (2019). Dietary lipids, gut microbiota and lipid metabolism. *Rev. Endo. Meta. Dis.* 20 (4): 461–472.

110 Ze, X., Duncan, S.H., Louis, P. et al. (2012). Ruminococcus bromii is a keystone species for the degradation of resistant starch in the human colon. *ISME J.* 6 (8): 1535–1543.

111 Tominaga, K., Kamimura, K., Takahashi, K. et al. (2018). Diversion colitis and pouchitis: a mini-review. *W. J. Gastro.* 24 (16): 1734–1747.

112 MacFabe, D.F. (2012). Short-chain fatty acid fermentation products of the gut microbiome: implications in autism spectrum disorders. *Micro. Eco. He. Dis.* 23.

113 Cherbut, C., Aubé, A.C., Blottière, H.M. et al. (1997). Effects of short-chain fatty acids on gastrointestinal motility. *Scan. J. Gastro., Supp.* 32 (222): 58–61.

114 Machate, D.J., Figueiredo, P.S., Marcelino, G. et al. (2020). Fatty acid diets: regulation of gut microbiota composition and obesity and its related metabolic dysbiosis. *Int. J. Mole. Sci.* 21 (11): 1–22.

115 Liu, R., Shu, Y., Qi, W. et al. (2021). Protective effects of almond oil on streptozotocin-induced diabetic rats via regulating Nrf2/HO-1 pathway and gut microbiota. *J. Food Qual.* 2021.

116 Miao, F., Shan, C., Shah, S.A.H. et al. (2021). Effect of walnut (*Juglans sigillata*) oil on intestinal antioxidant, anti-inflammatory, immunity, and gut microbiota modulation in mice. *J. Food Bio.* 45 (1).

117 Martinez, K.B., Leone, V., and Chang, E.B. (2017). Western diets, gut dysbiosis, and metabolic diseases: are they linked? *Gut Micr.* 8 (2): 130–142.

118 Rodríguez-García, C., Sánchez-Quesada, C., Algarra, I. et al. (2020). The high-fat diet based on extra-virgin olive oil causes dysbiosis linked to colorectal cancer prevention. *Nutrients* 12 (6): 1–17.

119 Gui, L., Chen, S., Wang, H. et al. (2019). ω-3 PUFAs alleviate high-fat diet–induced circadian intestinal microbes dysbiosis. *Mol. Nut. Food Res.* 63 (22).

120 Tomasello, G., Mazzola, M., Leone, A. et al. (2016). Nutrition, oxidative stress and intestinal dysbiosis: influence of diet on gut microbiota in inflammatory bowel diseases. *Biomed. Pap.* 160 (4): 461–466.

121 Wang, F., Zhu, H., Hu, M. et al. (2018). Perilla oil supplementation improves hypertriglyceridemia and gut dysbiosis in diabetic KKAy mice. *Mol. Nut. Food Res.* 62 (24).

122 Ye, Z., Xu, Y.J., and Liu, Y. (2021). Influences of dietary oils and fats, and the accompanied minor content of components on the gut microbiota and gut inflammation: a review. *Tren. Food Sci. Tech.* 113: 255–276.

123 Chung, W.S.F., Walker, A.W., Louis, P. et al. (2016). Modulation of the human gut microbiota by dietary fibres occurs at the species level. *BMC Bio.* 14 (1).

124 Jandhyala, S.M., Talukdar, R., Subramanyam, C. et al. (2015). Role of the normal gut microbiota. *W. J. Gastro.* 21 (29): 8836–8847.

125 Lattimer, J.M. and Haub, M.D. (2010). Effects of dietary fiber and its components on metabolic health. *Nutrients* 2 (12): 1266–1289.

126 Tojo, R., Suárez, A., Clemente, M.G. et al. (2014). Intestinal microbiota in health and disease: role of bifidobacteria in gut homeostasis. *W. J. Gastro.* 20 (41): 15163–15176.

127 Turnbaugh, P.J., Ley, R.E., Hamady, M. et al. (2007). The human microbiome project. *Nature* 449 (7164): 804–810.

128 Lee, P., Yacyshyn, B.R., and Yacyshyn, M.B. (2019). Gut microbiota and obesity: an opportunity to alter obesity through faecal microbiota transplant (FMT). *Dia., Obes. Metab.* 21 (3): 479–490.

129 De Palma, G., Lynch, M.D.J., Lu, J et al. (2017). Transplantation of fecal microbiota from patients with irritable bowel syndrome alters gut function and behavior in recipient mice. *Sci. Transl. Med.* 9 (379): eaaf6397. https://pubmed.ncbi.nlm.nih.gov/28251905/.

130 Allegretti, J.R., Mullish, B.H., Kelly, C. et al. (2019). Therapeutics: the evolution of the use of faecal microbiota transplantation and emerging therapeutic indications. *Lancet* 394.

131 Lopez, J., Grinspan, A., Mount, A.G. et al. (2016). Fecal microbiota transplantation for inflammatory bowel disease. *Gastro. Hepa.* 12 (6).

132 Icaza-Chávez, M.E. (2013). Gut microbiota in health and disease. *Rev. de Gastro. de México (English Ed.)* 78 (4): 240–248.

133 Mena, P. and Bresciani, L. (2020). Dietary fibre modifies gut microbiota: what's the role of (poly)phenols? *Int. J. Food Sci. Nut.* 71 (7): 783–784.

134 Swann, J. and Claus, S.P. (2014). Nutrimetabonomics: nutritional applications of metabolic profiling. *Sci. Pro.* 97 (1): 41–47.

135 Smirnov, K.S., Maier, T.V., Walker, A. et al. (2016). Challenges of metabolomics in human gut microbiota research. *Int. J. Med. Micro.* 306 (5): 266–279.

136 Miniello, V.L., Diaferio, L., Lassandro, C. et al. (2017). The importance of being eubiotic. *J. Pro. Hea.* 5 (1).

137 Morowitz, M.J., Carlisle, E.M., and Alverdy, J.C. (2011). Contributions of intestinal bacteria to nutrition and metabolism in the critically ill. *Sur. Clin. N. Am.* 91 (4): 771–785.

138 Valdes, A.M., Walter, J., Segal, E. et al. (2018). Role of the gut microbiota in nutrition and health. *BMJ (Online)* 361: 36–44.

139 Li, J., Zhang, A., Wu, F. et al. (2022). Alterations in the gut microbiota and their metabolites in colorectal cancer: recent progress and future prospects. *Front. Onc.* 12.

7

Composition of Gut Microbiota and *Clostridium difficile*

Jissin Mathew and Anu Jacob

Karunya Institute of Technology and Science, Coimbatore, India

7.1 Introduction

The term 'microbiota' encompasses a vast community of microbes that populate a certain area. This group of microbes includes bacteria as well as fungus, protozoans, viruses, and archaea [1]. One of the greatest interfaces (250–400 m^2) seen between host, external variables, and internal antigens in the human body is the gastrointestinal (GI) tract. Approximately 60 tonnes of food and numerous environmental microbes from the surroundings flow through the mammalian GI tract in a lifespan, representing a major threat to gut health. The term 'gut microbiota' refers to the group of bacteria, archaea, and eukarya that colonise the GI tract [2]. As the primary component of gut microecology, the intestinal microbiota play a crucial role in mediating both health and illness. The brain, lung, liver, bone, cardiovascular system, and other organ systems actively interact with the gut bacteria substances produced by the microbiota, such as the short chain fatty acid (SCFA) butyrate, and these systems seem to carry the main signals that connect the physiology to the gut microbiome [3]. According to a recently updated estimate, the proportion of mammalian to bacterial cells is probably closer to 1:1 [2]. The gut microbiota has been the subject of major research in the scientific community in recent years, and it has been linked to a wide range of human disorders, including luminal disease, metabolic disorders, autoimmune illnesses. and neurodevelopmental disabilities, despite these issues, the microbiota is not strong enough to cause lifelong infections [1]. The majority of gut microbes are not harmful to humans and live in harmony with enterocytes [4]. The primary functions such as intestinal barrier, nutrient and drug metabolism, and the restriction of the colonisation of harmful bacteria are supported by the gut commensals [1]. The microbiota also support the host in a variety of physiological ways, including enhancing gut integrity, modifying the intestinal epithelium, generating energy, and controlling host defences. When microbial content is changed it is called dysbiosis, and this has the ability to destabilise these systems [2].

The US Human Microbiome Project (HMP), the European Metagenomics of the Human Intestinal Tract (MetaHIT), and numerous other researchers have produced numerous high-quality data that have now proven the positive effects of the typical intestinal microbiota on health, even at the genome level [5]. The investigation of the gut microbiota currently involves many stages such as 16S rRNA-based sequencing of bacterial genes, and bioinformatics analysis. Since the bacterial 16S ribosomal RNA (rRNA) gene is involved in all bacteria and archaea and contains nine highly variable sections (V1–V9) that enable easy species differentiation, targeting of this domain is a common strategy. Although the use of smaller read lengths may cause mistakes, the focus of 16S rRNA sequencing has switched to examining shorter subareas of the gene in greater depth. Due to the greater specificity and accuracy of these approaches, whole-genome shotgun metagenomics may provide more accurate estimates of microbiota diversity and composition. The metabolomic study at molecular level of understanding on host-bacterial interrelationship provides the strongest correlation [2]. The combined data from the metabolome and intestinal microbiota provide the strongest evidence that shows the strongest correlation between healthy and unhealthy states [1].

Most experts agree that the growth of the microbiota starts at birth. The GI tract is quickly populated, and variations in food, antibiotic use, and sickness may all cause erratic alterations in the microbiota. When a newborn is delivered vaginally, their microbiota contains a high quantity of lactobacilli for their initial days, and reflects a high concentration of lactobacilli in the vaginal flora. This suggests that the mode of birth may also have an impact on the microbiota makeup. Contrarily, newborns delivered through C-section have a diminished microbiota and a delayed colonisation of the Bacteroides genus, but are colonised by microbial species such Clostridium. The prevalence of some microbial species in newborns intestinal microbiota may also be influenced by feeding practises. For instance, *Bifidobacterium longum* and numerous forms of Bacteroides can use the fucosylated oligosaccharides found in human milk to outcompete unrelated bacteria such as *E. coli* and *Clostridium perfringens*. While *Bifidobacterium* spp. are normally present in high concentrations in breast-fed infants' microbiome, there are significantly less in formula-fed newborns. Additionally, the microbiota of infants that consume formula exhibit higher variety and different concentrations of other species such *Lactobacilli, C. diff., Bacteroides fragilis*, and *E. coli* [2].

The ability to produce competitive elimination is one of the healthy gut microbiota's key defences against pathogens. It is common that the intestinal flora influences the control of intestinal disorders because it is concentrated in the gastrointestinal system. New research suggests that the microbiota may also play a role in extraintestinal organs because of the different microbial community composition. The host's physiological state is dominated by this changing intestinal microflora, which may be caused by diet or the atmosphere (cold, utilisation of antibiotics, consumption of probiotics, and the incidence of diseases) [3]. For more than 50 years antibiotic administration has been essential to treating bacterial infections, but it severely disrupts the gut's friendly bacteria and their function. Antibiotics have been shown to alter the mechanism of competitive elimination and lead to destruction of the elaborate system of interspecies interactions within the microbiota; which increases the quantity of host-derived sialic acid, which stimulate the development of pathogens like *Salmonella typhimurium* and *C. diff.* [1].

The use of antibiotics has indeed been linked to both short-term and long-term alterations in the intestinal microbiota. Most of these variations result in disease and are brought on by *Clostridium difficile*, an opportunistic human gastrointestinal bacterium belonging to the class Clostridia [6]. *C. diff.* is a gram-positive, exclusively anaerobic bacterium, which was first discovered in the microbiota of healthy babies in 1935, and was labelled as an 'effectively motile, heavy-bodied rod having extended subterminal or almost terminal spores.' A thorough analysis of the bacteria, then known as *C. difficile*, did not have a clear connection to human disease until the 1970s [7]. The fecal microbiota's barrier qualities hinder colonisation of these, and antibiotic use weakens this resistance, which is a key risk factor for illness [8]. The term *C. difficile*-associated disease/diarrhea (CDAD) was used to refer to this condition. More recently, the term *C. difficile* infection (CDI) has gained favour. Initially in the 2000s, there was a surge in chronic CDI cases in Canada, the US, and Europe, which were related to the introduction of a specific epidemic of *C. diff.* strains [9, 7]. Reported prevalence for CDI in India has ranged from 7.1% to 26.6% in the majority of earlier investigations. The likelihood of a *C. diff.* recurrence varies from 20% to 60%, and it increases after many past recurrences. It's possible that the consequences of recurrent infection are higher than those of original infection and is most frequently as a result of reactivation or re-exposure of spores in individuals with compromised colonic microbiota barrier function and decreased immunological resistance to infection [8].

There are numerous symptoms associated with CDI, ranging from moderate diarrhea to fulminant colitis, toxic megacolon, and even mortality. After receiving antibiotic therapy and the significant decline of the intestinal flora, the disease frequently becomes evident [10]. Ampicillin, amoxicillin, cephalosporins, clindamycin, and fluoroquinolones are the antibiotics that are most frequently associated with the disease [8]. The primary pathogenic components of *C. difficile* have been identified as toxin A (TcdA) and/or toxin B (TcdB), which are high molecular weight clostridial toxins [9]. As the first stage of the pathogenic process, antibiotics enable *C. diff.* to grow and colonise the gut. Subsequently, *C. diff.* releases TcdA and TcdB; its own toxins that cause cell damage and clinical symptoms. Colonisation is a crucial stage in the pathogenic phase of *C. diff.* that is dependent on both the microbiota colonisation resistance and *C. diff.* colonisation factors. Additional host factors, such as the host's immunological response, might also be involved in this process of causing infection [11]. TcdA and TcdB, which are inactivate components of the Rho group of guanosine triphosphatases (Rho GTPases), promote *C. diff.* diarrhea and cause neutrophilic colitis, colonocyte death, and intestinal barrier dysfunction. Infection outside the intestines is relatively uncommon, nor is the bacteria itself invasive. The pathogenicity of the infectious strain and the production of antibodies in host are the two elements that have the most effect on medical manifestation of the disease [8].

The risk factors for CDI have been extensively discussed in literature. Despite the fact that community-based infections are becoming increasingly frequent, CDI primarily affects hospitalised patients, particularly older multimorbid individuals [12]. A significant risk factor for CDI is age; it has been discovered that the chance of developing *C. diff.* disease when receiving medical care rises by about 2% for each year after the age of 18. The evidence shows that ageing also causes a slow change in the gut flora. Elderly people have a different core gut microbiota than younger individuals, with an elevation of the *Bacteroides* spp. and *Clostridium* genera. The second risk is taking medication for a short period of time, and healthy people's microbiotas experienced decrease of diversity and changes in the predominance of some taxa that persisted for up to two years. The term 'post-antibiotic dysbiosis' refers to this alteration in the condition of the gut microbiota and it is characterised by decreased diversity, loss of specific taxa, changes in metabolic capacity, and decreased colonisation resistance against invasive pathogens. The collapse of colonisation resistance against *C difficile* is the result of the many combined elements of post-antibiotic dysbiosis. Proton pump inhibitors (PPIs) are also thought to increase the risk of CDI. It is hypothesised that PPIs could affect the gut microbiota and stimulate the development of *C diff.* since they elevate gastric pH [13]. The alterations in the ecological and bacterial communities that take place in the intestine are little recognised, despite the fact that disrupting the normal faecal microbiota may foster an ecological state in which *C. diff.* may thrive. Both host and microbial community variables have a role in the infection of a dysbiotic intestinal population by *C. diff.* For growth and colonisation, *C. diff.* chooses particular settings, which seem to happen via complimentary pathways. Although there are various methods by which the native microbiota resists colonisation by harmful bacteria, the establishment of CDI may entail altered bile acid metabolism and competition between microbes for resources [9]. The human gut microbiota may stop pathogen invasion through a variety of common mechanisms, including direct inhibition (by secreting inhibitory substances called bacteriocins), nutrient deficiency (by ingesting nutrients that restrict growth), or inducing host immune defences. It is still unclear exactly how the microbiota defends towards *C. diff.* infection (CDI), inhibiting its proliferation and pathogenicity. Although *C. diff.* is a target of bacteriocin generated by an intestinal strain of *Bacillus thuringiensis*, effective antagonism was discovered in vitro in this aspect, because the intestinal microbiota actively engage in the breakdown of protein, amino acid, and lipid metabolism in the diet. Bile acid is transformed by gut microbes, which otherwise promote the germination and proliferation of *C. diff.* spores. Therefore, the loss of important taxa that fulfil these functions might lead to an anatomical and functional imbalance that allows for the colonisation of this infectious agent [6].

The US Center for Disease Control and Prevention (CDC) considers the multidrug-resistant (MDR) bacteria *C. diff.* to be an urgent concern for the antimicrobial resistance (AMR) threat. In recent years, there has been a rise in the frequency of CDI infection intensity, recurrences, and fatality rates [7]. While other highly virulent epidemic types such as ribotype (RT) 078 have progressively been recognised as a source of disease acquired in the subjects and genomic evaluation claims to support a potential zoonotic transfer of RT 078 strains between humans and pigs. The epidemiological variations have also been largely attributed to the rise of new, highly virulent *C. diff.* strains, in specific belonging towards the Polymerase Chain Reaction (PCR) RT 027 [14]. During the COVID-19 pandemic, changes in routine patient care procedures, adherence to antibiotic stewardship programmes (ASPs), and usage of personal protective equipment (PPE) had an impact on hospital-associated infections (HAI), including CDI. Data from January 2019 to September 2021 that are currently available show a general decline in the frequency of hospital-acquired CDI (HA-CDI) during the COVID-19 crisis. Despite the growing use of broad-spectrum antibiotics, with about 70% of patients with COVID-19 receiving antibiotic therapy primarily for the suspected acquisition of secondary bacterial infections, the barrier precautions, focused attention on cleanliness, environmental cleaning, patient isolation, and the increased usage of PPE have undoubtedly played a significant role in preventing *C. diff.* propagation [15].

One of the main mechanisms of CDI is disturbance of the intestinal microbiota, and earlier investigations adopting different techniques have consistently found a decline in species richness. More information on the microbial makeup of human CDI is still needed, and it is uncommon to compare overt CDI with coloniser CDI, or low-toxin gene load to high-toxin gene load. Qualitative TcdB gene positivity by PCR method cannot differentiate between asymptomatic colonisation and symptomatic infection when it comes to the diagnosis of CDI. Although there are conflicting findings about the relationship between toxin load and disease outcome, numerous recent research has revealed that toxin gene load (low Ct) is a predictor of free toxin positive [16].

Antibiotic medications, primarily metronidazole, are the most successful initial therapy for CDI, supported by vancomycin, which is frequently given orally or intravenously. However, a significant proportion of patients (between 20% and 35%) experience recurring infections many days to weeks after beginning antibiotic treatment [14]. Prebiotics and probiotics are an alternate strategy for maintaining and re-establishing the gut microbiota following antibiotic treatments. Although several studies on the use of probiotics to treat CDI have produced inconsistent findings, probiotics such as bifidobacteria and lactobacilli appear to counteract the antibiotic-associated diarrhea and recurrent CDI [17]. Fecal microbiota transplantation (FMT) for recurring CDI has been examined in recent research. FMT, which re-establish colon homeostasis by restoring microorganisms from healthy donor stool, has been successful in treating patients with severe CDI who are resistant to conventional antibiotic treatment. FMT has a better than 90% rate of success in treating individuals with recurrent CDI, even though its exact mechanism of action is uncertain [4]. Following the successful transplant, the fecal microbiota demonstrated significant increase in Bacteroidetes and a reduction in Proteobacteria. FMT successfully replaces the complete colonic microbiota with a healthier one in order to restore the disrupted intestinal homeostasis, as opposed to probiotic therapy, which only introduces a small bacterial population into the digestive tract. The efficacy of FMT in treating *C. diff.* infection, as seen in the recent research, also raises the possibility of using this method to treat various gastrointestinal conditions [11]. Whether the heterologous fecal microbiota transplants may be utilised to prevent or manage metabolic dysregulation with etiologies that are considerably more complicated than chronic illness brought on by *Clostridium difficile* is still up for debate. Lack of knowledge regarding the significance of nutrition for stool graft colonisation and survival, ideal anaerobic managing of donor feces, immunological compatibility with both donor and recipient, and the function of bacteriophages and fungi for an effective faecal microbiota transplantation are among the challenges [18].

Numerous disorders, including diabetes, colon cancer, obesity, and atherosclerosis, are shown to be related in studies to the gut flora. As the role of the gastrointestinal microbiota in health and disease becomes clearer through research in upcoming years, it may be able to regulate this population in ways that enhance desired effects and reduce unintentional impacts [9]. Improvements in personal hygiene, donning and doffing procedures, environmental cleanliness, and stricter visiting limitations may have prevented the spread of *C. diff.* in health facilities, as well as within similar locations during the days of the pandemic [15]. In this challenging period of COVID-19, CDI and the correlation of gut microbiota remains in research, prevention, and control methods, and proper diagnosis and therapy needs to be practiced for CDI in the near future.

References

1 Jandhyala, S.M., Talukdar, R., Subramanyam, C. et al. (2015). Role of the normal gut microbiota. *W. J. Gastroenterol.* 21 (29): 8836–8847.

2 Thursby, E. and Juge, N. (2017). Introduction to the human gut microbiota. *Biochem J.* 474 (11): 1823–1836.

3 Feng, Q., Chen, W.D., and Wang, Y.D. (2018 February). Gut microbiota: an integral moderator in health and disease. *Front. Microbiol.* 9: 1–8.

4 Theriot, C.M. and Young, V.B. (2015). Interactions between the gastrointestinal microbiome and clostridium difficile. *Ann. Rev. Microbiol.* 69 (1): 445–461.

5 Finucane, M.M., Sharpton, T.J., Laurent, T.J. et al. (2014). A taxonomic signature of obesity in the microbiome? Getting to the guts of the matter. *PLoS One* 9 (1): 1–5.

6 Pérez-Cobas, A.E., Artacho, A., Ott, S.J. et al. (2014 July). Structural and functional changes in the gut microbiota associated to Clostridium difficile infection. *Front. Microbiol.* 5: 1–15.

7 Smits, W.K., Lyras, D., Lacy, D.B. et al. (2016). Clostridium difficile infection. *Nat. Rev. Dis. Prim.* 2: 1–20.

8 Leffler, D.A. and Lamont, J.T. (2015). Clostridium difficile infection. *N. Eng. J. Med.* 372 (16): 1539–1548.

9 Britton, R.A. and Young, V.B. (2014). Role of the intestinal microbiota in resistance to colonization by Clostridium difficile. *Gastroenterology* 146 (6): 1547–1553.

10 Shankar, V., Hamilton, M.J., Khoruts, A. et al. (2014). Species and genus level resolution analysis of gut microbiota in Clostridium difficile patients following fecal microbiota transplantation. *Microbiome* 2 (1): 1–10.

11 Rousseau, C., Levenez, F., Fouqueray, C. et al. (2011). Clostridium difficile colonization in early infancy is accompanied by changes in intestinal microbiota composition. *J. Clin. Microbiol.* 49 (3): 858–865.

12 Milani, C., Ticinesi, A., Gerritsen, J. et al. (2016 March). Gut microbiota composition and Clostridium difficile infection in hospitalized elderly individuals: A metagenomic study. *Sci. Rep.* 6: 1–12.

13 Samarkos, M., Mastrogianni, E., and Kampouropoulou, O. (2018 February). The role of gut microbiota in Clostridium difficile infection. *Eur. J. Intern. Med.* 50: 28–32.

14 Zhang, L., Dong, D., Jiang, C. et al. (2015). Insight into alteration of gut microbiota in Clostridium difficile infection and asymptomatic C. difficile colonization. *Anaerobe* 34: 1–7.

15 Spigaglia, P. (2022 January). Clostridioides difficile infection (CDI) during the COVID-19 pandemic. *Anaerobe* 74.

16 Han, S.H., Yi, J., Kim, J.H. et al. (2019). Composition of gut microbiota in patients with toxigenic Clostridioides (Clostridium) difficile: comparison between subgroups according to clinical criteria and toxin gene load. *PLoS One* 14 (2): 1–12.

17 Pérez-Cobas, A.E., Moya, A., Gosalbes, M.J. et al. (2015). Colonization resistance of the gut microbiota against clostridium difficile. *Antibiotics* 4 (3): 337–357.

18 Fan, Y. and Pedersen, O. (2021). Gut microbiota in human metabolic health and disease. *Nat. Rev. Microbiol.* 19 (1): 55–71.

8

Gut Microbiota and Obesity

Shaimaa H. Negm

Department of Home Economic, Specific Education Faculty, Port Said University, Egypt

8.1 Introduction

Obesity is increasingly regarded as a worldwide epidemic that affects both industrialised and developing countries [1, 2]. The body mass index (BMI) is computed by dividing a person's weight in kilogrammes by their height in metres squared [3], and is used is used to identify obesity. For adults, a BMI of 25.0 to 29.9 kg/m^2 is defined as overweight and a BMI of 30 kg/m^2 or higher is defined as obese.

8.2 Obesity Epidemic: Statistics and General Background

Obesity prevalence has increased 27.5% in adults and 47.1% in children in the previous three decades [4]. Obesity or overweight is expected to affect 81% of males and 74.9% of females in the United States by 2030 [5]. Obesity in children is a serious problem (BMI-for-age more than 95%) is a significant risk factor for adult obesity [6]. Obesity has a complicated aetiology [4], as can be seen in Table 8.1.

8.3 Gut Microbiota and Obesity

The makeup of the gut microbiome has been proven to boost dietary energy intake and thereby promote the obesity phenotype [4]. The human gastrointestinal tract allows the absorption of nutrients to meet metabolic needs. It harbors a complex microbial ecosystem including around 100 trillion (10^{14}) microorganisms that perform nutritional, metabolic, and protective functions. Accordingly, Gut microbiome (GM) contributes to modulating gut health [7], behavior [8], and immunity [9]. The human GM is mainly composed of bacteria belonging to the Firmicutes and Bacteroidetes phyla, the vast majority being strictly anaerobic [10]. Other subdominant phyla are *Actinobacteria*, *Proteobacteria*,

The Gut Microbiota in Health and Disease, First Edition. Edited by Nimmy Srivastava, Salam A. Ibrahim, Jayeeta Chattopadhyay, and Mohamed H. Arbab.
© 2023 John Wiley & Sons Ltd. Published 2023 by John Wiley & Sons Ltd.

Table 8.1 Primary and secondary disease-related causes of obesity.

Primary Causes of Obesity	Secondary Causes of Obesity
Genetic causes	Neurologic
Monogenic disorders	Brain injury, brain tumor
Melanocortin-4 receptor mutation	Consequences of cranial irradiation
Deficiency of leptin and leptin receptors	Hypothalamic obesity
Prohormoneconvertase deficiency	Endocrine
BDNF and TrkB insufficiency	Hypothyroidism[a]
SIM 1 insufficiency	Cushing syndrome
Proopiomelanocortin deficiency	Growth hormone deficiency
Syndromes	Pseudohypoparathyroidism
Prader–Willi	Psychological
Bardet–Biedl	Eating disorders, depression[b]
Cohen	Drug-induced
Alstrom	Tricyclic antidepressants, antipsychotics
Beckwith-Wiedemann	Oral contraceptives
Froehlich	Anticonvulsants
Carpenter	Glucocorticoids, Sulfonylureas, Glitazones, Beta-blockers

Note:
a) Controversial whether hypothyroidism causes obesity or exacerbates obesity.
b) Depression associated with overeating or binging [4].

Fusobacteria, and *Verrucomicrobia* [11]. Some bacterial taxa, including *Lactobacillus* spp., *Bifidobacterium* spp., and *Akkermansiamuciniphila*, or butyrate-producing bacteria such as *Faecalibacterium prausnitzii* are considered beneficial to health; while others such as the genera *Staphylococcus*, *Fusobacterium*, and *Pseudomonas* are considered as pathobionts that may create chemicals linked to diarrhea, infections, liver damage, and cancer [12, 13].

GM diversity is influenced by various factors such as diet, xenobiotic intake, host's genetic background, physical activity, and lifestyle [14]. GM is in balance with the host under healthy conditions, but this balance can be affected by obesity and other diseases (Figure 8.1a) [15]. In their first study, Ley et al. [16] reported an increased Firmicutes/Bacteroidetes ratio in obese (ob/ob) mice in addition to obese humans, compared with normal weight individuals. However, later investigations showed the presence of gut dysbiosis in obese people, despite conflicting findings about the Firmicutes/Bacteroidetes ratio, which is why this component is not currently recognised as a marker of obesity in humans [17]. Backhed et al. [18] showed that germ-free mice, despite consuming 30% more food than conventional animals of the same age and weight, had 42% less body fat. When normal weight, germ-free mice were conventionalised with the GM of obese mice they accumulated more body fat and added more weight than mice who were genetically modified to be normal weight (Figure 8.1b).

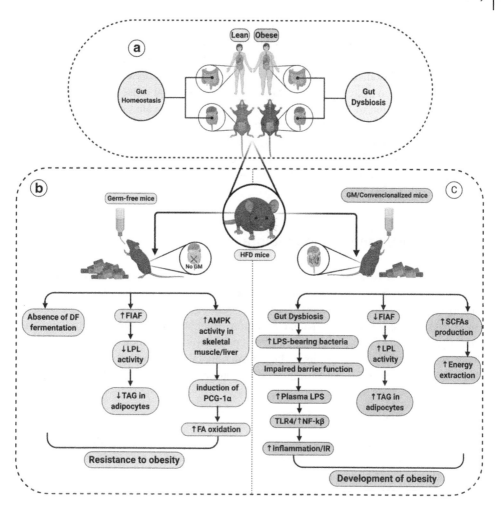

Figure 8.1 Obesity and dysbiosis of the gut microbiota. (a) Obesity has been linked to gut microbial dysbiosis in both humans and animal models. (b) Germ-free mice fed an HFD are less likely to acquire obesity because fibre fermentation is absent and FIAF levels are higher. In addition, these animals have increased AMPK activity in skeletal muscle and liver, as well as stimulation of PGC1-, resulting in a faster rate of oxidation of fatty acids in these organs. When germ-free mice are fed the gut microbiota of obese mice (fed a high-fat diet), they become obese. Obese mice have higher LPS levels in their blood, which triggers TLR4 and leads to the establishment characterised by a pro-inflammatory condition that promotes the appearance of insulin resistance. (c) Adenosine monophosphate-activated protein kinase (AMPK); fatty acids (FA); fasting-induced adipocyte factor (FIAF); lipoprotein lipase (LPL); lipopolysaccharide (LPS); Toll-like receptor 4 (TLR-4); nuclear factor kappa (NF-K); peroxisome proliferator-activated receptor gam (PGC1-). *Source:* Reproduced with permission from Duarte, L., et al. 2021 [22]/ Springer Nature.

On the other hand, according to reports, the activity of lipoprotein lipase (LPL), an enzyme involved in the adipocyte accumulation of triacylglycerides, increased in adipose tissue and cardiac tissue of conventionalised mice, resulting in larger size adipocytes, compared with germ-free animals [18]. This increased LPL activity may be explained by the GM-mediated inhibition of fasting-induced adipocyte factor (FIAF), a hormone constitutively expressed in the gastrointestinal tract mucosa of axenic mice that acts as a circulating LPL inhibitor [19]. Due to the absence of fibre fermentation and higher FIAF levels, germ-free mice fed a high-fat diet HFD are resistant to the progress of obesity (Figure 8.1b,c) [20]. Other factors explaining the resistance of these animals to obesity is the increase in Adenosine mono-phosphate-activated protein kinase (AMPK) activity in skeletal muscle and liver, together with the introduction of PGC1-α (peroxisome proliferator-activated receptor gam), which generates a higher rate of oxidation of fatty acids in these tissues. Cani et al. [21] demon-strated that the administration of HFD to mice for four weeks alters their GM, increasing LPS-bearing gram-negative bacteria at the expense of gram-positive bacteria, and affects their intestinal barrier function by inhibiting the expression of tight junction proteins in the intestinal epithelium.

8.4   Adiposity and Gut Microbiota

One of the key activities of the gut microbiota is the enzymatic conversion of primary bile acids into secondary bile acids, which has a direct impact on the emulsification and absorption properties of bile acids [23, 24]. Throughout this process, the gut microbiota has an impact on bile acid enterohepatic circulation. Their seondary form binds to G-proteins and stimulates the release of glucagon-like peptide 1 (GLP1), which decreases blood and liver triglyceride levels. Variations in the gut microbiota, both qualitative and quantitative, may affect this pathway by encouraging fat formation in the body [23, 24].

8.4.1   Short Chain Fatty Acids (SCFAs)

Saccharolytic microorganisms in the caecum and colon are required for the digestion and fermentation of dietary polysaccharides into SCFAs. Different types of bacteria produce three different SCFAs: butyric acid is a source for colonic epithelial cells and a suppressor of appetite through central hypothalamic mechanisms; propionic acid is a precursor for protein synthesis, gluconeogenesis, and liponeogenesis in the liver, an inhibitor of fatty acid production, and a low-grade inflammation-reducing agent in the gut; and butyric acid is a source for colonic epithelial cells and a suppressor of appetite through central hypothala [25].

SCFAs created during fermentation could serve as both an energy source and a metabolic regulator. Furthermore, investigations in G-protein-coupled receptors GPR41-knockout mice revealed that SCFAs activate GPR41, causing the release of peptide YY (PYY), an anorexigenic peptide. Additionally, some research on GPR43-deficient animals has dem-onstrated that metabolic abnormalities, such as increased fat buildup may occur, when antibiotics are used, the condition can be reversed. One study found that GPR43-deficient mice had a lower body mass and a higher lean mass than wild-type mice fed a high-carbo-hydrate/high-fat diet [25–28].

The microbiota may alter peripheral adipose tissue storage, and thus host adiposity, adenosine monophosphate kinase inhibition (AMPc) in the liver and muscles, and influence fatty acid oxidation, resulting in increased energy storage in these tissues. Furthermore, inhib-iting the microbiota that produces fasting-induced adipocyte factor (FIAF, or angiopoietin-like protein 4 ANGPTL4) may result in an increase in lipoprotein lipase (LPL) levels, boosting the storage of circulating triglycerides in adipocytes [23, 24]. Obese phenotype is associated with different SCFA profiles than the nonobese phenotype, and the gut microbiota may directly or indirectly affect processes related to obesity. However, there is an internal paradox in the fat model: the excess of substrates does not, as expected, result in a rise in anorexic hormonal response. This dichotomy could point to the presence of additional bacteria or bacterial components/metabolites that could activate regulatory pathways [24, 26, 27, 29].

8.4.2   AMPK and FIAF

The gut microbiota may impair hepatic fatty acid oxidation by lowering adenosine monophosphate kinase (AMPK) and fasting-induced adipose factor (FIAF), a circulating lipoprotein lipase inhibitor, resulting in increased fat accumulation [30]. Bacterial suppression of FIAF and AMPK expression in the liver and skeletal muscle causes weight gain from a carbohydrate and fat-rich diet [31].

The colon, liver, and adipose tissue all create FIAF. LPL's activity, which facilitates cellular absorption of triglycerides and triglyceride buildup in adipocytes, is increased when FIAF is inhibited. The bacteria that have been shown to be the most frequently in the digestive tracts of conventionalised mice were *Bacteroides* and *Clostridium*. *B. thetaiotaomicron* colonisation changed the expression of lipid-related host genes breakdown and absorption, as well as polysaccharide metabolism in germ-free mice [32].

Backhed et al. [33] found that mice fed a high-fat diet supplemented with *Lactobacillus paracasei* had lower body fat and higher FIAF activity. In addition, germ-free mice have more phosphorylated AMPK in their muscle and liver, which protects them from diet-induced obesity. AMPK enhances fatty acid oxidation in peripheral tissues by activating mitochondrial fatty acid oxidation enzymes such as acetyl-CoA carboxylase and carnitine-palmitoyltransferase I. There was a decrease in AMPK and adiponectin activity, as well as a decrease in fatty acid oxidation and an increase in the input of free fatty acids into the liver, in both normal and obese mice [34].

8.4.3   Bile Acids

Bile acids are metabolised by the gut microbiota into primary and secondary bile acids, which bind to the FXR receptor and promote the release of gut-derived hormones such as fibroblast growth factor FGF-19. Bile acids and the gut bacteria contribute to host metabolism via this route within FXR signalling. FGF-19, in turn, regulates the synthesis of bile acids as well as lipid and glucose metabolism. Increased bile acid synthesis stimulates brown adipose tissue and skeletal muscle via TGR5, a membrane-bound G protein-coupled bile acid receptor, and activates type 2 deiodinase, resulting in increased energy expenditure in the host [35].

8.4.4   Lipopolysaccharides (LPS)

The absorption and transport of dietary triglycerides is aided by lipoproteins,which may cause an inflammatory response and lead to insulin resistance in obese people. In healthy people LPS concentrations are low, but in obese people they can reach dangerously high levels, resulting in metabolic endotoxemia [36].

By causing systemic inflammation, gut bacteria may play a role in metabolic issues in obese patients. Gramnegative microbes in the gut microbiota produce LPSs, which bind to immunological transmembrane proteins called toll-like receptors (TLRs), notably TLR4. If inflammatory cytokines and chemokines are upregulated, and intracellular signalling pathways are activated, they have the potential to change the structure, magnitude, and duration of inflammatory responses [30]. Proinflammatory cytokines such as interleukin 6 (IL-6) and tumour necrosis factor α (TNF-α) are released into the body when LPS binds to the TLR4 receptor [37].

Changes in the gut microbiota may have a role in the pathogenesis of obesity and the development of obesity-related metabolic illnesses such as type 2 diabetes, NAFLD, metabolic syndrome, and cardiovascular disease according to current data. Obesity treatments such as calorie-restricted diets and/or bariatric surgery affect the gut microbiota in ways that have been associated to health benefits, reinforcing the idea that changing gut microbiota composition could provide another route to long-term weight loss [38].

8.5 Gut Microbiota Modification

Changes in the gut microbiota's makeup can be triggered by a variety of factors; diet, age, antibiotic use, and environmental influences are the most important [39].

8.5.1 Diet

Depending on foods eaten, the gut flora changes significantly. The gut microbiota has been demonstrated to change statistically significantly when people eat a diet with various levels of carbs, fat, and fibre [39, 40]. Furthermore, the microbiota composition varies by culture, which may be related to dietary variances [40].

8.5.2 Age

Age-related changes in the gastrointestinal environment, as well as decreased immune system reactivity and increased drug usage, will affect the composition of the gut microbiota [40].

8.5.3 Antibiotics

Antibiotic use causes the eradication of symbiotic microflora as well as pathogenic microorganisms, potentially resulting in a major microbiota imbalance [41]. Because of their direct toxicity to the gastrointestinal epithelium and the growth of antibiotic-resistant bacteria, antibiotics alter the composition of the gut microbiota [42].

8.5.4 Probiotics

Gut flora may be affected by dietary supplements containing probiotics and prebiotics [40]. The World Health Organisation defines probiotics as 'live bacteria that, when consumed in adequate amounts, exert a health effect on the host' [43]. The most widely used bacterial genera are *Lactobacillus* and *Bifidobacterium*. Probiotics may have a favourable effect on a host's intestines [44].

8.6 The Microbiota and Obesity Interactions

Obesity has been linked to specific bacterial species, according to research. These microbes promote a variety of molecular pathways that all contribute to fat maintenance [45].

8.6.1 Immune System

Increased intestinal permeability is caused by an excess of specific gram-negative bacteria interacting with the protein structure of endothelial 'tight junctions' in obese patients. In addition, intestinal dysbiosis enhances the absorption of LPS (bacterial endotoxin) via the CD14 receptor. Plasma LPS functions as a trigger for immunological cascades, causing pro-inflammatory cytokines to be produced. As a result, obesity maintenance is linked to a pro-inflammatory phenotype [38].

8.6.2 Lipid Metabolism

Bacteria in the gut microbiome create bile salt hydrolase enzymes, which allow non-conjugated and secondary bile acids to be formed. The TGR5 G protein-coupled receptor may bind to these bile acids, lowering pro-inflammatory phenotype and lipopro-tein absorption. Furthermore, because bacterial cells assimilate cholesterol and assemble it into bacterial walls, lipid metabolism interacts with the gut microbiome. Both of these patterns are critical in preventing the development of atherosclerosis, and they may be affected by changes in microbiota composition in obese patients [45]. By stimulating endothelial CB1 receptors, an unbalanced microbiota affects the integrity of the intestinal epithelium and increases metabolic endotoxemia by increasing the activity of the gut endo-cannabinoid system. By promoting the synthesis of activin A, this method promotes the proliferation of adipose precursor cells and adipocyte hyperplasia [45].

8.6.3 Satiety Hormones

Enteroendocrine cells are stimulated to create satiety hormones by chemicals excreted in the gut microbiome. This method is most likely linked to commensal bacteria's release of propionate. The microbiota makeup of obese patients has a tendency to boost ghrelin pro-duction, and this is linked to a greater food consumption. Obese adults, on the other hand, were found to have lower amounts of GLP-1 and PYY. Intestinal L cells emit GLP-1 and PYY, which influence satiety and may regulate food intake [45].

8.6.4 Nutrient Metabolism

The most essential mechanism involving gut bacteria in food metabolism is what is known as short chain fatty acids (SCFAs). Bacteria in the intestines releases enzymes that help in glucose metabolism. They convert dietary fibres into SCFAs, a type of energy that can be stored as lipids or glucose [38].

8.6.5 Lymphoid Structures

The gut-associated lymphoid tissue (GALT) is made up of Peyer's patches, isolated lymphoid follicles, and crypt plaques.The gut microbiota interacts with GALT formation because pattern recognition receptors, nucleotide-binding oligomerisation domain-containing protein 1, and toll-like receptors recognise the bacterial peptidoglycan.When these receptors are activated, the expression of Camu-Camu (CC) chemokine ligand 20 and defensin 3 ligand increases, and this results in the creation of new lymphoid follicles that are isolated. A pathogenic inflammatory response in the gastrointestinal tract may emerge if this mechanism is disrupted due to an imbalance in the gut flora [45].

8.6.6 Microbiota–Adipose Tissue Axis

Gut microbiota metabolites drive adipogenesis by causing LPS-induced inflammation and SCFA-induced adipocyte differentiation [46]. LPS, which is found in gram-negative bacteria cell membranes, functions as a trigger, creating low-grade chronic inflammation and insulin resistance. Inflammation in the intestinal mucosa causes both the breakdown of intestinal barrier integrity and the increased transfer of LPS into the blood by chylomicrons [47].

Increased SCFA production by gut bacteria offers more calories to the host, causing weight gain. They can bind to GPR41 (also known as FFAR3), causing the enteroendocrine hormone peptide YY (PYY) to be produced in gut epithelial L-cells, decreasing gut motility and enhancing energy harvest in mice. Furthermore, in mice35, binding of SCFAs to GPR41 or GPR43 (FFAR2) causes intestinal L-cells to generate the hormone glucagon-like peptide (GLP-1), which has a major impact on pancreatic function and insulin release, as well as cerebral effects regulating hunger. When the feces of overweight people and thin people were compared, overweight people's feces included higher SCFAs [48].

The microbiota affect lipoprotein lipase function via changing the expression of FIAF, a lipoprotein lipase inhibitor that causes triglyceride (TG) buildup in adipocytes. Hypertrophy is caused by an increase in TG, which leads to chronic inflammation, prevents additional TG deposition, and promotes ectopic TG accumulation in other organs, resulting in insulin resistance [49].

References

1 Tokarek, J., Gadzinowska, J., Młynarska, E. et al. (2022). What is the role of gut microbiota in obesity prevalence? A few words about gut microbiota and its association with obesity and related diseases. *Microorganisms* 10: 52.

2 Kwaifa, I.K., Bahari, H., Yong, Y.K. et al. (2020). Endothelial dysfunction in obesity induced inflammation: molecular mechanisms and clinical implications. *Biomolecules* 10: 291.

3 Binkley, J.K., Eales, J., and Jekanowski, M. (2000). The relation between dietary change and rising US obesity. *Int. J. Obes.* 24: 1032–1039.

4 Apovian, C.M. (2016). Obesity: definition, comorbidities, causes, and burden. *Am. J. Manag. Care* 22: S176–S185.

5 Wang, Y., Beydoun, M.A., Min, J. et al. (2020). Has the prevalence of overweight, obesity and central obesity levelled off in the United States? Trends, patterns, disparities, and future projections for the obesity epidemic. *Int. J. Epidemiol.* 49: 810–823.

6 Maffeis, C. and Tatò, L. (2001). Long-term effects of childhood obesity on morbidity and mortality. *Horm. Res. Paediatr.* 55 (Suppl. S1): 42–45.

7 Clemente, J.C., Ursell, L.K., Parfrey, L.W. et al. (2012). The impact of the gut microbiota on human health: an integrative view. *Cell* 148 (6): 1258–1270.

8 Dinan, T.G. and Cryan, J.F. (2017). Microbes, immunity, and behavior: psychoneuroimmunology meets the microbiome. *Neuropsychopharmacology* 42 (1): 178–192.

9 Hill, D.A. and Artis, D. (2010). Intestinal bacteria and the regulation of immune cell homeostasis. *Annu. Rev. Immunol.* 28: 623–67.

10 Ringel-Kulka, T., Cheng, J, Ringel, Y. et al. (2013). Intestinal microbiota in healthy U.S. young children and adults–a high throughput microarray analysis. *PLoS One* 8 (5): e64315.

11 Eckburg, P.B., Bik, E.M., Bernstein, C.N. et al. (2005). Diversity of the human intestinal microbial flora. *Science* 308 (5728): 1635–8.

12 Gibson, G.R. and Roberfroid, M.B. (1995). Dietary modulation of the human colonic microbiota: introducing the concept of prebiotics. *J. Nutr.* 125 (6): 1401–1412.

13 Kim, E., Coelho, D., and Blachier, F. (2013). Review of the association between meat consumption and risk of colorectal cancer. *Nutr. Res.* 33 (12): 983–994.

14 Fujio-Vejar, S., Vasquez, Y., Morales, P. et al. (2017). The gut microbiota of healthy Chilean subjects reveals a high abundance of the phylum Verrucomicrobia. *Front. Microbiol.* 8: 1221.

15 Harakeh, S.M., Khan, I., Kumosani, T. et al. (2016). Gut microbiota: a contributing factor to obesity. *Front. Cell Infect. Microbiol.* 6: 95.

16 Ley, R.E., Backhed, F., Turnbaugh, P. et al. (2005). Obesity alters gut microbial ecology. *Proc. Natl. Acad. Sci. USA* 102 (31): 11070–11075.

17 Magne, F., Gotteland, M., Gauthier, L. et al. (2020). The Firmicutes/Bacteroidetes ratio: a relevant marker of gut dysbiosis in obese patients? *Nutrients* 12 (5).

18 Backhed, F., Ding, H., Wang, T. et al. (2004). The gut microbiota as an environmental factor that regulates fat storage. *Proc. Natl. Acad. Sci. USA* 101 (44): 15718–15723.

19 Mandard, S., Zandbergen, F., van Straten, E. et al. (2006). The fasting-induced adipose factor/angiopoietinlike protein 4 is physically associated with lipoproteins and governs plasma lipid levels and adiposity. *J. Biol. Chem.* 281 (2): 934–944.

20 Backhed, F., Manchester, J.K., Semenkovich, C.F. et al. (2007). Mechanisms underlying the resistance to diet-induced obesity in germ-free mice. *Proc. Natl. Acad. Sci. USA* 104 (3): 979–984.

21 Cani, P.D., Bibiloni, R., Knauf, C. et al. (2008). Changes in gut microbiota control metabolic endotoxemia-induced inflammation in high-fat diet-induced obesity and diabetes in mice. *Diabetes* 57 (6): 1470–1481.

22 Duarte, L., Gasaly, N., Poblete-Aro, C. et al. (2021). Polyphenols and their anti-obesity role mediated by the gut microbiota: a comprehensive review. *Rev. Endocr. Metab. Disord.* 22: 367–388.

23 Musso, G., Gambino, R., and Cassader, M. (2010). Obesity, diabetes, and gut microbiota: the hygiene hypothesis expanded? *Diab. Care* 33: 2277–2284.

24 Khan, M.J., Gerasimidis, K., Edwards, C.A. et al. (2016). Role of gut microbiota in the aetiology of obesity: proposed mechanisms and review of the literature. *J. Obes.* 2016: 7353642.

25 Bjursell, M., Admyre, T., Göransson, M. et al. (2011). Improved glucose control and reduced body fat mass in free fatty acid receptor 2-deficient mice fed a high-fat diet. *Am. J. Physiol. Endocrinol. Metab.* 300: 211–220.

26 Murugesan, S., Nirmalkar, K., Hoyo-Vadillo, C. et al. (2018). Gut microbiome production of short-chain fatty acids and obesity in children. *Eur. J. Clin. Microbiol. Infect. Dis.* 37: 621–625.

27 Koh, A., De Vadder, F., Kovatcheva-Datchary, P. et al. (2016). From dietary fiber to host physiology: short-chain fatty acids as key bacterial metabolites. *Cell* 165: 1332–1345.

28 Samuel, B.S., Shaito, A., Motoike, T. et al. (2008). Effects of the gut microbiota on host adiposity are modulated by the short-chain fatty-acid binding G protein-coupled receptor, GPR41. *Proc. Natl. Acad. Sci. USA* 105: 16767–16772.

29 Payne, A.N., Chassard, C., Zimmermann, M. et al. (2011). The metabolic activity of gut microbiota in obese children is increased compared with normal-weight children and exhibits more exhaustive substrate utilization. *Nutr. Diab.* 1: e12.

30 Cerdó, T., García-Santos, J.A., Bermúdez, M.G. et al. (2019). The role of probiotics and prebiotics in the prevention and treatment of obesity. *Nutrients* 11: 635.

31 John, G.K. and Mullin, G.E. (2016). The gut microbiome and obesity. *Curr. Oncol. Rep.* 18: 45.

32 Cardinelli, C.S., Sala, P.C., Alves, C.C. et al. (2015). Influence of intestinal microbiota on body weight gain: a narrative review of the literature. *Obes. Surg.* 25: 346–353.

33 Bäckhed, F., Ding, H., Wang, T. et al. (2004). The gut microbiota as an environmental factor that regulates fat storage. *Proc. Natl. Acad. Sci. USA* 101: 15718–15723.

34 Kobyliak, N., Virchenko, O., and Falalyeyeva, T. (2016). Pathophysiological role of host microbiota in the development of obesity. *Nutr. J.* 15: 43.

35 Lee, C.J., Sears, C.L., and Maruthur, N. (2020). Gut microbiome and its role in obesity and insulin resistance. *Ann. N.Y. Acad. Sci.* 1461: 37–52.

36 Gomes, A.C., Hoffmann, C., and Mota, J.F. (2018). The human gut microbiota: metabolism and perspective in obesity. *Gut Microb.* 9: 308–325.

37 da Silva, S.T., Santos, C.A.D., and Bressan, J. (2013). Intestinal microbiota; relevance to obesity and modulation by prebiotics and probiotics. *Nutr. Hosp.* 28: 1039–1048.

38 Muscogiuri, G., Cantone, E., Cassarano, S. et al. (2019). Gut microbiota: a new path to treat obesity. *Int. J. Obes. Suppl.* 9: 10–19.

39 Schoeler, M. and Caesar, R. (2019). Dietary lipids, gut microbiota and lipid metabolism. *Rev. Endocr. Metab. Disord.* 20: 461–472.

40 Lozupone, C.A., Stombaugh, J.I., Gordon, J.I. et al. (2012). Diversity, stability and resilience of the human gutmicrobiota. *Nature* 489: 220–230.

41 Li, X., Liu, L., Cao, Z. et al. (2020). Gut microbiota as an "invisible organ" that modulates the function of drugs. *Biomed. Pharm.* 121: 109653.

42 Ianiro, G., Tilg, H., and Gasbarrini, A. (2016). Antibiotics as deep modulators of gut microbiota: between good and evil. *Gut* 65: 1906–1915.

43 Food and Agriculture Organization of the United Nations; World Health Organization. (2006). *Probiotics in Food: Health and NutritionalProperties and Guidelines for Evaluation.*

Rome, Italy: Food and Agriculture Organization of the United Nations; Geneva, Switzerland: World Health Organization.

44 Butel, M.-J. (2014). Probiotics, gut microbiota and health. *Med. Mal. Infect.* 44: 1–8.

45 Gomes, A.C., Hoffmann, C., and Mota, J.F. (2018). The human gut microbiota: metabolism and perspective in obesity. *Gut Microb.* 9: 308–325.

46 Sivamaruthi, B.S., Kesika, P., Suganthy, N. et al. (2019). A review on role of microbiome in obesity and antiobesity properties of probiotic supplements. *Bio. Med. Res. Int.* 2019: 3291367.

47 Park, S.-E., Kwon, S.J., Cho, K.-M. et al. (2020). Intervention with kimchimicrobial community ameliorates obesity by regulating gut microbiota. *J. Microbiol.* 58: 859–867.

48 Sun, L., Ma, L., Ma, Y. et al. (2018). Insights into the role of gut microbiota in obesity: pathogenesis, mechanisms,and therapeutic perspectives. *Prot. Cell* 9: 397–403.

49 Schroeder, B. and Bäckhed, F. (2016). Signals from the gut microbiota to distant organs in physiology and disease. *Nat. Med.* 22: 1079–1089.

9

Gut Microbiota and Cardiovascular Disease

Shaimaa H. Negm

Department of Home Economic, Specific Education Faculty, Port Said University, Egypt

9.1 Introduction

Cardiovascular disease (CVD) is a chronic, progressive disease that causes permanent vascular damage in the form of atherosclerosis, as well as negative clinical outcomes such as arterial thrombosis, myocardial infarction (MI), and stroke. Hypercholesterolemia, or high levels of serum cholesterol, especially low-density lipoprotein cholesterol (LDL-C), is a well-known risk factor for CVD. LDL-C causes plaque build-up in artery walls, which can lead to atherosclerosis [1, 2], which is estimated to cause 12 million coronary deaths per year by 2030. [3].

The World Health Organisation (WHO) estimates that over 75% of premature CVD is preventable, and that improving risk factors may help reduce the rising incidence of CVD [4]. Several studies have linked gut microbiota and metabolites to CVD such risk factors as hyperlipidemia, obesity, inflammation, hypertension, and platelet hyperactivity [5, 6], showing the complex interaction between food, gut microbiota, and CVD [7, 8].

The human microbiota is made up of trillions of different bacteria that live in the human body, and the gut has the largest microbe population, with 100 trillion germs from at least 1000 different bacterial species. There is enough evidence to suggest that the gut microbiome influences a variety of physiological activities, including the immune system, cardiovascular system, intestinal function, nutritional absorption, and metabolism. Atherosclerosis, hypertension, platelet hyperactivity, aberrant lipid metabolism, and vascular dysfunction have all been linked to gut dysbiosis in investigations [9]. Important CVD risk factors such as atherosclerosis, hypertension, and platelet hyperactivity are all linked to gut dysbiosis [10].

Targeting the gut microbiota and their metabolites may be a beneficial strategy in the treatment and prevention of CVD, according to new findings [10–12]. Various gut microbiota species create a variety of metabolites that affect human health, depending on the diet and microbiome composition. Short-chain fatty acids (SCFAs), secondary metabolites of bile acid, and trimethyl-N-oxide (TMAO) are significant modulatory factors for a variety of

The Gut Microbiota in Health and Disease, First Edition. Edited by Nimmy Srivastava, Salam A. Ibrahim, Jayeeta Chattopadhyay, and Mohamed H. Arbab.

disorders produced by the gut microbiota. Platelet hyperactivity, aberrant plasma lipids, obesity, and insulin resistance are all linked to high levels of TMAO in the blood [5, 9].

9.2 Gut Microbiota and CVD

Many metabolites in the human body are produced by gut microorganisms, and there is mounting evidence that these metabolites are linked to the development of CVD. The gut microbiota influences host metabolic pathways such as cholesterol metabolism, as well as inflammatory reactions and oxidative stress, through these metabolites. Gut microbe-dependent metabolites may enter the circulation via the intestinal epithelium, influencing the function of various organs and physiological systems [13, 17, 18].

9.2.1 Role of TMAO in Coronary Heart Disease

The gut microbiota's generation of metabolic TMAO is a major mechanism in cardiovascular disease. Cholesterol and sterol metabolism, cholesterol transport, and bile acid levels have all been found to be affected by TMAO [14–16, 19]. TMAO levels in the blood are linked to early atherosclerosis, the severity of peripheral arterial disease, and a high risk of CVD death [20, 21] .Increased plasma levels of TMAO were linked to an increased risk of death, MI, and stroke over the course of a three year trial of 4007 individuals receiving elective coronary angiography [16].

TMAO supplementation inhibited the expression of Cyp7a1, the major bile acid synthase enzyme and rate-limiting step in cholesterol catabolism, resulting in a substantial reduction in cholesterol transport. The gut metabolites choline, TMAO, and betaine were found to have correlations with coronary artery disease (CAD), peripheral vascular disease, and MI in research by Wang et al. [15] A TMAO-enriched diet increased the size of atherosclerotic lesions in atherosclerosis-prone mice (C57BL/6J Apoe/-), but gut microbiota suppression reduced dietary-choline-enhanced atherosclerosis in atherosclerosis-prone mice.

A recent mouse investigation shows that both good and bad diets may raise plasma levels of TMAO, with the gut being a major location for oxidative TMAO formation [22]. This study is significant because it reconciles some inconsistent results on TMAO by revealing that while there is no direct link between plasma TMAO and atherosclerosis severity, there is a definite link between TMAO levels and atherosclerotic plaque instability [23]. This shows that TMAO is a cardiovascular risk indicator.

In animal experiments, a high-choline diet resulted in elevated TMAO levels and atherosclerosis. The available data indicate modulation of the gut microbial TMAO generating a pathway that attenuates atherosclerosis and platelet hyperactivity and in vivo thrombosis potential in animal models; however, the effective treatment modality has yet to be established. Lowering TMAO levels may be as simple as changing one's lifestyle, which includes exercise, diet, functional foods, and modifying one's microbiota [24].

The inflammatory reactions of the vascular wall are exacerbated by TMAO, which causes the generation of reactive oxygen species (ROS) and hinders cholesterol reverse transport [25]. The effects of TMAO on cholesterol and sterol metabolism have been linked to the development of atherosclerosis [26]. Despite increasing macrophage reverse cholesterol transfer, flavin monooxygenase (FMO3) knockout mice showed lower circulating TMAO levels and decreased atherosclerotic plaque formation [27]. TMAO-produced l-carnitine and -butyro-betaine, as well as gut microbial dietary phosphatidylcholine metabolites, were linked to CVD risk [28].

SCFAs bind to G protein-coupled receptors, with the free fatty acid receptors FFAR2 and FFAR3 being the most well-studied [29]. By limiting the action of liver adipose synthetase, SCFAs regulate cholesterol distribution in the liver and circulation. Reduced SCFA synthesis has been linked to dyslipidaemia because SCFAs have a function in lowering serum cholesterol levels. In patients with atherosclerotic vascular disease or hypertension, SFCA concentrations have also been found to be decreased [30].

Increased BA production and the presence of extra BAs in the gut are caused by a high saturated fat consumption. Primary BAs, such as deoxycholic acid (DCA), are transformed to hydrophobic secondary Bas [31, 32]. Bile acid secretion irregularities have been linked to the development of atherosclerosis and other cardiometabolic diseases [31, 33]; they may produce blood lipid abnormalities and have been linked to the development of atherosclerosis and other cardiometabolic diseases.

Endotoxemia has been linked to the development of a number of diseases, including atherosclerosis, obesity, and insulin resistance [34]; in particular, it has been linked to an increased risk of developing atherosclerosis in smokers and people with infectious diseases [35].

The gut lumen is responsible for external intake via cholesterol absorption and plays an important role in controlling the body's cholesterol equilibrium [36]. The primary sources of luminal cholesterol are our diet, bile via the hepatobiliary pathway [37], and de novo cholesterol via the transintestinal cholesterol efflux (TICE) pathway [38, 39] (see Figure 9.1a).

Cholesterol is converted into bile acid in the liver and released into bile through the hepatobiliary pathway, where the ATP-binding cassette transporter G5/ABCG5/G8 (ABCG5/G8) plays a major role in cholesterol efflux from hepatocytes into bile [40]. TICE is an alternative to the hepatobiliary pathway, in which cholesterol from the blood enters enterocytes directly via LDL receptors (LDL-R) and is effluxed into the lumen by ABCG5/G8 and the ATP binding cassette transporter B1 (ABCB1a/b) [41]. The cholesterol in the lumen is either absorbed into enterocytes via Niemann-Pick C1-like 1 (NPC1L1) and incorporated into chylomicrons for entry into the circulatory system [36], or it is reduced by the gut microbiota to poorly absorbable coprostanol (5BCholestan-3B-ol) [40, 41], which is mostly excreted.

9.3 Gut Microbiota Composition in Cardiovascular Disease

The gut microbiota has been linked to the development of obesity, a major risk factor for cardiovascular disease. The gut microbiome was first proposed by Bäckhed et al. as an essential environmental component that influences predisposition to energy storage and fat mass growth [42]. The gut bacteria can potentially play a role in lipid dysregulation. GF mice have lower plasma triglyceride and LDL-C levels than control mice, according to Martinez Guryn et al. [43]. According to Karlsson et al., there is a positive link between

(a)

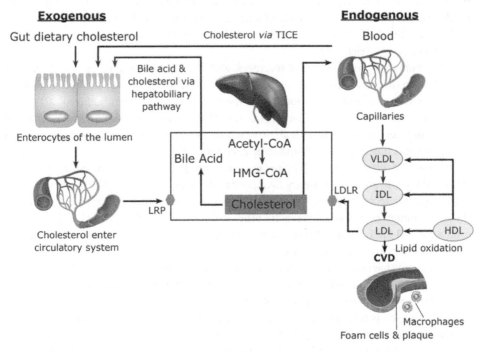

(b)

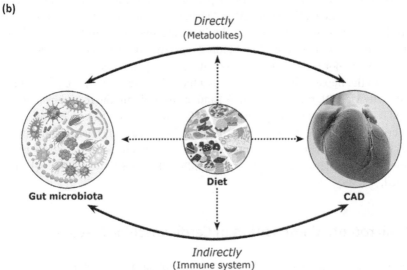

Figure 9.1 Cholesterol, gut microbiota, and CAD. (a) Exogenous and endogenous sources of luminal cholesterol. (b) The multifaceted mechanisms involved in CAD development. The gut microbiota may directly (via metabolites) and indirectly (via the immune system) lead to CAD. *Source*: Negin Kazemian et al. (2020) / Springer Nature / CC BY 4.0.

HDL-C and Clostridium species, but a negative correlation between serum triglycerides and Clostridium species [44]. Rebolledo et al. reviewed the variations in gut microbial makeup between hypercholesterolemics and healthy people [45], and the richness and diversity of bacterial communities in hypercholesterolemic patients were lower than in controls. Fu et al. looked at the gut microbiota composition in 893 people from the Life Lines DEEP population cohort [46]. BMI and blood lipids were linked to 34 different bacterial taxa. Eggerthella was linked to higher triglycerides and lower HDL-C, while the Pasteurellaceae family was linked to lower triglycerides.

The microbiome had no influence on LDL-C or total cholesterol (TC), according to the scientists. A study published in 2021 found that Lachnospiraceae genera are inversely associated with lipid CVD risk variables such as body fat, LDL-C, and TC [42]. When compared to a high-fat diet (HFD) alone, Liang et al. found that a high-fat and high-cholesterol diet (HFHCD) dramatically reduced the alpha diversity of the gut microbiota in mice [47]. In addition, as compared to HFD mice, HFHCD animals had lower levels of Oscillospira, Odoribacter, Bacteroides, and Prevotella, but higher levels of Ruminococcus and Akkermansia. Zhang et al. found that mice given an HFHCD exhibited higher levels of Mucispirillum, Desulfovibrio, Anaerotruncus, and Desulfovibrionaceae, but lower levels of Bacteroides and Bifidobacterium [48], and this observation was confirmed in patients with hypercholesterolemia.

In CAD patients, Emoto et al. found a drop in the *phylum Bacteroidetes* and an increase in the order *Lactobacillales* when compared to controls [49]. Symptomatic and asymptomatic atherosclerotic plaques have different microbial compositions, according to Mitra et al. [50], *Porphyromonadaceae, Bacteroidaceae, Micrococcaceaea*, and *Streptococcacaea* were found in greater number in asymptomatic atherosclerotic plaques [51]. In a recent study by Zhu et al., lower variety and richness were seen in patients with coronary artery disease [52]. In CAD patients, *Escherichia coli, Subdoligranulum, Roseburia*, and *Eubacteriumrectale* were highly enriched, while *Faecalibacterium, Subdoligranulum, Roseburia*, and *Eubacteriumrectale* were significantly reduced. In fecal samples from patients with atherosclerotic CVD, Jie et al. found that relative abundances of *Escherichia coli, Enterobacteraerogenes, Klebsiella*, and *Streptococcus* were higher than in healthy controls [53]. *Streptococcus, Lactobacillus salivarius, Solobacteriummoorei*, and *Atopobiumparvulum* bacteria commonly found in the mouth, were also shown to be more abundant in atherosclerotic patients than in healthy controls. Periodontal disease has been linked to atherosclerosis, implying that oral bacteria may play a role in atherosclerosis development [54].

9.4 Gut Microbiota Function in Cardiovascular Disease

Many metabolites in the human body are produced by intestinal microorganisms, and there is mounting evidence that these metabolites are linked to the development of CVD [13]. High-fat diet (HFD)-induced changes in 19 metabolites in the liver and 43 metabolites in the fecal contents of mice were identified as possible biomarkers for obesity in a study published in 2021 [55]. The HFD was linked to higher lipid profiles and total bile acid levels.

9.5 Gut Microbiota as Therapeutic Strategies for Cardiovascular Disease

9.5.1 Probiotics

The FAO/WHO defines probiotics as 'live microorganisms that impart a health benefit on the host when administered in suitable levels' [56]. Probiotic supplementation has been shown to have positive health effects, and it could be used as a possible CVD therapeutic strategy, according to a growing body of research. The use of probiotic microorganisms as a therapy to enhance lipid profiles has been investigated. By deconjugating bile acids (BAs) and boosting their excretion, probiotic bacteria with bile salt hydrolase activity may lower serum cholesterol levels [57]. This raises the necessity for de novo bile synthesis, which results in greater cholesterol conversion to BAs in the liver, lowering serum cholesterol levels. SCFAs have been demonstrated to inhibit hepatic cholesterol production and modulate cholesterol metabolism [58]. Other possible mechanisms of action include probiotic-driven cholesterol assimilation and increased cholesterol binding to probiotic cell walls in the small intestine, resulting in less cholesterol being absorbed by the body [59]. In a 2021 investigation, *L. plantarum* K50 supplementation lowered blood triglyceride levels and raised HDL-C levels in HFD-induced obese mice [60].

Probiotic treatment resulted in a considerable reduction of serum triglycerides by 20% and a 25% increase in apolipoprotein A-V (apo A-V). Total cholesterol (TC), LDL-C, and electronegative LDL concentrations were all improved when the probiotic soy product with isoflavone was consumed. High-density lipoproteincholesterol (HDL-C) levels were unaffected [61]. At the end of treatment, the probiotic group, which included *Lactobacillus acidophilus* and *Bifidobacteriumbifidum*, had lower TC, HDL-C, and LDL-C levels than the control group [62]. Pregnant women who consumed probiotic yogurt had significantly lower TC, LDL-C, and HDL-C values, as well as lower blood triglyceride levels. Serum lipid profiles, on the other hand, revealed no significant alterations [63].

9.5.2 Fecal Microbiota Transplantation

Fecal microbiota transplantation (FMT) is gaining traction as a promising treatment option for a variety of microbiota-related diseases. Eisman et al. were the first to describe the use of FMT as an adjuvant in the treatment of pseudomembranous colitis through fecal enema [64]. The use of FMT in the treatment of recurrent *Clostridium difficile* infection, in particular, has proven to be exceedingly beneficial and has been shown to be much more effective than typical treatment methods such vancomycin antibiotic therapy [65]. FMT is also showing promise as a treatment for various microbiota-related diseases such as ulcerative colitis, Crohn's disease, obesity, type 2 diabetes, and cardiovascular disease.

References

1 Stewart, J., Manmathan, G., and Wilkinson, P. (2017). Primary prevention of cardiovascular disease: a review of contemporary guidance and literature. *JRSM Cardiovasc. Dis.* 6: 2048004016687211.

2 Linton, M.R.F., Yancey, P.G., Davies, S.S. et al. (2019). The role of lipids and lipoproteins in atherosclerosis. In: *Endotext* (eds. K.R. Feingold). South Dartmouth, MA, USA: MDText. com, Inc.

3 Cassar, A., Holmes, D.R., Rihal, C.S. et al. (2009). Chronic coronary artery disease: diagnosis and management. *Mayo Clinic. Proc.* 84: 1130–1146.

4 WHO (2021). *The challenge of cardiovascular disease-quick statistics.* https://www.who.int/news-room/fact-sheets/detail/cardiovascular-diseases-(cvds).

5 Zhu, W., Gregory, J.C., Org, E. et al. (2016). Gut microbial metabolite TMAO enhances platelet hyperreactivity and thrombosis risk. *Cell* 165: 111–124.

6 Wang, H., Zhang, W., Zuo, L. et al. (2014). Intestinal dysbacteriosis contributes to decreased intestinal mucosal barrier function and increased bacterial translocation. *Lett. Appl. Microbiol.* 58: 384–392.

7 Michelson, A.D. (2010). Antiplatelet therapies for the treatment of cardiovascular disease. *Nat. Rev. Drug Discov.* 9: 154–169.

8 Jackson, S.P., Nesbitt, W.S., and Westein, E. (2009). Dynamics of platelet thrombus formation. *J. Thromb. Haemost.* 7 (Suppl. 1): 17–20.

9 Wang, Z., Klipfell, E., Bennett, B.J. et al. (2011). Gut flora metabolism of phosphatidylcholine promotes cardiovascular disease. *Nature* 472: 57–63.

10 Lau, K., Srivatsav, V., Rizwan, A. et al. (2017). Bridging the gap between gut microbial dysbiosis and cardiovascular diseases. *Nutrients* 9: 859.

11 Anbazhagan, A.N., Priyamvada, S., and Priyadarshini, M. (2017). Gut microbiota in vascular disease: therapeutic target? *Curr. Vasc. Pharm.* 15: 291–295.

12 Santisteban, M.M., Qi, Y., Zubcevic, J. et al. (2017). Hypertension-linked pathophysiological alterations in the gut. *Circ. Res.* 120: 312–323.

13 McCarville, J.L., Chen, G.Y., Cuevas, V.D. et al. (2020). Microbiota metabolites in health and disease. *Annu. Rev. Immunol.* 38: 147–170.

14 Koeth, R.A., Wang, Z., Levison, B.S. et al. (2013). Intestinal microbiota metabolism of L-carnitine, a nutrient in red meat, promotes atherosclerosis. *Nat. Med.* 19: 576–585.

15 Wang, Z., Klipfell, E., Bennett, B.J. et al. (2011). Gut flora metabolism of phosphatidylcholine promotes cardiovascular disease. *Nature* 472: 57–63.

16 Tang, W.H., Wang, Z., Levison, B.S. et al. (2013). Intestinal microbial metabolism of phosphatidylcholine and cardiovascular risk. *N. Engl. J. Med.* 368: 1575–1584.

17 Kasahara, K. and Rey, F.E. (2019). The emerging role of gut microbial metabolism on cardiovascular disease. *Curr. Opin. Microbiol.* 50: 64–70.

18 Velmurugan, G., Dinakaran, V., Rajendhran, J. et al. (2020). Blood microbiota and circulating microbial metabolites in diabetes and cardiovascular disease. *Trends Endocrinol. Metab.* 31: 835–847.

19 Warrier, M., Shih, D.M., Burrows, A.C. et al. (2015). The TMAO-generating enzyme lavin Monooxygenase 3 is a central regulator of cholesterol balance. *Cell Rep.* 10: 326–338.

20 Senthong, V., Wang, Z., Li, X.S. et al. (2016). Intestinal microbiota-generated metabolite Trimethylamine-N-Oxide and 5-year mortality risk in stable coronary artery disease: the contributory role of intestinal microbiota in a COURAGE-like patient cohort. *J. Am. Heart Assoc.* 5.

21 Roncal, C., Martinez-Aguilar, E., Orbe, J. et al. (2019). Trimethylamine-N-Oxide (TMAO) predicts cardiovascular mortality in peripheral artery disease. *Sci. Rep.* 9: 15580.

22 Koay, Y.C., Chen, Y.C., Wali, J.A. et al. (2021). Plasma levels of trimethylamine-N-oxide can be increased with 'healthy' and 'unhealthy' diets and do not correlate with the extent of atherosclerosis but with plaque instability. *Cardiovasc. Res.* 117: 435–449.

23 Witkowski, M., Weeks, T.L., and Hazen, S.L. (2020). Gut microbiota and cardiovascular disease. *Circ. Res.* 127 (4): 553–570.

24 Janeiro, M.H., Ramirez, M.J., Milagro, F.I. et al. (2018). Implication of Trimethylamine N-Oxide (TMAO) in disease: potential biomarker or new therapeutic target. *Nutrients* 10: 1398.

25 Sun, X., Jiao, X., Ma, Y. et al. (2016). Trimethylamine N-oxide induces inflammation and endothelialdys function in human umbilical vein endothelial cells via activating ROS-TXNIP-NLRP3 inflammasomes. *Biochem. Biophys. Res. Commun.* 481: 63–70.

26 Koeth, R.A., Wang, Z., Levison, B.S. et al. (2013). Intestinal microbiota metabolism of L-carnitine, a nutrient in red meat, promotes atherosclerosis. *Nat. Med.* 19: 576–585.

27 Shih, D.M., Wang, Z., Lee, R. et al. (2015). Flavin containing monooxygenase 3 exerts broad effects on glucose and lipid metabolism and atherosclerosis. *J. Lipid Res.* 56: 22–37.

28 Chen, K., Zheng, X., Feng, M. et al. (2017). Gut microbiota-dependent metabolite Trimethylamine N-Oxide contributes to cardiac dysfunction in Western diet-induced obese mice. *Front. Physiol.* 8: 139.

29 Sina, C., Gavrilova, O., Forster, M. et al. (2009). G protein-coupled receptor 43 is essential for neutrophil recruitment during intestinal inflammation. *J. Immunol.* 183: 7514–7522.

30 Gerdes, V., Gueimonde, M., Pajunen, L. et al. (2020). How strong is the evidence that gut microbiota composition can be influenced by lifestyle interventions in a cardio-protective way? *Atherosclerosis* 311: 124–142.

31 Ridlon, J.M., Harris, S.C., Bhowmik, S. et al. (2016). Consequences of bile salt biotransformations by intestinal bacteria. *Gut Microb.* 7: 22–39.

32 Brown, J.M. and Hazen, S.L. (2018). Microbial modulation of cardiovascular disease. *Nat. Rev. Microbiol.* 16: 171–181.

33 Tang, W.H., Kitai, T., and Hazen, S.L. (2017). Gut microbiota in cardiovascular health and disease. *Circ. Res.* 120: 1183–1196.

34 Ghanim, H., Sia, C.L., Upadhyay, M. et al. (2010). Orange juice neutralizes the proinflammatory effect of a high-fat, high-carbohydrate meal and prevents endotoxin increase and Toll-like receptor expression. *Am. J. Clin. Nutr.* 91: 940–949.

35 Wiedermann, C.J., Kiechl, S., Dunzendorfer, S. et al. (1999). Association of endotoxemia with carotid atherosclerosis and cardiovascular disease: prospective results from the Bruneck Study. *J. Am. Coll. Cardiol.* 34: 1975–1981.

36 Morgan, A.E., Mooney, K.M., Wilkinson, S.J. et al. (2016). Cholesterol metabolism: a review of how ageing disrupts the biological mechanisms responsible for its regulation. *Ageing Res. Rev.* 27: 108–24.

37 Grundy, S.M. (2016). Does dietary cholesterol matter? *Curr. Atheroscler. Rep.* 18: 68.

38 Van der Velde, A.E., Brufau, G., and Groen, A.K. (2010). Transintestinal cholesterol efflux. *Curr. Opin. Lipidol.* 21: 167–171.

39 Le May, C., Berger, J.M., Lespine, A. et al. (2013). Transintestinal cholesterol excretion is an active metabolic process modulated by PCSK9 and statin involving ABCB1. *Arterioscler. Thromb. Vasc. Biol.* 33: 1484–1493.

40 Yu, L., Hammer, R.E., Li-Hawkins, J. et al. (2002). Disruption of Abcg5 and Abcg8 in mice reveals their crucial role in biliary cholesterol secretion. *Proc. Natl. Acad. Sci. USA* 99: 16237–16242.

41 Gerard P, Béguet, F., Lepercq, P. et al. (2004). Gnotobiotic rats harboring human intestinal microbiota as a model for studying cholesterol-to coprostanol conversion. *FEMS Microbiol. Ecol.* 47: 337–343.

42 Backhed, F., Ding, H., Wang, T. et al. (2004). The gut microbiota as an environmental factor that regulates fat storage. *Proc. Natl. Acad. Sci. USA* 101: 15718–15723.

43 Martinez-Guryn, K., Hubert, N., Frazier, K. et al. (2018). Small intestine microbiota regulate host digestive and absorptive adaptive responses to dietary lipids. *Cell Host Microbe.* 23: 458–469.

44 Karlsson, F.H., Tremaroli, V., Nookaew, I. et al. (2013). Gut metagenome in European women with normal, impaired and diabetic glucose control. *Nature* 498: 99–103.

45 Rebolledo, C., Cuevas, A., Zambrano, T. et al. (2017). Bacterial community profile of the gut microbiota differs between hypercholesterolemic subjects and controls. *Biomed. Res. Int.* 2017: 8127814.

46 Fu, J., Bonder, M.J., Cenit, M.C. et al. (2015). The gut microbiome contributes to a substantial proportion of the variation in blood lipids. *Circ. Res.* 117: 817–824.

47 Liang, H., Jiang, F., Cheng, R. et al. (2021). A high-fat diet and high-fat and high cholesterol diet may affect glucose and lipid metabolism differentially through gut microbiota in mice. *Exp. Anim.* 70: 73–83.

48 Zhang, X., Coker, O.O., Chu, E.S. et al. (2021). Dietary cholesterol drives fatty liver-associated liver cancer by modulating gut microbiota and metabolites. *Gut* 70: 761–774.

49 Emoto, T., Yamashita, T., Sasaki, N. et al. (2016). Analysis of gut microbiota in coronary artery disease patients: a possible link between gut microbiota and coronary artery disease. *J. Atheroscler. Thromb.* 23: 908–921.

50 Mitra, S., Drautz-Moses, D.I., Alhede, M. et al. (2015). In silico analyses of metagenomes from human atherosclerotic plaque samples. *Microbiome* 3: 38.

51 Karlsson, F.H., Fak, F., Nookaew, I. et al. (2012). Symptomatic atherosclerosis is associated with an altered gut metagenome. *Nat. Commun.* 3: 1245.

52 Zhu, Q., Gao, R., Zhang, Y. et al. (2018). Dysbiosis signatures of gut microbiota in coronary artery disease. *Physiol. Genom.* 50: 893–903.

53 Jie, Z., Xia, H., Zhong, S.L. et al. (2017). The gut microbiome in atherosclerotic cardiovascular disease. *Nat. Commun.* 8: 845.

54 Bale, B.F., Doneen, A.L., and Vigerust, D.J. (2017). High-risk periodontal pathogens contribute to the pathogenesis of atherosclerosis. *Postgrad. Med. J.* 93: 215–220.

55 Cai, H., Wen, Z., Meng, K. et al. (2021). Metabolomic signatures for liver tissue and cecum contents in high-fat diet-induced obese mice based on UHPLC-Q-TOF/MS. *Nutr. Metab.* 18: 69.

56 Hill, C., Guarner, F., Reid, G. et al. (2014). Expert consensus document. The International Scientific Association for Probiotics and Prebiotics consensus statement on the scope and appropriate use of the term probiotic. *Nat. Rev. Gastroenterol. Hepatol.* 11: 506–514.

57 Tsai, C.C., Lin, P.P., Hsieh, Y.M. et al. (2014). Cholesterol-lowering potentials of lactic acid bacteria based on bile-salt hydrolase activity and effect of potent strains on cholesterol metabolism in vitro and in vivo. *Sci. World J.* 2014: 690752.

58 Ishimwe, N., Daliri, E.B., Lee, B.H. et al. (2015). The perspective on cholesterol-lowering mechanisms of probiotics. *Mol. Nutr. Food Res.* 59: 94–105.

59 Pereira, D.I. and Gibson, G.R. (2002). Cholesterol assimilation by lactic acid bacteria and bifidobacteria isolated from the human gut. *Appl. Environ. Microbiol.* 68: 4689–4693.

60 Joung, H., Chu, J., Kim, B.K. et al. (2021). Probiotics ameliorate chronic low-grade inflammation and fat accumulation with gut microbiota composition change in diet-induced obese mice models. *Appl. Microbiol. Biotechnol.* 105: 1203–1213.

61 Cavallini, D.C., Manzoni, M.S., Bedani, R. et al. (2016). Probiotic soy product supplemented with isoflavones improves the lipid profile of moderately hypercholesterolemic men: a randomized controlled trial. *Nutrients* 8: 52.

62 Rerksuppaphol, S. and Rerksuppaphol, L. (2015). A randomized double-blind controlled trial of *Lactobacillus acidophilus* plus *Bifidobacteriumbifidum* versus placebo in patients with hypercholesterolemia. *J. Clin. Diagn. Res.* 9: KC01-04.

63 Asemi, Z., Samimi, M., Tabasi, Z. et al. (2012). Effect of daily consumption of probiotic yoghurt on lipid profiles in pregnant women: a randomized controlled clinical trial. *J. Matern. Fetal. Neonatal. Med.* 25: 1552–1556.

64 Eiseman, B., Silen, W., Bascom, G.S. et al. (1948). Fecal enema as an adjunct in the treatment of pseudomembranous enterocolitis. *Surgery* 44: 854–859.

65 Khan, M.Y., Dirweesh, A., Khurshid, T. et al. (2018). Comparing fecal microbiota transplantation to standard-of-care treatment for recurrent Clostridium difficile infection: a systematic review and meta-analysis. *Eur. J. Gastroenterol. Hepatol.* 30: 1309–1317.

10

Gut Microbiota and Inflammatory Bowel Diseases

Anu Jacob and Jissin Mathew

Department of Biotechnology, Karunya Institute of Technology and Science, Coimbatore, India

10.1 Introduction

With more than 6.9 million people on a global scale currently living with the complications of inflammatory bowel disease (IBD) [1], it is essential to understand it and formulate successful strategies for its treatment and prevention. Most of the IBD cases are observed in North America and Europe [2] while the cases in Africa, Asia, and South America are on the rise [3]. The current prevalence of IBD in the industrialised society [4] reveals the contributing factors such as lifestyle, diet, and environment for the occurrence of disease in genetically susceptible individuals.

Inflammatory bowel disease (IBD) is the non-infectious chronic inflammation of the gastrointestinal (GI) tract with an unclear aetiology, and several factors are assumed to be the causal factors. The foremost factor is genetic predisposition and several researchers have presented the role of the microbiome in the onset of IBD [5]. On the other hand, stress factors including exposure to stress from environmental or psychological factors, or pathologic bacteria [6] also contribute to the development of IBD.

The two subtypes, Crohn's disease (CD) and ulcerative colitis (UC) are collectively called IBD (Figure 10.1). The former affects any segment of the GI tract from mouth to anus, whereas the latter affects colonic mucosa. Histologically, inflammation in UC is superficial, while CD is transmural with severe difficulties [7]. The clinical symptoms shown by IBD patients are diarrhea, anemia, abdominal pain, abdominal distension, weight loss, and bloody stool [8]. The emergence of the disease is usually diagnosed in the 20's to 30's, but also among children and adolescents [9]. IBD is detected in patients with clinical symptoms by using endoscopy, biopsy, or imaging techniques [10].

The Gut Microbiota in Health and Disease, First Edition. Edited by Nimmy Srivastava, Salam A. Ibrahim, Jayeeta Chattopadhyay, and Mohamed H. Arbab.
© 2023 John Wiley & Sons Ltd. Published 2023 by John Wiley & Sons Ltd.

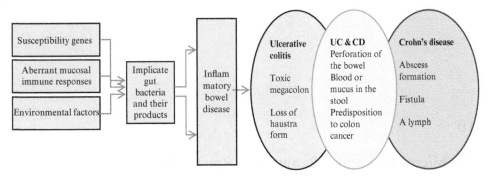

Figure 10.1 Complications in CD and UC.

10.2 Intestinal Microbiome in IBD Patients

The microbiota refers to the association of microorganisms present on or within the human tissues or biofluids. Alternatively, the microbiome is the complete collection of the genomic materials of the microbiota. These microbial consortiums are highly dynamic and play a significant role in the host (Figure 10.2).

Over the large intestine lays a thick mucus layer composed of a large number of microbes that form the gut microbiota [11]. The human gut houses most of the microbiota and estimates of more than 1000 different species [12], the gut microbiome consists of more than 5 million different genes [13]. The most represented phyla in gut microbiota are Firmicutes (38.8%), Bacteroidetes (27.8%), Actinobacteria (8.2%), Proteobacteria (2.1%) [14]. Fungi in gut microbiota are approximately 0.1% [15], and the gut biome is typically comprised of

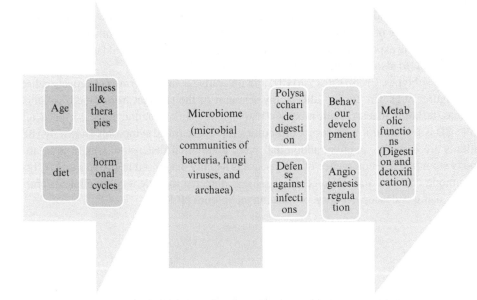

Figure 10.2 The dynamic nature and functions of microbiota.

bacteriophages that influence human health [16]. The greatest fungal phyla are *Ascomycota* and *Basidiomycota* [17]. In the gut microbiome, 99.1% is of bacterial origin, while the fungal genome accounts for about 0.02% of the whole mucosa-associated microbiota [15]. Since the microbiota is remarkable in the physical, chemical, and immunological interactions of the host with the environment, any alterations of this interface can lead to disease development [18]. Experimental IBD trials with germ-free conditions revealed the absence of disease onset or a considerably reduced intensity [19]. The unbalanced association among gut microbiota and the mucosal immune system bring about IBD.

While the gut microbiota has significant physiological functions, it may disturb the immune homeostasis in the host. A failure in the defensive mechanism, the layer of epithelial cells above the bowel wall, leads to inflammatory immune reactions against the bacteria that are present in people with IBD [20, 21].

10.2.1 Dysbiosis in IBD

In healthy individuals, the numerous and diverse gut microbial community exists in a relative balance, although the microbiome among healthy individuals is different [22, 23]. The imbalance in the gut microbial species that occur due to IBD is termed dysbiosis and results in functional changes within the host [24]. The bacterial diversity is decreased in CD and UC, while the fungal species is reduced in UC alone, specifying that the CD gut environment prefers fungi to bacteria. The equilibrium among bacterial and fungal diversity changed during IBD and was found to escalate the fungi-to-bacteria diversity ratio [25] (see Table 10.1).

10.2.2 Genetic Factors of the Host Affecting the Pathogenesis of IBD

Genetic factors have a vital impact on the susceptibility of IBD, as studies proved that about 12% of IBD patients have a family history of IBD [31]. The population-based Genome-wide association studies (GWAS) next-generation sequencing techniques and other analyses have significantly expanded the number of known IBD associated loci to more than 240

Table 10.1 Gut microbiota variation in inflammatory bowel diseases.

Dysbiosis	Decrease	Increase	Reference
Bacterial Dysbiosis	*Clostridium* groups IV and XIVa, *Bacteroides, Suterella, Roseburia, Bifidobacterium* species, and *Faecalibacterium prausnitzii*	Proteobacteria members (including invasive and adherent *Escherichia coli*), *Veillonellaceae, Pasteurellaceae, Fusobacterium* species, *Ruminococcusgnavus*	[26]
Fungal Dysbiosis	*Saccharomyces cerevisiae*	*Candida albicans, Clavisporalusitaniae, Kluyverpmycesmarxianus, Candida tropicalls, Cyberlindnerajadini, Basidomycota*	[25, 27]
Viral Dysbiosis		*Caudovirales*	[28, 29]
Archaeal Dysbiosis	*Methanobrevibactersmithii*	*Methanosphaerastastmanae*	[30]

non-overlapping genetic risk loci, of which about 30 genetic loci are common for Crohn's disease and ulcerative colitis [32]. These loci are linked with three mechanisms, foremost is involved in innate immunity and autophagy (e.g., *NOD2, ATG161*), the second is involved in adaptive immunity of interleukin-23 signalling and T-helper 17 cells (*IL23R, STAT3*). The final mechanism is involved in the epithelial barrier role that retains against microbial entry (e.g., *ECM1, HNF4A*). The first mechanism occurs in CD while the third in UC only. The second mechanism is associated with both CD and UC [30]. A study on the identified genes show that they are responsible for significant constituents for recognising and acclimatising to alterations in the gut microbiome [33]. The intestinal homeostasis is modulated by the interaction between the pathways and environmental factors as well.

The Nucleotide-binding oligomerisation domain 2 (NOD2) is often mutated in patients with Crohn's disease, and is the first gene detected to be involved in Crohn's disease. The gene is associated with the autophagy pathway that plays a vital role in identifying and eliminating to screen the accurate microbes that continue in the host. Mutations in the gene interrupt the essential host defences and immune mechanisms such as reduced epithelial elimination of intrusive bacteria, malfunction of Paneth cells, and declined antimicrobial peptide synthesis.[34] Patients with 1007fs mutation in the NOD2 gene express a considerably higher severity in CD, whereas R702W and G908R mutations are associated with increased inflammatory cytokine responses [35].

Additionally, polymorphisms in the IBD susceptibility genetic factor change the gut microbes and induce imbalances in the host–microbiota interfaces that increase the possibility of IBD onset. The susceptible gene identified so far constitutes <25% of the predicted heritability of the disease [33]. Additional genetic analysis is required to completely identify the rare loci to exploit susceptibility loci as predictive biomarkers.

10.2.3 Environmental Factors in the Disruption of Gut Microbiota and Development of IBD

IBD is a heterogeneous disease which develops in a genetically susceptible person, influenced by environmental factors. Genetics pose a relatively lower risk potential while environmental factors are vital in the disease pathogenicity. A rapid emergence of IBD reported in Asia, where it was considered a rare disease twenty years ago. Recent studies have shown an increased prevalence of IBD in countries such as Taiwan, Hong Kong, South Korea, India and China [36]. The mutualistic interaction between microbiota and the host benefits the microbiota with the nutrient-rich human intestine; yet, the host lifestyle including diet, hygiene, or antibiotic intake creates quick and continuous deviations in gut microbiota biodiversity.

10.2.3.1 Early Life Environmental Exposure
The mode of birth influences the occurrence of IBD as the biodiversity of microbiota in newborns born by cesarean section is considerably altered compared to that of those born by vaginal delivery. Likewise, profuse pathogenic bacteria have been known in breastfed infants, indicating a health benefit of breastfeeding with transmission to the infant of antibacterial compounds and maternal antibodies [37, 38]. However, a recent population-based study showed no effect on the mode of birth, formula feed, and the development of

pediatric IBD [39]. Childhood hygiene is another factor associated with the risk of development of IBD. Cholapranee and Ananthakrishnan [40] demonstrated that practices such as consuming tap water and acquaintance with farm animals or household pets have prevented the onset of IBD.

10.2.3.2 Diet

The dietary variations directed towards westernisation are frequent in human culture and result in variations in the populations of the gut microbiota and lead to an irregular intestinal immune response and, ultimately, IBD [41]. The intake of a high-fat diet has the likelihood of developing IBD as evident in the western diet with high amounts of Omega-6 (ω-6) to Omega-3 (ω-3) resulting in IBD [42]. In addition, the long-chain triglycerides increase the pro-inflammatory mediators and the high-fat diet intensifies the intestinal permeability and modifies intestinal microbiota [43]. The protein of fish or meat was shown to amplify the IBD progress, as these animal proteins decomposed in the gut resulting in substrates that supported pathobionts [44]. Carbohydrates in the diet create differential sugar profiles being accessible in the intestinal lumen and support the proliferation of certain pathobionts. A low fibre diet has also been related to higher IBD prevalence [45].

10.2.3.3 Lifestyle Factors

Cigarette smoking was identified to intensify the emergence of CD and result in a severe state, whereas smoking termination intensifies the risk of UC emergence and relapse [46].

10.3 Interventions for the Treatment of IBD

There have been many approaches in the management of IBD that have proved to relieve the patients with the complexities associated with the disease (Table 10.2). One of the major advances is the use of anti-tumour necrosis factor (anti-TNF) agents that reduce surgical requirements and upgrade the health conditions of moderate to severe IBD [47]. Conversely, the treatment failure rates showing about 30% of patients not responding to the treatment and about 40% of patients losing the response during the disease course [48] is a challenge in this approach. In the current scenario, with a rise in the occurrence of IBD, there is a need for further safe and effective therapeutic alternatives to address unmet treatment needs in IBD patients.

10.3.1 Microbiome-modulating Approach in the Treatment of IBD

10.3.1.1 Antibiotics

The impact of gut microbiota in the emergence and progress of IBD indicates the significance of the manipulation of the microbial community in the cure of IBD. Antibiotics reduce the concentration and composition of pro-inflammatory bacteria present and thereby support the beneficial bacteria in the intestinal lumina [54]. Additionally, antibiotics may reduce bacterial tissue invasion, cure microabscesses, weaken bacterial

Table 10.2 Traditional interventions in treatment of IBD.

Intervention	Mechanism	Medication	Reference
Anti-inflammatory drugs; corticosteroids and aminosalicylates	Decrease inflammation and avoid damage to the intestinal tract	5-ASA class of medications, including sulfasalazine, mesalamine, and diazo-bonded 5-ASA	[49]
Immunomodulators	Lessen the tissue impairment and release of chemicals such as cytokines, that cause inflammation of the intestinal lining	azathioprine, mercaptopurine, cyclosporine, and methotrexate.	[50]
Biologics	Reduce inflammatory cytokines	infliximab, adalimumab, and golimumab	[51]
Antibiotics	Prevent postoperative recurrence in CD, decrease luminal bacterial concentrations and altering the gut microflora population	ciprofloxacin, metronidazole, azithromycin, and rifaximin	[52]
Anti-adhesion agent	Prevent lymphocyte infiltration of the intestines by selectively targeting the adhesion molecules involved	Natalizumab, Vedolizumab	[53]

adhesion, reduce bacterial translocation, and inhibit systemic dissemination [55]. Moreover, antibiotics have immunomodulatory [56] and anti-inflammatory properties [57]. Long term ciprofloxacin treatment enhanced clinical outcomes when administered as adjuvant therapy to steroids and salicylates, for the induction and maintenance of disease remission [58]. An amalgamation of diverse antibiotics such as metronidazole, amoxicillin, doxycycline, and vancomycin was effective in children with moderate-severe UC [59]. Despite the lack of proof for the application of antibiotics in treating IBD, experts still recommend its administration [52].

10.3.1.2 Prebiotics and Probiotics

Prebiotics are nondigestible by the host and are fermentable carbohydrates such as oligosaccharides, lactitol, lactulose, and inulin and are appended by the consumption of beans, fruits, and vegetables [60]. Prebiotics regulate the bacterial flora in the intestine as it triggers the growth of beneficial bacteria [61].

Probiotics are living microorganisms which, when administered, may help the host by altering the microbial diversity, increasing the gut barrier function, and controlling the immune response. Examples of the frequently used microorganisms are *Lactobacillus*, *Bifidobacterium*, *Escherichia coli* Nissle 1917 (EcN), *Enterococcus*, and *Saccharomyces boulardii* [62].

Administration of pre- and probiotics benefit the host by reinforcing the intestinal integrity, preventing the disease and invasion of pathogens, regulating the cytokine synthesis, and retaining gut microbiota [63–65]. Probiotics stimulate the synthesis of anti-inflammatory factors by supporting the immune system, and also inhibit or repair the damage to the mucosal wall caused by pathogens [66]. Probiotic administration with *Lactobacillus* and

Bifidobacterium or in combinations at a dose of 10^{10}–10^{12} CFU per day is suitable for IBD remission [67]. Probiotics are nontoxic and benefit the host as a therapeutic technique for the treatment of IBD, while prebiotics are effective in patients with lower clinical activity of disease [68]. The effectiveness of probiotics on reduction in IBD is studied more in UC compared to CD. Further studies are required to confirm probiotics are beneficial for the remission of IBD [69].

10.3.1.3 Fecal Microbiota Transplantation

Fecal microbiota transplantation (FMT) implicates transferring feces from a healthy bene-factor into the gastrointestinal tract of a patient with a particular chronic disease to restore the normal intestinal microbiome and recover from a pathological state [70]. The treatment of a patient with IBD by FMT exhibited better colon microbiota diversity in the patient and it alters the benefactor profile [71]. The approach has been successful (cure rate >90%) in dealing with refractory and recurrent *Clostridium difficile* infection [72]. FMT is a safe and effective approach to treating CD and improves gut microbial population and diversity [73] at a clinical remission rate of 0.62. A recurrent therapy is recommended [74], as the micro-biome response to a single FMT is temporary [75]. However, the outcome of the FMT treatment is not consistent [76] and requires more randomised controlled studies.

10.4 Conclusion

The gut microbiota has a significant role in IBD development and thus should be further utilised for the development of treatments. However, more studies are required to under-stand the involvement of the specific species in the IBD pathogenesis so that better preven-tion and treatment may be carried out. More studies are required on the viral and fungal microbiota as limited investigations are available. The microbiota-based diagnostic tool development is also desirable for better management of the disease.

References

1 Alatab, S., Sepanlou, S.G., Ikuta, K. et al. (2020). The global, regional, and national burden of inflammatory bowel disease in 195 countries and territories, 1990–2017: a systematic analysis for the Global Burden of Disease Study 2017. *Lancet Gastroenterol. Hepatol.* 5 (1): 17–30.

2 Wang, C., Liu, H., Mu, G. et al. (2019). Effects of traditional Chinese medicines on immunity and culturable gut microflora to Oncorhynchus masou. *Fish Shell. Immunol.* 93: 322–327.

3 Shamoon, M., Martin, N.M., and O'Brien, C.L. (2019). Recent advances in gut microbiota mediated therapeutic targets in inflammatory bowel diseases: emerging modalities for future pharmacological implications. *Pharmacol. Res.* 148: 104344.

4 Kaplan, G.G. and Ng, S.C. (2017). Understanding and preventing the global increase of inflammatory bowel disease. *Gastroenterology* 152 (2): 313–21.

5 Ryan, F.J., Ahern, A.M., Fitzgerald, R.S. et al. (2020). Colonic microbiota is associated with inflammation and host epigenomic alterations in inflammatory bowel disease. *Nat. Commun.* 11 (1): 1–12.

6 Sgambato, D., Miranda, A., Ranaldo, R. et al. (2017). The role of stress in inflammatory bowel diseases. *Curr. Pharm. Des.* 23 (27): 3997–4002.

7 Qin, X. (2013). Why is damage limited to the mucosa in ulcerative colitis but transmural in Crohn's disease? *World J. Gastrointest. Pathophysiol.* 4 (3): 63–64.

8 Hedin, C., Rioux, J.D., and D'Amato, M. (eds.) (2019). *Molecular genetics of inflammatory bowel disease.* Second. Springer Nature. Switzerland; 3–25 p.

9 Rubalcava, N.S. and Gadepalli, S.K. (2021). Inflammatory bowel disease in children and adolescents. *Adv. Pediatr.* 68: 121–42.

10 Tontini, G.E., Vecchi, M., Pastorelli, L. et al. (2015). Differential diagnosis in inflammatory bowel disease colitis: state of the art and future perspectives. *W. J. Gastroenterol.* 21 (1).

11 Rodrıguez-Pineiro, A.M. and Johansson, M.E.V. (2015). The colonic mucus protection depends on the microbiota. *Gut Microbes.* 6 (5): 326–330.

12 Consortium HMP. (2012). Structure, function and diversity of the healthy human microbiome. *Nature* 486: 207–214.

13 Cosortium HMP (2012). A framework for humanmicrobiome research. *Nature* 486: 215–221.

14 D'Argenio, V. and Salvatore. F. (2015). The role of the gut microbiome in the healthy adult status. *Clin. Chim. Acta.* 451: 97–102.

15 Qin, J., Li, R., Raes, J. et al. (2010). A human gut microbial gene catalogue established by metagenomic sequencing. *Nature* 464 (7285): 59–65.

16 Shkoporov, A.N., Clooney, A.G., Sutton, T.D.S. et al. (2019). The human gut virome is highly diverse, stable, and individual specific. *Cell. Host. Microbe.* 2 (4): 527–541.e5.

17 Chehoud, C., Albenberg, L.G., Judge, C. et al. (2015). Fungal signature in the gut microbiota of pediatric patients with inflammatory bowel disease. *Inflamm. Bowel Dis.* 21 (8): 1948–1956.

18 Santana, P.T., Rosas, S.L.B., Ribeiro, B.E. et al. (2022). Dysbiosis in inflammatory bowel disease: pathogenic role and potential therapeutic targets. *Int. J. Mol. Sci.* 23 (3464): 1–25.

19 Sartor, R.B. (2004). Therapeutic manipulation of the enteric microflora in inflammatory bowel diseases: antibiotics, probiotics, and prebiotics. *Gastroenterology* 126 (6): 1620–1633.

20 Goto, Y. and Kiyono, H. (2011). Epithelial barrier: an interface for the cross-communication between gut flora and immune system. *Immunol. Rev.* 245 (1): 147–163.

21 Cario, E. (2012). Commensal-innate immune miscommunication in IBD pathogenesis. *Dig. Dis.* 30: 334–340.

22 Mobeen, F., Sharma, V., and Prakash, T. (2018). Enterotype variations of the healthy human gut microbiome in different geographical regions. *Bioinformation* 14 (9): 560–573.

23 Aldars-García, L., Chaparro, M., and Gisbert, J.P. (2021). Systematic review: the gut microbiome and its potential clinical application in inflammatory bowel disease. *Microorganisms* 9: 1–43.

24 McIlroy, J., Ianiro, G., Mukhopadhya, I. et al. (2018). Review article: the gut microbiome in inflammatory bowel disease—avenues for microbial management. *Ali. Pharmacol. Ther.* 47 (1): 26–42.

25 Sokol, H., Leducq, V., Aschard, H. et al. (2017). Fungal microbiota dysbiosis in IBD. *Gut* 66 (6): 1039–1048.

26 Pittayanon, R., Lau, J.T., Leontiadis, G.I. et al. (2020). Differences in gut microbiota in patients with vs without inflammatory bowel diseases: a systematic review. *Gastroenterology* 158 (4): 930–946.e1.

27 Mckenzie, H., Main, J., Pennington, C.R. et al. (1990). Antibody to selected strains of Saccharomyces cerevisiae (baker's and brewer's yeast) and Candida albicans in Crohn's disease. *Gut* 31: 536–538.

28 Zuo, T., Lu, X.J., Zhang, Y. et al. (2019). Gut mucosal virome alterations in ulcerative colitis. *Gut* 68 (7): 1169–1179.

29 Imai, T., Inoue, R., Kawada, Y. et al. (2019). Characterization of fungal dysbiosis in Japanese patients with inflammatory bowel disease. *J. Gastroenterol.* 54 (2): 149–159.

30 Scanlan, P.D., Shanahan, F., and Marchesi, J.R. (2008). Human methanogen diversity and incidence in healthy and diseased colonic groups using mcrA gene analysis. *BMC Microbiol.* 8 (1): 1–8.

31 Turpin, W., Goethel, A., Bedrani, L. et al. (2018). Determinants of IBD heritability: genes, bugs, and more. *Inflamm. Bowel Dis.* 24 (6): 1133–1148.

32 Mirkov, M.U., Verstockt, B., and Cleynen, I. (2017). Genetics of inflammatory bowel disease: beyond NOD2. *Lancet Gastroenterol. Hepatol.* 2 (3): 224–234.

33 Lee, M. and Chang, E.B. (2021). Inflammatory Bowel Diseases (IBD) and the microbiome—searching the crime scene for clues. *Gastroenterology* 160 (2): 524–537.

34 Kobayashi, K.S., Chamaillard, M., Ogura, Y. et al. (2005). Nod2-dependent regulation of innate and adaptive immunity in the intestinal tract. *Science* 307 (80): 731–734.

35 Yamamoto, S. and Ma, X. (2009). Role of Nod2 in the development of Crohn's disease. *Microbes. Infect.* 11 (12): 912–918.

36 Mak, W.Y., Zhao, M., Ng, S.C. et al. (2020). The epidemiology of inflammatory bowel disease: East meets West. *J. Gastroen. Hepatol.* 35 (3): 380–389.

37 van den Elsen, L.W.J., Garssen, J., Burcelin, R. et al. (2019). Shaping the gut microbiota by breastfeeding: the gateway to allergy prevention? *Front. Pediatr.* 7 (47): 1–10.

38 Xu, L., Lochhead, P., Ko, Y. et al. (2017). Systematic review with meta-analysis: breastfeeding and the risk of Crohn's disease and ulcerative colitis. *Aliment Pharmacol. Ther.* 46 (9): 780–789.

39 Burgess, C.J., Schnier, C., Wood, R. et al. (2022). Prematurity, delivery method and infant feeding type are not associated with paediatric-onset inflammatory bowel disease risk: a Scottish retrospective birth cohort study. *J. Crohn's Colitis.* 16 (8): 1235–1242.

40 Cholapranee, A. and Ananthakrishnan, A.N. (2016). Environmental hygiene and risk of inflammatory bowel diseases. *Inflamm. Bowel Dis.* 22 (9): 2191–2199.

41 Lewis, J.D. and Abreu, M.T. (2017). Diet as a trigger or therapy for inflammatory bowel diseases. *Gastroenterology* 152 (2): 398–414.e6.

42 Hou, J.K., Abraham, B., and El-Serag, H. (2011). Dietary intake and risk of developing inflammatory bowel disease: a systematic review of the literature. *Am. J Gastroenterol.* 106 (4): 563–573.

43 Pendyala, S., Walker, J.M., and Holt, P.R. (2012). A high-fat diet is associated with endotoxemia that originates from the gut. *Gastroenterology* 142 (5): 1100–1101.

44 Jowett, S.L., Seal, C.J., Pearce, M.S. et al. (2004). Influence of dietary factors on the clinical course of ulcerative colitis: a prospective cohort study. *Gut* 53 (10): 1479–1484.

45 Octoratou, M., Merikas, E., Malgarinos, G. et al. (2012). A prospective study of pre-illness diet in newly diagnosed patients with Crohn's disease. *Rev. Med. Chir. Soc. Med. Nat. Iasi.* 116 (1): 40–49.

46 Vedamurthy, A. and Ananthakrishnan, A.N. (2019). Influence of environmental factors in the development and outcomes of inflammatory bowel disease. *Gastroenterol. Hepatol.* 15 (2): 72–82.

47 Sokol, H., Seksik, P., and Cosnes, J. (2014). Complications and surgery in the inflammatory bowel diseases biological era. *Curr. Opin. Gastroenterol.* 30 (4): 378–384.

48 Ben-Horin, S. and Chowers, Y. (2011). Loss of response to anti-TNF treatments in Crohn's disease. *Aliment Pharmacol. Ther.* 33 (9): 987–995.

49 Ko, C.W., Singh, S., Feuerstein, J.D. et al. (2019). AGA clinical practice guidelines on the management of mild-to-moderate ulcerative colitis. *Gastroenterology* 156 (3): 748–764.

50 Mishra, J., Stubbs, M., Kuang, L. et al. (2022). Inflammatory bowel disease therapeutics: a focus on probiotic engineering. *Mediators Inflamm.* 9621668: 1–15.

51 Peyrin-Biroulet, L. (2010). Anti-TNF therapy in inflammatory bowel diseases: a huge review. *Minerva Gastroenterol. Dietol.* 56 (2): 233–243.

52 Ledder, O. and Turner, D. (2018). Antibiotics in IBD: still a role in the biological era? *Inflamm. Bowel Dis.* 24 (9): 1676–1688.

53 Chudy-Onwugaje, K.O., Christian, K.E., Farraye, F.A. et al. (2019). A state-of-the-art review of new and emerging therapies for the treatment of IBD. *Inflamm. Bowel Dis.* 25 (5): 820–830.

54 Gao, J., Gillilland, M.G., and Owyang, C. (2014). Rifaximin, gut microbes and mucosal inflammation: unraveling a complex relationship. *Gut Microbes.* 5 (4): 571–575.

55 Sartor, R.B. (2016). The potential mechanisms of action of rifaximin in the management of inflammatory bowel diseases. *Aliment Pharmacol. Ther.* 43: 27–36.

56 Wani, Y.C., Li, T., Han, Y.D. et al. (2015). Effect of Pregnane Xenobiotic receptor activation on inflammatory bowel disease treated with Rifaximin. *J. Biol. Regul. Homeo. Agen.* 29 (2): 401–410.

57 Huckle, A.W., Fairclough, L.C., and Ma, I.T. (2018). Prophylactic antibiotic use in COPD and the potential anti-inflammatory activities of antibiotics. *Respir. Care* 63 (5): 609–619.

58 Turunen, U.M., Färkkilä, M.A., Hakala, K. et al. (1998). Long-term treatment of ulcerative colitis with ciprofloxacin: a prospective, double-blind, placebo-controlled study. *Gastroenterology* 115 (5): 1072–1078.

59 Turner, D., Levine, A., Kolho, K.L. et al. (2014). Combination of oral antibiotics may be effective in severe pediatric ulcerative colitis: a preliminary report. *J. Crohn's Col.* 8 (11): 1464–1470.

60 Mohanty, D., Misra, S., Mohapatra, S. et al. (2018 November). Prebiotics and synbiotics: recent concepts in nutrition. *Food Biosci.* 26: 152–160.

61 Markowiak, P. and Ślizewska, K. (2017). Effects of probiotics, prebiotics, and synbiotics on human health. *Nutrients* 9 (1021): 1–30.

62 Cruz, B.C., Sarandy, M.M., Messias, A.C. et al. (2020). Preclinical and clinical relevance of probiotics and synbiotics in colorectal carcinogenesis: a systematic review. *Nutr. Rev.* 78 (8): 667–687.

63 Vemuri, R., Shinde, T., Gundamaraju, R. et al. (2018). Lactobacillus acidophilus DDS-1 modulates the gut microbiota and improves metabolic profiles in aging mice. *Nutrients* 10 (9): 1255.

64 Camilleri, M. (2019). Leaky gut: Mechanisms, measurement and clinical implications in humans. *Gut* 68 (8): 1516–1526.

65 Wong, W.Y., Chan, B.D., Leung, T.W. et al. (2022). Beneficial and anti-inflammatory effects of formulated prebiotics, probiotics, and synbiotics in normal and acute colitis mice. *J. Funct. Foods* 88: 104871.

66 Shen, Z.H., Zhu, C.X., Quan, Y.S. et al. (2018). Relationship between intestinal microbiota and ulcerative colitis: mechanisms and clinical application of probiotics and fecal microbiota transplantation. *W. J. Gastroenterol.* 24 (1): 5–14.

67 Zhang, X.F., Guan, X.X., Tang, Y.J. et al. (2021). Clinical effects and gut microbiota changes of using probiotics, prebiotics or synbiotics in inflammatory bowel disease: a systematic review and meta-analysis. *Eur. J. Nutr.* 60 (5): 2855–2875.

68 Hansen, J.J. and Sartor, R. (2015). Therapeutic manipulation of the microbiome in IBD: current results and future approaches. *Curr. Treat. Options Gastroenterol.* 13: 105–120.

69 Darb Emamie, A., Rajabpour, M., Ghanavati, R. et al. (2021). The effects of probiotics, prebiotics and synbiotics on the reduction of IBD complications, a periodic review during 2009–2020. *J. Appl. Microbiol.* 130 (6): 1823–1838.

70 Akutko, K. and Stawarski, A. (2021). Probiotics, prebiotics and synbiotics in inflammatory bowel diseases. *J, Clin. Med.* 10 (11).

71 Sood, A., Singh, A., Midha, V. et al. (2020). Fecal microbiota transplantation for ulcerative Colitis: an evolving therapy. *Crohn's Col. 360* 2 (4): otaa067.

72 Kassam, Z., Lee, C.H., Yuan, Y. et al. (2013). Fecal microbiota transplantation for Clostridium difficile infection: systematic review and meta-analysis. *Off. J. Am. Coll. Gastroenterol. ACG* 108 (4): 500–508.

73 Cheng, F., Huang, Z., Wei, W. et al. (2021). Fecal microbiota transplantation for Crohn's disease: a systematic review and meta-analysis. *Tech. Coloproctol.* 25 (5): 495–504.

74 Sudarshan, P., Kamm, M.A., Kaakoush, N.O. et al. (2017). Multidonor intensive faecal microbiota transplantation for active ulcerative colitis: a randomised placebo-controlled trial. *Lancet* 389 (10075): 1218–1228.

75 Goyal, A., Yeh, A., Bush, B.R. et al. (2018). Safety, clinical response, and microbiome findings following fecal microbiota transplant in children with inflammatory. *Inflamm. Bowel Dis.* 24 (2): 410–421.

76 Rossen, N.G., MacDonald, J.K., De Vries, E.M. et al. (2015). Fecal microbiota transplantation as novel therapy in gastroenterology: a systematic review. *W. J. Gastroenterol.* 21 (17): 5359–5371.

11

Gut Microbiota and Diabetes

Ankita Dey[1], Ridashisha Rymbai[1], Hriiziini Monica[2], and Jutishna Bora[3]

[1] Department of Biochemistry, North Eastern Hill University, Shillong, Meghalaya
[2] Department of Botany, Plant Biotechnology Laboratory, North Eastern Hill University, Shillong, Meghalaya
[3] Amity Institute of Biotechnology, Amity University Jharkhand, Ranchi, Jharkhand, India

11.1   Introduction

Diabetes mellitus, a complex metabolic disorder characterised by hyperglycemia, has been a global threat to approximately 420 million people, and this number may substantially increase in the near future. By 2045, the prevalence of diabetes is expected to affect approximately 630 million people. Furthermore, its impact on public health care expenditure is estimated to hit $827 billion worldwide [1]. The pathogenesis of diabetes mellitus is not completely understood yet, and it is broadly classified into two major types: Type 1 diabetes mellitus and Type 2 diabetes mellitus.

Type 1 diabetes mellitus: Type 1 diabetes (T1D), commonly known as insulin dependent diabetes, is an autoimmune disorder which is mainly caused when an individual's antibodies attack its own pancreatic cells, leading to organ damage, destruction of pancreatic β-cells, and impairment in the production of insulin [2].

Type 2 diabetes mellitus: Type 2 diabetes (T2D), commonly known as non-insulin dependent diabetes, is a chronic metabolic disorder caused primarily due to impaired insulin secretion by the pancreas, increased production of hepatic glucose, improper insulin signaling, and insulin resistance [3].

Various factors such as diet, lifestyle, gender, ageing, genetics, and epigenetics play a crucial role in the development of the disease [4]. However, many studies have shown that the composition of the gut microbiota also has great impact both positively and negatively on the development of various metabolic diseases including diabetes mellitus [5]. Hence, this chapter is framed to illustrate the relationship between the gut microbiota and diabetes and the mechanism of action involved.

11.2   Gut Microbiota

Gut microbiota encompasses diverse microorganisms inhabiting the human gastro-intestinal tract. The dynamic community of gut microbiota is predominantly populated by species from the prokaryotic domain which are dominated by bacteria. Additionally, fungi, parasites, archae, and viruses also constitute the environment to lesser extent. Together, they work in harmony to carry out various biological functions in the host body such as

The Gut Microbiota in Health and Disease, First Edition. Edited by Nimmy Srivastava, Salam A. Ibrahim, Jayeeta Chattopadhyay, and Mohamed H. Arbab.
© 2023 John Wiley & Sons Ltd. Published 2023 by John Wiley & Sons Ltd.

metabolism of nutrients, conserving the metabolic and immune homeostasis, protecting the host against pathogens, modulating cognitive functions of the brain, and regulating host immunity [6]. Any alteration in the gut microbiota leads to an unbalanced ecosystem, which causes a condition known as dysbiosis, which further acts as the causal link for the onset of various disorders and diseases. The process of microbial colonisation is dependent on numerous host factors. In addition, the vicinity of the gastro-intestinal tract with different chemical environments is a vital deciding factor that allows certain microbes to thrive better than others [7]. There are various internal and external factors and life events which modulate the composition that may bring about greater diversity [8]. Every individual's gut microbiota is characterised by distinct taxonomy and functions, growth, and development processes such as infant transitions (mode of delivery and feeding), age, body mass index (BMI), altered lifestyle, dietary patterns, ethnicity, cultural habits, and oxidative stress [6]. Anatomical intestinal regions and further environmental factors such as antibiotic use bring about substantial changes in gut microbiota. The physiological gut microbiota variations have wide implications in intestinal and extra-intestinal disorders. It is often difficult to precisely predict whether the changes are beneficial or detrimental to the host. Some of the disorders are also caused by external stimulations which may be stressful and disruptive for gut microbiome; some of which are irritable bowel syndrome (IBS), inflammatory bowel diseases (IBD), celiac disease (CD), colorectal cancer, obesity, diabetes central nervous system (CNS) related disorders, Alzheimer's, Parkinson's, hepatic encephalopathy, and autism spectrum disorders [9].

11.3 Role of Gut Microbiota in Diabetes

Dysbiosis of the host microbiota equilibrium leads to the disruption of gut barrier function and increase in gut permeability, which leads to an influx of inflammatory bacterial fragments. Elevated gut permeability ultimately leads to increased translocation of bacterial endotoxins, primarily lipopolysaccharide (LPS) which is an essential component of gram-negative bacteria [10]. The higher level of metabolic endotoxemia drives to low-grade systemic inflammation that consequently promotes insulin resistance, hyperglycemia, and hyperinsulinemia [11]. Gut microbiota activate host inflammation and insulin resistance through the activity of lipopolysaccharide (LPS) [3]. The role of LPS is important as it aids in increasing the level of pro-inflammatory cytokines via toll-like receptors (TLRs), thereby portraying an essential role in causing pancreatic beta-cell failure in susceptible individuals [12]. On reaching systemic circulation, LPS binds the plasma LPS-binding protein (LBP), which ultimately leads to the activation of a receptor protein CD14, which is positioned in the plasma membrane of macrophages. This complex in turn binds to toll-like receptor 4 (TLR4) on the macrophages membrane, activating the synthesis of several inflammatory effectors, namely, nuclear factor κB (NF-κB) [13], which are categorised by increased production of inflammatory factors such as TNF-γ, IL-1β, IL-6, and TNF-α. Subsequently, abnormal phosphorylation of insulin receptor substrate and insulin resistance follows [14] (see Figure 11.1).

Unhealthy dietary habits, such as high-sugar and high-fat diet, alter the composition of the gut microbiota. This disruption increases the permeability, which leads to an influx of

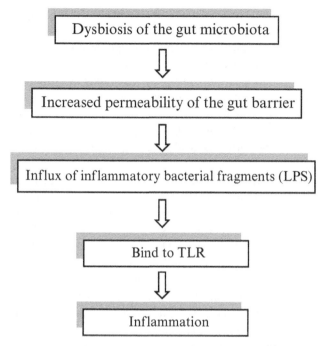

Figure 11.1 Disruption of the gut barrier is an important cause of metabolic inflammation in the body.

inflammatory bacterial fragments. Successively, the bacterial component LPS binds to TLR on the surface of the intestinal epithelial cells, recruiting immune cells in the intestine, which cause other proinflammatory cytokines to be released, resulting to inflammation.

Gut microbiota yields energy from hydrolysis and fermentation of non-digestible polysaccharides. Further, they generate monosaccharides and short chain fatty acids (SCFAs). SCFAs are one of the prominent primary end-products of bacterial fermentation, which impose huge effects on the physiology of the host and function as signaling molecules between intestinal microbiota and the host. SCFAs generated by the gut microbiota are predominantly acetate, butyrate, and propionate, which are beneficial for different metabolic processes such as regulation of proper function, motility, and integrity of the gastrointestinal tract [15], and are eventually taken up by the intestinal epithelial cells. *Bacteroidetes* mainly generate acetate and propionate, and *Firmicutes* produce butyrate. Acetate enters systemic circulation and reaches peripheral tissue, which is an important source of energy for intestinal cells. As an intestinal nutrient, it may increase the total cholesterol. Propionate also enters peripheral tissues, where both are used for lipogenesis and gluconeogenesis. These may increase glucose in the blood and reduce the hypercholesterolemia response caused by acetate [16]. On the other hand, butyrate may be degraded into glutamate, glutamine, and acetoacetate in the liver. Butyrate is used by intestinal epithelium, where it stimulates the regeneration of intestinal cells by repairing the intestinal mucosa, initiating the differentiation, apoptosis of normal intestinal cells, stimulates the production of intestinal mucin glycoprotein, and strengthening the defensive outcome of the mucous layer [17]. An adequate amount of butyrate, produced mainly by *Firmicutes*, leads to appropriate mucin synthesis and enhances tight junctions in the intestine. Butyrate also shows anti-inflammatory properties and decreases bacterial transport through the epithelial cells [18]. Lactate producers (*Bifidobacterium, Lactobacillus, Lactococcus*, and *Streptococcus*) were more common in contrast to butyrate producers (*Anaerostipes, Eubacterium, Fusobacterium, Faecalibacterium, Roseburia*, and *Subdoligranulum*) which were more abundant in controls. Butyrate-producing species of *Clostridium* reduce bacterial translocation, improve the organisation of tight junctions, and stimulate the synthesis of mucin, a glycoprotein maintaining the integrity of the gut epithelium, with beneficial effects against inflammation in the intestinal tissues [19].

Remarkably, complex metabolic processes occur in the host gut microbiota where colonic bacteria break down the complex carbohydrates consumed by the host into simpler monosaccharides and oligosaccharides. Furthermore, they are fermented into SCFAs and gases (hydrogen, methane, and carbon dioxide) [20]. Great amounts of SCFA acetate are produced by genus *Bifidobacterium*, belonging to *Actinobacteria* in addition to the production of lactate, which is processed by other bacteria to obtain butyrate. They perhaps improve glucose homeostasis and have a vital role in strengthening the satiety by enhancing the production of the glucagon-like peptide-1 (GLP-1) in the intestine [18]. Interestingly, the SCFAs, which are secreted by some important probiotic bacteria such as *Lactobacilli, Bifidobacteria*, and the butyrate-producing species, are found to be efficient against T1D, most possibly through the induction of apoptosis in the macrophages infiltrating the pancreatic islets. Additionally, they may lessen the progression of T2D by inducing pancreatic insulin secretion, simultaneously reducing insulin resistance while enhancing β-cell survival. GLP-1, secreted due to the SCFAs, ultimately improves the blood glucose levels in type I diabetes T1D and insulin resistance is reduced while enhancing insulin secretion in T2D. Thus, the extensively documented disruption of the SCFA producing species in both T1D and T2D results in the loss of the beneficial effects of the SCFAs and incretins [21] (see Figure 11.2).

11.4 Alteration in Gut Microbiota Composition in T1 and T2 Diabetes

11.4.1 T1D

Various studies conducted have shown that with the onset of T1D, there has been drastic shift in the *Bacteroidetes* (gram-negative):*Firmicutes* (gram-positive) ratio leading to an imbalance in its ecosystem [22]. Individuals with T1D have less diverse gut microbiota with elevated levels of microbes belonging to the genus *Bacteriodetes* (mainly *Bacteroides ovatus*), *Parabacteroides*, and decreased levels of *Firmicutes* [3, 23, 24], which facilitates the production of harmful inflammatory cytokines, such as interleukin (IL)-6, maintaining poor blood glycemic control [12]. Certain lactic acid-producing pathogenic bacteria such as *Bifidobacterium* and *Lactobacillus* were predominantly present at the later stage of T1D mellitus, leading to an increase in lactate levels and decrease in butyrate levels in the host, for which lactate-utilising and non-butyrate producing bacteria flourished, while the concentration of butyrate producing bacteria is significantly decreased, affecting the mucin

Figure 11.2 Increase in butyrate-producing bacteria enhances SCFAs (e.g., butyrate) production, which leads to increase in glucagon like peptide-1 (GLP-1), and decreases insulin resistance.

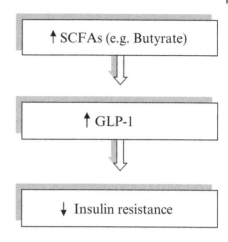

synthesis in the gut, which depleted the gut integrity and also caused β-cell auto immunity in T1D individuals [25]. Such an unbalanced environment in the gut with T1D negatively affects the growth of some beneficial bacterial genera such as *Ruminococcaceae, Lactococcus, Streptococcus,* and *Akkermansia,* which further averts the production of SCFAs, increasing gut permeability and elevating the blood glucose level [3, 22], as seen in Table 11.1.

11.4.2 Type 2 Diabetes

As mentioned earlier, individuals with T2D mellitus lack uniformity in the gut microbiota, which gives rise to a number of complications. Many studies have illustrated that the amount of beneficial butyrate and SCFA-producing bacteria, probiotics such as *Faecalibacterium (Faecalibacterium prausnitzii), Roseburia (Roseburia intestinalis, Roseburia inulinivorans),* and *Eubacterium (Eubacterium rectal)* [26], *Bifidobacterium* [12], *Firmicutes (Lactobacillus, Ruminococcus)* [27], and mucin-degrading bacteria such as *Akkermansia muciniphila* [18]

Table 11.1 Changes in the concentration of gut microbiota in Type I diabetes.

SL. No.	Gut Microbiota	Concentration in the gut during T1D mellitus	Reference
1	*Bacteroidetesi, Bacteroides ovatus*	↑	[22–24]
2	*Firmicutes*	↓	[24]
3	*Parabacteroides*	↑	[3]
4	*Bifidobacterium*	↑	[22, 25]
5	*Lactobacillus*	↑	[22, 25]
6	*Ruminococcaceae*	↓	[3]
7	*Lactococcus*	↓	[3]
8	*Streptococcus*	↓	[3]
9	*Akermansia*	↓	[3]

are remarkably reduced [3, 22, 26, 28]. Conversely, some opportunistic bacterial population such as *Actinobacteria, Bacteroidetes (Prevotella, Xylanibacter), Lactobacillus, Bacteroides (Bacteroidescaccae)* [10], *Clostridium (Clostridium clostridioforme, Clostridium hathewayi, Clostridium ramosum, Clostridium symbiosum, and Clostridium coccoides), Escherichia coli, Eggerthell asp, Proteobacteria (Betaproteo bacteria)* [1, 26], and the sulfate-reducing species *Desulfovibrio* [22] are seen to flourish in individuals suffering from T2D mellitus. Due to loss of the butyrate-producing bacteria and increase in the pathogenic bacteria population, there were complications such as elevated blood glucose levels, and increased gut permeability (leaky gut with high LPS endotoxins), which facilitates translocation of harmful pathogens across the gut epithelium into the bloodstream [26] and triggers metabolic endotoxemia. Due to the presence of metabolic endotoxemia, the production of SCFAs [29] and incretin hormone [25] are greatly reduced, insulin resistance and low-grade inflammation seem to exist, and raised level of macrophages and TNF-α were exhibited, which up-regulates the transcription of the suppressor of cytokine signaling-3 (SOCS-3). This then pairs up to the tyrosine-960 of the insulin receptor and prevents the binding of IRS-1 to the insulin receptor. This phenomenon then causes disruption of the insulin-signaling pathway by degrading the IRS-1. It is worth mentioning that Interleukin-1 (IL-1), a type of inflammatory cytokine belonging to the interleukin family, also has a potential effect to suppress the expression or gene transcription of IRS-1, peroxisome proliferator-activated receptors (PPARs), reduce the translocation of GLUT-4 into the plasma membrane and inhibit insulin-stimulated tyrosine phosphorylation and insulin-stimulated glucose uptake, which is associated with lower glucose tolerance, enhanced islet dysfunction, and increased insulin resistance in the individual with T2D [3]. Several others factors such as SCFAs, bile acids, LPS, BCAAs, and imidazole propionate are also associated with gut microbiota and have been elucidated in T2D [14], as seen in Table 11.2.

Table 11.2 Changes in the concentration of gut microbiota in Type 2 diabetes.

S L. No.	Gut Microbiota	Concentrat ion in the gut during Type 2 diabetes mellitus	Reference
1	*Faecalibacterium, Faecalibacterium prausnitzii*	↓	[26]
2	*Roseburia, Roseburia intestinalis, Roseburia inulinivorans*	↓	[26]
3	*Eubacterium, Eubacterium rectal*	↓	[26]
4	*Bifidobacterium*	↓	[12]
5	*Firmicutes, Lactobacillus, Ruminococcus*	↓	[27]
6	*Akkermansia muciniphila*	↓	[18]
7	*Actinobacteria*	↑	
8	*Bacteroidetes, Prevotella, Xylanibacter*	↑	[27]

(Continued)

Table 11.2 (Continued)

S L. No.	Gut Microbiota	Concentrat ion in the gut during Type 2 diabetes mellitus	Reference
9	*Lactobacillus*	↑	[12]
10	*Bacteroides, Bacteroides caccae*	↑	[13]
10	*Clostridium, Clostridium clostridioforme, Clostridium hathewayi, Clostridium ramosum, Clostridium symbiosum, Clostridium coccoides*	↑	[26]
11	*Escherichia coli*	↑	[26]
12	*Eggerthell asp*	↑	[26]
13	*Proteobacteria, Betaproteobacteria*	↑	[26]
14	*Desulfovibrio*	↑	[22]

11.5 Diabetic Complications

11.5.1 Diabetic Retinopathy

Diabetic retinopathy (DR) is one of the most common microvascular complications and a major cause of blindness and vision impairment in the working age population worldwide [30], and usually develops 10 to 15 years after initial diagnosis of diabetes. Globally, it is estimated that the number of individuals with DR will be approximately 191 million by 2030. The commencement and development of DR is complicated and has been related to various factors, including disease duration, glycemia, and blood pressure control. However, the ultimate molecular mechanisms in DR pathogenesis remain inadequate and indistinct [31].

Diabetic retinopathy is a complication of poorly controlled diabetes, in which eye pressure increases and elevated levels of glucose in blood vessels may affect the normal conditions of the eye. In addition, complications such as retinal microglia activation increases and infiltration of immune cells into the retina were found with diabetic retinopathy. DR also results due to the variations of overall gut microbiota. Approximately 87% of microorganisms in the eye are *Actinobacteria*, *Firmicutes*, and *Proteobacteria*; and a drastic decrease in the proportion of *Actinobacteria* and *Bacteroidetes* was observed in diabetic retinopathy individuals as compared to healthy individuals. On the other hand, significant enhancement in the proportion of *Acidaminococcus* was observed. In bacterial diabetic retinopathy, species such as *Escherichia* and *Enterobacter* also appears in the microbiota of patients [32].

11.5.2 Diabetic Nephropathy

Diabetic nephropathy (DN), a common microvascular complication of diabetes mellitus, is characterised by proteinuria, hypertension, and reduction in kidney function, leading to the cause of end-stage renal disease (ESRD). Almost one-third of diabetic individuals have

DN and its prevalence is increasing globally. Some species of gut microbiota are found to be detrimental in DN viz., *Alistipes*, *Bacteroides*, *Subdoligranulum*, *Lachnoclostridium*, and *Ruminococcus*. In DN individuals, *Enterobacteriaceae* and *Proteobacteriaceae* could enhance production of pro-inflammatory substances [33]. Hyperglycemic condition stimulates numerous events that lead to destruction of kidneys, both structurally and functionally. In the pathogenesis of diabetic kidney disease (DKD), prominent factors such as renal hemodynamics change, renin–angiotensin–aldosterone system, oxidative stress, inflammatory responses, and fibrosis play a crucial role [34]. Subsequently, DN extensively enhances the risk of developing cardiovascular disease and end-stage kidney disease (ESKD), which eventually necessitates dialysis or kidney transplantation [12]. The gut microbial ecosystem of DN individuals was drastically different from that of non-DN individuals, and remarkable increases in *Proteobacteria*, *Selenomonadales*, *Neosynechococcus*, *Shigella*, *Bilophila*, *Acidaminococcus*, *Escherichia coli*, *Bacteroidesplebeius*, *Megasphaera elsdenii*, *Acidaminococcus*, and *Bilophila wadsworthia* were reported.

11.5.3 Diabetic Neuropathy

Diabetic neuropathy, a neuro degenerative disease associated with chronic uncontrolled diabetes, damages the peripheral nerves triggering pain and numbness. Diabetic neuropathy also leads to the alteration of the gut microbiota. In diabetic neuropathy, an individuals' upsurge in *Firmicutes* and *Actinobacteria* and decline in *Bacteroidetes* was prevalent, contrary to individuals with diabetes without diabetic neuropathy and healthy individuals (see Figure 11.3). Likewise, at the genus level, a reduction of *Bacteroides* and *Faecalibacterium*, and rise of *Escherichia shigella*, *Lachnoclosridium*, *Blautia*, *Megasphaera*, and *Ruminococcus torques* were observed [20].

11.6 Therapeutic Approaches

Diabetes mellitus is a complex multi-system disorder associated with a number of life changing complications with no cure, so proper diagnosis and treatment play an important role in managing the disease appropriately. As described in this chapter, we have seen that the gut microbiota heavily contributes to the cause and consequence of the disease. Hence, alteration of the gut microbiota with beneficial microbes may be adopted as a potential

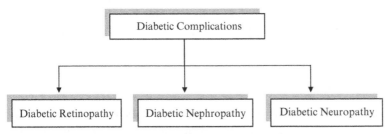

Figure 11.3 Diabetes mellitus is associated with various diabetic complications such as diabetic nephropathy, diabetic retinopathy, and diabetic neuropathy.

therapeutic strategy in controlling the disease. Some of the best-known and safe therapeutic methods which are put into application for altering the gut microbiome are shown here:

1) Balanced diet.
2) Probiotics: Used for prevention of dysbiosis when the patient is susceptible to predisposing factors (chronic disorder and diseases such as diabetes, obesity, physical and mental stress, and extended antibiotic therapies) and may also act as therapeutic agents to rebalance prolonged condition of dysbiosis [35].
3) Prebiotics: Usually non-digestible food substances which are used along with probiotics to increase their efficacy and produce beneficial physiological effects. Some well-known, characterised, and frequently used prebiotics are fructo-oligosaccharide supplements (FOS), galacto-oligosaccharides (GOS), inulin, lactulose, breast milk oligosaccharides, and xylooligosaccharide (XOS) [35].
4) Synbiotics: Combinations of pre-biotics and probiotics which have synergistic impacts in improving the gut health [35].
5) Fecal microbiota transplant (FMT): A process by which the fecal matter or feces from a healthy donor are used for therapeutic purpose to restore eubiosis in patients with gut dysbiosis. Although it is a very simple technique, FMT must be done with care, and selection of a donor should be done only after conducting necessary precautionary tests [35].
6) Bacterial consortium transplantation (BCT): The use of BCT is similar to FMT, but BCT only uses characterised microbial populations of specific fecal bacteria from the healthy donor [35].
7) Phage therapy: Utilises phages, which are actually viruses that infect bacteria. Genetically modified phages can be used as 'gene carriers,' a potential therapeutic agent to carry out for various processes such as synthesis and degradation of nutrients as well as genetic modulation of the intestinal microbiota [35].
8) Administration of predatory bacteria: Predatory bacteria are a class of microorganism which is smaller than their prey; this feature allows them to penetrate inside its prey and destroy it and replicate [35].

These are some effective and relevant agents in controlling the desired bacterial populations in the gut to bring about eubiosis.

11.7 Conclusion

Since the incidence of diabetes mellitus has increased during the past few decades, it has led to several negative impacts on the health status of human population on a global scale. With growing evidence, it has been proposed that the gut microbiota not only play a major role in absorption of nutrients, energy homeostasis, building up host immune system, modulation of inflammatory processes, and making alterations in expression of human genome, but also acts as one of the most important environmental factors, which has both positive and negative impact over the onset of diabetes. Throughout the chapter we have discussed the gut microbiota, its alterations during diabetic condition, its impact on health and disease, the possible mechanisms involved in association with diabetes, and the complications it leads to. The concept of using gut microbiota and its alterations as a potential therapeutic agent in managing diabetes and other disorders has also been well documented. Hence, the details provided in this chapter produces a better insight in understanding how strongly the gut microbes are linked to diabetes mellitus and how it is worthy for future investments and efforts.

References

1 Salgaço, M.K., Oliveira, L.G.S., Costa, G.N. et al. (2019). Relationship between gut microbiota, probiotics, and type 2 diabetes mellitus. *Appl. Microbio. Biotech*. Springer 103: 9229–9238.

2 Zheng, H., Xu, P., Jiang, Q. et al. (2021). Depletion of acetate-producing bacteria from the gut microbiota facilitates cognitive impairment through the gut-brain neural mechanism in diabetic mice. *Microbiome* 9 (1).

3 Cunningham, A.L., Stephens, J.W., and Harris, D.A. (2021). Gut microbiota influence in type 2 diabetes mellitus (T2DM). *Gut Patho. BioMed Cent. Ltd*. 13.

4 Yang, G., Wei, J., Liu, P. et al. (2021). Role of the gut microbiota in type 2 diabetes and related diseases. In: *Metabolism: Clinical and Experimental*, 117. W.B. Saunders.

5 Alvarez, S.C., Kashani, A., Hansen, T.H. et al. (2021). Trans-ethnic gut microbiota signatures of type 2 diabetes in Denmark and India. *Geno. Med*. 13 (1).

6 Jabbehdari, S. and Sallam, A.B. (2022). Gut microbiome and diabetic retinopathy. *Euro. J. Ophthal*. 32. SAGE Publications Ltd.

7 Bander, Z., Nitert, M.D., Mousa, A. et al. (2020). The gut microbiota and inflammation: an overview. *Int. J. Enviro. Res. Pub. Health*, MDPIAG 117: 1–22.

8 Gilbert, J.A., Blaser, M.J., Caporaso, J.G. et al. (2018). Current understanding of the human microbiome. *Nat. Med*. 24 (4): 392–400.

9 Rinninella, E., Raoul, P., Cintoni, M. et al. (2019). What is the healthy gut microbiota composition? A changing ecosystem across age, environment, diet, and diseases. *Microorganisms* 7 (1).

10 Duan, L., An, X., Zhang, Y. et al. (2021). Gut microbiota as the critical correlation of polycystic ovary syndrome and type 2 diabetes mellitus. In: *Biomed. Pharmaco.*, 142. Elsevier Massons.

11 Howard, E.J., Lam, T.K.T., and Duca, F.A. (2021). *The gut microbiome: connecting diet, glucose homeostasis, and disease*. https://doi: 10.1146/annurev-med-042220-012821.

12 Zaky, A., Glastras, S.J., Wong, M.Y.W. et al. (2021). The role of the gut microbiome in diabetes and obesity-related kidney disease. *Int. J. Molec. Sci*. 22.

13 Moffa, S., Mezza, T., Cefalo, C.M.A. et al. (2019). The interplay between immune system and microbiota in diabetes. *Medi. Inflam*. Hindawi Limited.

14 Zhang, L., Chu, J., Hao, W. et al. (2021). Gut microbiota and type 2 diabetes mellitus: association, mechanism, and translational applications. *Medi. Inflam*. Hindawi Limited.

15 Alagiakrishnan, K. and Halverson, T. (2021). Holistic perspective of the role of gut microbes in diabetes mellitus and its management. *World J. Diab*. 12 (9): 1463–1478.

16 Woldeamlak, B., Yirdaw, K., and Biadgo, B. (2019). Role of gut microbiota in type 2 diabetes mellitus and its complications: novel insights and potential intervention strategies. *Korean J. Gastroent*. 74: 314–320.

17 Upadhyaya, S. and Banerjee, G. (2015). Type 2 diabetes and gut microbiome: at the intersection of known and unknown. In: *Gut Microbes*, 6, 85–92. Taylor & Francis Inc.

18 Bielka, W., Przezak, A., and Pawlik, A. (2022). The role of the gut microbiota in the pathogenesis of diabetes. *Int. J. Molec. Sci.* 23.

19 Bibbò, S., Dore, M.P., Pes, G.M. et al. (2017). Is there a role for gut microbiota in type 1 diabetes pathogenesis? In: *Annals of Medicine*, 49, 11–22. Taylor & Francis Ltd.

20 Tanase, D.M., Gosav, E.M., Neculae, E. et al. (2020). Role of gut microbiota on onset and progression of microvascular complications of type 2 diabetes (T2DM). *Nutrients* 12: 1–26.

21 Kanbay, M., Onal, E.M., Afsar, B. et al. (2018). The crosstalk of gut microbiota and chronic kidney disease: role of inflammation, proteinuria, hypertension, and diabetes mellitus. In: *International Urology and Nephrology*, 50, 1453–1466. Springer Netherlands.

22 Patterson, E.E., Ryan, P.M., Cryan, J.F. et al. (2016). Gut microbiota, obesity and diabetes. In: *Postgraduate Medical Journal*, 92, 286–300. BMJ Publishing Group.

23 Dedrick, S., Sundaresh, B., Huang, Q. et al. (2020). The role of gut microbiota and environmental factors in type 1 diabetes pathogenesis. *Front. Endocrin.* 11.

24 Han, H., Li, Y., Fang, J. et al. (2018). Gut microbiota and type 1 diabetes. *Int. J. Molec. Sci.* 19.

25 Baothman, O.A., Zamzami, M.A., Taher, I. et al. (2016). The role of gut microbiota in the development of obesity and diabetes. In: *Lipids in Health and Disease*, 15. Bio. Med. Central Ltd.

26 Bordalo, T.L., dos Santos, K.M.O., de Luces Fortes Ferreira, C.L. et al. (2017). Gut microbiota and probiotics: focus on diabetes mellitus. *Crit. Rev. Food Sci. Nutri.* 57 (11): 2296–2309.

27 Hasain, Z., Mokhtar, N.M., Kamaruddin, N.A. et al. (2020). Gut microbiota and gestational diabetes mellitus: a review of host–gut microbiota interactions and their therapeutic potential. *Front. Cell. Infec. Microbio.* 10.

28 Que, Y., Cao, M., He, J. et al. (2021). Gut Bacterial characteristics of patients with type 2 diabetes mellitus and the application potential. *Front. Imm.* 12.

29 Aw, W. and Fukuda, S. (2018). Understanding the role of the gut ecosystem in diabetes mellitus. *J. Diab. Investin.* 9: 5–12.

30 Ye, P., Zhang, X., Xu, Y. et al. (2021). Alterations of the gut microbiome and metabolome in patients with proliferative diabetic retinopathy. *Front. Microbio.* 1.

31 Jiao, J., Yu, H., Yao, L. et al. (2021). Recent insights into the role of gut microbiota in diabetic retinopathy. *J. Inflam. Res.* 14 (692): 9–38.

32 Iatcu, C.O., Steen, A., and Covasa, M. (2022). Gut microbiota and complications of type-2 diabetes. *Nutrients* 14.

33 He, X., Sun, J., Liu, C. et al. (2022). Compositional alterations of gut microbiota in patients with diabetic kidney disease and type 2 diabetes mellitus. *Dia., Meta. Synd. Obesity: Tar. Ther.* 15: 755–765.

34 Fang, Q., Liu, N., Zheng, B. et al. (2021). Roles of Gut Microbial Metabolites in Diabetic Kidney Disease. *Front. Endocrin.* 12.

35 Gagliardi, A., Totino, V., Cacciotti, F. et al. (2018). Rebuilding the gut microbiota ecosystem. *Int. J. Enviro. Res. Pub. Health* 15 (8): 1679.

12

Novel Therapeutic Strategies Targeting Gut Microbiota to Treat Diseases

Shaimaa H. Negm

Department of Home Economic, Specific Education Faculty, Port Said University, Egypt

12.1   Introduction

Diabetes is a category of metabolic illnesses defined by hyperglycemia due to insulin insufficiency, either directly or indirectly. T1D is an autoimmune illness in which antibodies are created against numerous parts of pancreatic cells, causing the islets that produce insulin to degrade and eventually die, resulting in a lack of insulin [1]. Insulin resistance (IR) causes T2D by increasing the demand for insulin in peripheral tissues, and as a result, causing the functional failure of cells [2]. Inadequate metabolic control of diabetes may result in major long-term consequences such as retinopathy, chronic renal disease, neuropathy, and cardiovascular disease, as well as an elevated mortality rate [3].

Humans rely on the gut bacteria functioning properly [4], and changes in the makeup of gut bacteria have a role in the aetiology of diseases such as obesity, diabetes, and heart failure [5, 6], which are all on the rise worldwide. As a result, it is critical to decipher whether microorganisms play a role in the development of civilisation's ailments, as it can not only help to alter their course or delay the emergence of complications, but also help to prevent the disorders from occurring initially. We describe the differences in the gut microbiota in patients with T1D and T2D compared to healthy individuals in this chapter, explain the potential impact of altered bacterial composition on the host organism, and suggest potential therapeutic targets aimed at the microbiota that may influence the course of diabetes.

12.2   Changes in the Composition of the Gut Microbiota in Patients with T1D

It is believed that T1D is linked to the stability, connection, quantity, and composition of the gut microbiota [7]. Several studies have found that T1D patients have a different gut microbiome than healthy people. A high Firmicutes to Bacteroidetes ratio and microbiome instability may be one of the early diagnostic markers of emerging autoimmune illnesses such as T1D, according to Giongo et al. [8]. De Goffau et al. investigated the gut microbiota composition during the beginning of T1D in young children. *Bacteroidetes* and *Streptococcus mitis* were shown to be more prevalent in diabetic youngsters, while the butyrate makers

Lactobacillus plantarum and *Clostridium clusters* IV and XIVa were found to be more prevalent in healthy controls [9]. Meja-León et al. came to similar results; T1D patients showed a Bacteroides dominance upon diagnosis, whereas controls had a higher amount of *Prevotella*, but after 2 years of insulin treatment, the gut microbiota of patients and controls were identical [10]. In the TEDDY longitudinal investigation, the fecal microbiota of people with early-onset T1D were also examined using metagenomic sequencing. According to Vatanen et al., the levels of *Roseburia hominis*, *Alistipes shahii*, and *Bifidobacterium pseudocatenulatum* were greater in stool samples from children with T1D, whereas *Lactococcus lactis* and *Streptococcus thermophilus* were higher in controls without T1D. The youngsters in the control group had more species found in dairy products, as well as more genera involved with short chain fatty acid (SCFA) production and fermentation in their microbiota. This study backs up the idea that SCFAs protect against T1D [11]. In the duodenal mucosa of T1D patients, Pellegrini et al. discovered a distinct inflammatory profile and microbiome. Increased inflammation and monocyte/macrophage lineage infiltration were found in mucosa samples. Firmicutes levels and the Firmicutes/Bacteroidetes ratio were higher in T1D patients, but *Proteobacteria* and *Bacteroidetes* levels were lower [12].

12.3 The Potential Role of the Gut Microbiota in the Development of T1D

T1D is described as a pro-inflammatory state mediated by cells that is caused by both innate and adaptive immunity [13]. The primary causes of a genetic propensity to T1D development are specific human leucocyte antigen (HLA) genotypes such as DQ2, DQ8, DR3, and some DR4 alleles [14].

Environmental factors such as feeding habits, food, and early childhood viral exposure are all critical contributors in disease initiation [15]. Furthermore, changing gut bacterial composition has been linked to insulin dysregulation and T1D development [16]. Such processes as immune system development, gut microbiota maturation, and the appearance of the first autoantibodies linked to T1D occur during early childhood [12].

Breastfeeding, diet, delivery method, antibiotic usage, and exposure to bacteria in the environment are all factors that may alter the composition of the gut microbiota [17]. Their actions may cause intestinal barrier disturbance and delayed immune response maturation, which may lead to T1D progression later in life [18]. Furthermore, the host's genetic make-up may interact with the gut microbiota, resulting in alterations in microbial composition, immune activation, and vulnerability to T1D [19].

Dysbiosis-induced intestinal inflammation and a decrease in SCFAs may be important in the aetiology of T1D [20]. Increased intestinal permeability is thought to precede the clinical onset of T1D [21]. A butyrate-rich diet increased the number and function of regulatory T cells [22], whereas acetate- and butyrate-rich diets reduced serum levels of diabetogenic cytokines such IL-21 and improved gut integrity. In non-obese diabetic (NOD) mice, this sort of diet reduced the incidence of diabetes, while female NOD mice also had a higher number of pancreatic islets that were free of invasion [23]. Because Lipopolysaccharides (LPSs) decrease pancreatic cell function and raise levels of pro-inflammatory cytokines, they may play a role in the development of diabetes [24]. Figure 12.1 depicts the potential impact of dysbiosis on T1D progression.

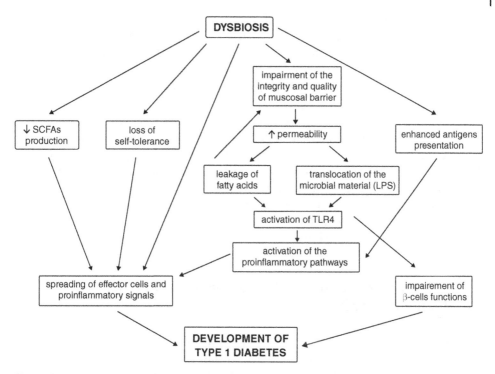

Figure 12.1 The possible influence of dysbiosis on type 1 diabetes development. *Source:* [25] / MDPI/ CC BY 4.0.

12.4 Changes in the Composition of the Gut Microbiota in Patients with T2D

T2D patients' microbiome differs from healthy people's microbiota in the same way that T1D patients' microbiota differs from healthy people's microbiota [16]. According to numerous studies, the main alteration is an increase in opportunistic infections and a decrease in bacteria generating butyrate, one of the SCFAs [24]. Larsen et al. found lower levels of the phylum Firmicutes and the class Clostridia in one of the first studies on the microbiota of T2D patients. Furthermore, the Bacteroidetes/Firmicutes ratio was favourably linked with plasma glucose levels, as was the Bacteroidetes–Prevotella/*C. coccoides E.* rectal ratio. Furthermore, the Betaproteo bacteria class was elevated and was linked with decreased glucose tolerance [26].

According to Qin et al. and Karlsson et al., the gut microbiota of people with T2D is characterised by higher levels of opportunistic pathogens and lower levels of butyrate makers Faecalibacterium and Roseburia [27, 28]. In T2D patients, Zhang et al. found a lower level of Akkermansia muciniphila [29]. Allin et al. made a similar observation, finding that people with prediabetes have fewer Clostridium and Akkermansia muciniphila species than do healthy people [30]. Sedighi et al., in contrast to Larsen et al., found a lower level of Bacteroidetes and a higher level of Firmicutes and Proteobacteria, resulting in a higher Firmicutes/Bacteroidetes ratio [31]. Zhao et al. later corroborated these findings, but they also revealed that the increased Firmicutes/Bacteroidetes ratio was much larger in T2D-affected people with illness problems than in those without issues [32].

The injection of *B. acidifaciens* and *B. uniformis* to diabetic rodents improved their glucose tolerance and IR in animal tests [33]. Bacteroides appear to have a possibly favourable influence on glucose metabolism, which could explain the negative connection between Bacteroides and T2D. Firmicutes includes the genera *Roseburia, Faecalibacterium, Lactobacillus, Ruminococcus,* and *Blautia. Roseburia* levels have been observed to be lower in T2D patients than in healthy people [34–36]. *R. intestinalis* was positively related with diabetes, while *R. inulinivorans* and *Roseburia* 272 were negatively associated [28, 35, 37]. Fecal bacterium levels were shown to be lower in T2D patients, although *F. prausnitzii* was found to be inversely linked with the disease at the species level [28, 35, 36, 38]. Some Lactobacillus species, such as *L. acidophilus* or *L. salivarius,* are favourably related with T2D, whereas others, such as *L. amylovorus,* are negatively connected with diabetes [28, 34, 39]. Bifidobacterium species, which belong to the Actinobacteria family, are closely linked to T2D [34, 38, 40]. *Bifidobacterium* spp. improved glucose tolerance in diabetic mice in animal trials, suggesting a protective role for bifidobacteria in T2D [41].

12.5 The Potential Role of the Gut Microbiota in the Development of T2D

T2D is primarily caused by insufficient insulin secretion by cells in the pancreas and a condition known as 'insulin resistance,' which is defined as the inability of insulin-sensitive tissues to respond appropriately to insulin [42]. Insulin secretion is reduced when cells are dysfunctional, resulting in higher glucose levels in the blood. IR elevates glycemia via stimulating glucose synthesis in the liver and impairing glucose absorption in the liver, muscle, and adipose tissue. Chronic hyperglycemia develops because of this scenario, affecting many organs and tissues, and causing harmful micro- and macrovascular problems [43]. Chronic low-grade inflammation is linked to the onset of IR and, as a result, T2D develops [44].

Genetic predisposition, ethnicity, and family history of diabetes, as well as metabolic and environmental factors such obesity, low-grade physical activity, and diet are all risk factors for T2D. Obesity is the most significant risk factor, as it is linked to metabolic alterations that lead to IR [45].

Much of our knowledge of the importance of the gut microbiota is based on studies involving germ-free animals who are born and raised without exposure to bacteria, but may be exposed to specific germs during the research. These rodents are resistant to diet-induced obesity [46], and exposure to *Enterobacter cloacae*, a bacterium linked to obesity, or bacteria obtained from obese donors causes increased energy harvesting capacity, weight gain, and decreased glucose tolerance [47].

These findings point to a possible link between the gut microbiome and obesity. T2D is marked by a reduction in the generation of butyrate [24], one of the SCFAs that helps cells in the pancreas function properly, especially after food consumption [48]. Butyrate plays a role in immune system regulation and protection against pathogen invasion [49], and it stimulates intestinal gluconeogenesis, which has a positive impact on glucose homeostasis [50]. Sanna et al. found that a host genetically-driven increase in gut butyrate production is linked to a better insulin response after an oral glucose test, and that anomalies in propionate production or absorption are causally linked to an increased risk of T2D [48]. Figure 12.2 depicts the potential impact of dysbiosis on the progression of T2D.

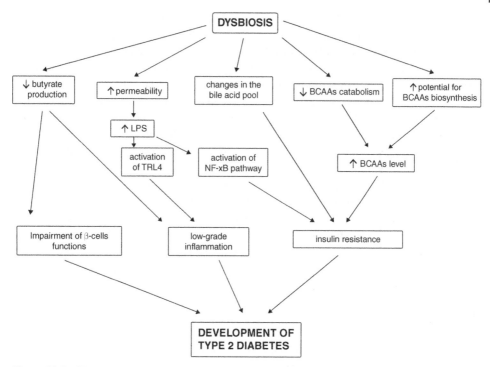

Figure 12.2 The possible influence of dysbiosis on type 2 diabetes development. *Source:* [25] / MDPI/ CC BY 4.0.

12.7 Preventive and Therapeutic Perspectives Including the Gut Microbiota

The gut microbial community may be influenced by a balanced diet and physical activity, among other things. *Roseburia hominis*, *Akkermansia muciniphila*, and *Faecalibacterium prausnitzii* were shown to be more abundant in active women than in sedentary women [51]. The Mediterranean diet, as well as the use of dietary substances including green tea, caffeine, and omega-3 polyunsaturated fatty acids aid in the restoration of the altered intestinal bacterial composition [52]. Obese patients who follow a carbohydrate- or fat-restricted low-calorie diet have seen their Firmicutes/Bacteroidetes ratio shift again [53]. Furthermore, a fibre-rich diet is linked to higher levels of Prevotella, and a protein-rich diet is linked to higher levels of Bacteroides [54]. Six obese individuals with T2D and/or hypertension had significantly lower HbA1c and triglyceride levels, decreased body weight, and better fasting and postprandial glucose levels after one month on a strict vegetarian diet. This diet is linked to a lower Firmicutes/Bacteroidetes ratio and higher levels of *Clostridium* and *Bacteroides fragilis*, resulting in lower intestinal inflammation and SCFA levels [55].

Probiotics are live bacteria that may modify the gut microbiota when consumed as food or as a supplement [56], and the principal probiotics with glucose-lowering potential are *Lactobacillus* species [56]. A daily dose of *Lactobacillus reuteri* increases insulin and incretin secretion in persons with normal glucose tolerance, although the impact is linked to improved cell activity [57]. Furthermore, a study found that early oral exposure to probiotics may reduce the incidence of islet autoimmunity in children with the high-risk HLA DR3/4 genotype, which is linked to T1D susceptibility [58]. Prebiotics and probiotics are combined in synbiotics; a diet supplemented with either prebiotics or synbiotics has the ability to maintain glucose homeostasis and enhance lipid metabolism in people with T2D [59].

A gluten-free diet may aid in the protection of cell function by affecting the gut microbiome, which has been linked to diabetes [60]. Furthermore, a high-fat diet may alter the composition of the gut microbiota, mostly by reducing Bifidobacterium. Prebiotics may help prevent high-fat diet-induced diabetes by improving glucose tolerance, insulin secretion, lowering intestinal endotoxin levels, and reducing inflammation [61]. Vitamin A deficiency raises the Firmicutes/Bacteroidetes ratio and lowers the number of bacteria that produce butyrate [62]. Furthermore, retinoic acid, a vitamin A metabolite, may decrease pro-inflammatory Th17 cell differentiation while promoting anti-inflammatory Treg cell differentiation [63], and these systems help to prevent the onset of T1D. Zinc deficiency also affects the inflammatory response and metabolic regulation, which can increase the risk of T1D [64].

References

1 Bluestone, J.A., Herold, K., and Eisenbarth, G. (2010). Genetics, pathogenesis and clinical interventions in type 1 diabetes. *Nat. Cell Biol.* 464: 1293–1300.
2 Kahn, S.E., Cooper, M.E., and Del Prato, S. (2014). Pathophysiology and treatment of type 2 diabetes: perspectives on the past, present, and future. *Lancet* 383: 1068–1083.
3 Orchard, T., Nathan, D.M., Zinman, B. et al. (2015). Association between 7 years of intensive treatment of Type 1 Diabetes and long-term mortality. *JAMA J. Am. Med. Assoc.* 313: 45–53.
4 Vrancken, G., Gregory, A.C., Huys, G.R.B. et al. (2019). Synthetic ecology of the human gut microbiota. *Nat. Rev. Genet.* 17: 754–763.
5 Faith, J.J., Guruge, J.L., Charbonneau, M. et al. (2013). The long-term stability of the human gut microbiota. *Science* 341: 1237439.
6 Tang, W.W., Kitai, T., and Hazen, S.L. (2017). Gut microbiota in cardiovascular health and disease. *Circ. Res.* 120: 1183–1196.
7 Han, H., Li, Y., Fang, J. et al. (2018). Gut microbiota and Type 1 Diabetes. *Int. J. Mol. Sci.* 19: 995.
8 Giongo, A., Gano, K.A., Crabb, D.B. et al. (2011). Toward defining the autoimmune microbiome for type 1 diabetes. *ISME J.* 5: 82–91.
9 de Goffau, M., Fuentes, S., Bogert, B.V.D. et al. (2014). Aberrant gut microbiota composition at the onset of type 1 diabetes in young children. *Diabetologia* 57: 1569–1577.
10 Mejía-León, M.E., Petrosino, J.F., Ajami, N.J. et al. (2015). Fecal microbiota imbalance in Mexican children with type 1 diabetes. *Sci. Rep.* 4: 3814.
11 Vatanen, T., Franzosa, E.A., Schwager, R. et al. (2018). The human gut microbiome in early-onset type 1 diabetes from the TEDDY study. *Nature* 562: 589–594.

12 Pellegrini, S., Sordi, V., Bolla, A.M. et al. (2017). Duodenal mucosa of patients with type 1 diabetes shows distinctive inflammatory profile and microbiota. *J. Clin. Endocrinol. Metab.* 102: 1468–1477.

13 Devaraj, S., Dasu, M.R., and Jialal, I. (2010). Diabetes is a proinflammatory state: a translational perspective. *Expert Rev. Endocrinol. Metab.* 5: 19–28.

14 Hu, Y., Wong, F.S., and Wen, L. (2017). Antibiotics, gut microbiota, environment in early life and type 1 diabetes. *Pharmacol. Res.* 119: 219–226.

15 Rewers, M. and Ludvigsson, J. (2016). Environmental risk factors for type 1 diabetes. *Lancet* 387: 2340–2348.

16 Bachem, A., Makhlouf, C., Binger, K.J. et al. (2019). Microbiota-derived short-chain fatty acids promote the memory potential of antigen-activated CD8+ T Cells. *Immunity* 51: 285–297.e5.

17 Milani, C., Duranti, S., Bottacini, F. et al. (2017). The first microbial colonizers of the human gut: composition, activities, and health implications of the infant gut microbiota. *Microbiol. Mol. Biol. Rev.* 81: e00036–00017.

18 Zhou, H., Sun, L., Zhang, S. et al. (2021). The crucial role of early-life gut microbiota in the development of type 1 diabetes. *Acta Diabetol.* 58: 249–265.

19 Bonder, M.J., Kurilshikov, A., Tigchelaar, E.F. et al. (2016). The effect of host genetics on the gut microbiome. *Nat. Genet.* 48: 1407–1412.

20 Ma, Q., Li, Y., Wang, J. et al. (2020). Investigation of gut microbiome changes in type 1 diabetic mellitus rats based on high-throughput sequencing. *Biomed. Pharmacother.* 124: 109873.

21 Bosi, E., Molteni, L., Radaelli, M.G. et al. (2006). Increased intestinal permeability precedes clinical onset of type 1 diabetes. *Diabetologia* 49: 2824–2827.

22 Li, W.-Z., Stirling, K., Yang, J.-J. et al. (2020). Gut microbiota and diabetes: from correlation to causality and mechanism. *W. J. Diab.* 11: 293–308.

23 Mariño, E., Richards, J.L., McLeod, K.H. et al. (2017). Gut microbial metabolites limit the frequency of autoimmune T cells and protect against type 1 diabetes. *Nat. Immunol.* 18: 552–562.

24 Allin, K.H., Nielsen, T., and Pedersen, O. (2015). Mechanisms in endocrinology: gut microbiota in patients with type 2 diabetes mellitus. *Eur. J. Endocrinol.* 172: R167–R177.

25 Bielka, W., Przezak, A., and Pawlik, A. (2022). The role of the gut microbiota in the pathogenesis of diabetes. *Int. J. Mol. Sci.* 23: 480.

26 Festi, D., Schiumerini, R., Eusebi, L.H. et al. (2014). Gut microbiota and metabolic syndrome. *W. J. Gastroenterol.* 20: 16079–16094.

27 Qin, J., Li, Y., Cai, Z. et al. (2021). A metagenome-wide association study of gut microbiota in type 2 diabetes. *Nature* 490: 55–60.

28 Karlsson, F.H., Tremaroli, V., Nookaew, I. et al. (2013). Gut metagenome in European women with normal, impaired and diabetic glucose control. *Nature* 498: 99–103.

29 Zhang, Y. and Zhang, H. (2013). Microbiota associated with type 2 diabetes and its related complications. *Food Sci. Hum. Well.* 2: 167–172.

30 Allin, K.H., Tremaroli, V., Caesar, R. et al. (2018). Aberrant intestinal microbiota in individuals with prediabetes. *Diabetologia* 61: 810–820.

31 Sedighi, M., Razavi, S., Navab-Moghadam, F. et al. (2017). Comparison of gut microbiota in adult patients with type 2 diabetes and healthy individuals. *Microb. Pathog.* 111: 362–369.

32 Zhao, L., Lou, H., Peng, Y. et al. (2019). Comprehensive relationships between gut microbiome and faecal metabolome in individuals with type 2 diabetes and its complications. *Endocrine* 66: 526–537.

33 Yang, J.-Y., Lee, Y.-S., Kim, Y. et al. (2017). Gut commensal Bacteroides acidifaciens prevents obesity and improves insulin sensitivity in mice. *Mucosal Immunol.* 10: 104–116.

34 Candela, M., Biagi, E., Soverini, M. et al. (2016). Modulation of gut microbiota dysbioses in type 2 diabetic patients by macrobiotic Ma-Pi 2 diet. *Br. J. Nutr.* 116: 80–93.

35 Zhang, X., Shen, D., Fang, Z. et al. (2013). Human gut microbiota changes reveal the progression of glucose intolerance. *PLoS ONE* 8: e71108.

36 Salamon, D., Sroka-Oleksiak, A., Kapusta, P. et al. (2018). Characteristics of the gut microbiota in adult patients with type 1 and 2 diabetes based on the analysis of a fragment of 16S rRNA gene using next-generation sequencing. *Pol. Arch. Intern. Med.* 128: 336–343.

37 Murphy, R., Tsai, P., Jüllig, M. et al. (2016). Differential changes in gut microbiota after gastric bypass and sleeve gastrectomy bariatric surgery vary according to diabetes remission. *Obes. Surg.* 27: 917–925.

38 Gao, R., Zhu, C., Li, H. et al. (2018). Dysbiosis signatures of gut microbiota along the sequence from healthy, young patients to those with overweight and obesity. *Obesity* 26: 351–361.

39 Forslund, K., Hildebrand, F., Nielsen, T. et al. (2017). Disentangling type 2 diabetes and metformin treatment signatures in the human gut microbiota. *Nature* 545: 116.

40 Sedighi, M., Razavi, S., Navab-Moghadam, F. et al. (2017). Comparison of gut microbiota in adult patients with type 2 diabetes and healthy individuals. *Microb. Pathog.* 111: 362–369.

41 Kikuchi, K., Ben Othman, M., and Sakamoto, K. (2018). Sterilized bifidobacteria suppressed fat accumulation and blood glucose level. *Biochem. Biophys. Res. Commun.* 501: 1041–1047.

42 Roden, M. and Shulman, G.I. (2019). The integrative biology of type 2 diabetes. *Nature* 576: 51–60.

43 DeFronzo, R.A. (2009). Banting Lecture. From the triumvirate to the ominous octet: a new paradigm for the treatment of type 2 diabetes mellitus. *Diabetes* 58: 773–795.

44 Gregor, M.F. and Hotamisligil, G.S. (2011). Inflammatory mechanisms in obesity. *Annu. Rev. Immunol.* 29: 415–445.

45 Bellou, V., Belbasis, L., Tzoulaki, I. et al. (2018). Risk factors for type 2 diabetes mellitus: an exposure-wide umbrella review of meta-analyses. *PLoS ONE* 13: e0194127.

46 Rabot, S., Membrez, M., Bruneau, A. et al. (2010). Germ-free C57BL/6J mice are resistant to high-fat-diet-induced insulin resistance and have altered cholesterol metabolism. *FASEB J.* 24: 4948–4959.

47 Ridaura, V.K., Faith, J.J., Rey, F.E. et al. (2013). Gut microbiota from twins discordant for obesity modulate metabolism in mice. *Science* 341: 1241214.

48 Sanna, S., Van Zuydam, N.R., Mahajan, A. et al. (2019). Causal relationships among the gut microbiome, short-chain fatty acids and metabolic diseases. *Nat. Genet.* 51: 600–605.

49 Macfarlane, G.T. and Macfarlane, S. (2011). Fermentation in the human large intestine: Its physiologic consequences and the potential contribution of prebiotics. *J. Clin. Gastroenterol.* 45: S120–S127.

50 De Vadder, F., Kovatcheva-Datchary, P., Goncalves, D. et al. (2014). Microbiota generated metabolites promote metabolic benefits via gut-brain neural circuits. *Cell* 156: 84–96.

51 Bressa, C., Bailen, M., Pérez-Santiago, J. et al. (2017). Differences in gut microbiota profile between omen with active lifestyle and sedentary women. *PLoS ONE* 12: e0171352.

52 Pascale, A., Marchesi, N., Marelli, C. et al. (2018). Microbiota and metabolic diseases. *Endocrine* 61: 357–371.

53 Bouter, K.E., van Raalte, D.H., Groen, A.K. et al. (2017). Role of the gut microbiome in the pathogenesis of obesity and obesity-related metabolic dysfunction. *Gastroenterology* 152: 1671–1678.

54 Hartstra, A.V., Bouter, K.E., Bäckhed, F. et al. (2014). Insights into the role of the microbiome in obesity and type 2 diabetes. *Diab. Care* 38: 159–165.

55 Kim, M.-S., Hwang, S.-S., Park, E.-J. et al. (2013). Strict vegetarian diet improves the risk factors associated with metabolic diseases by modulating gut microbiota and reducing intestinal inflammation. *Environ. Microbiol. Rep.* 5: 765–775.

56 Vallianou, N., Stratigou, T., Christodoulatos, G.S. et al. (2019). Understanding the role of the gut microbiome and microbial metabolites in obesity and obesity-associated metabolic disorders: current evidence and perspectives. *Curr. Obes. Rep.* 8: 317–332.

57 Simon, M.-C., Strassburger, K., Nowotny, B. et al. (2015). Intake of Lactobacillus reuteri improves incretin and insulin secretion in glucose-tolerant humans: a proof of concept. *Diab. Care* 38: 1827–1834.

58 Uusitalo, U., Liu, X., Yang, J. et al. (2016). Association of early exposure of probiotics and islet autoimmunity in the TEDDY Study. *JAMA Pediatr.* 170: 20–28.

59 Mahboobi, S., Rahimi, F., and Jafarnejad, S. (2018). Effects of prebiotic and synbiotic supplementation on glycaemia and lipid profile in type 2 diabetes: a meta-analysis of randomized controlled trials. *Adv. Pharm. Bull.* 8: 565–574.

60 Marietta, E.V., Gomez, A.M., Yeoman, C. et al. (2013). Low incidence of spontaneous type 1 diabetes in non-obese diabetic mice raised on gluten-free diets is associated with changes in the intestinal microbiome. *PLoS ONE* 8: e78687.

61 Cani, P.D., Neyrinck, A., Fava, F. et al. (2007). Selective increases of bifidobacteria in gut microflora improve high-fat-diet-induced diabetes in mice through a mechanism associated with endotoxaemia. *Diabetologia* 50: 2374–2383.

62 Tian, Y., Nichols, R., Cai, J. et al. (2018). Vitamin A deficiency in mice alters host and gut microbial metabolism leading to altered energy homeostasis. *J. Nutr. Biochem.* 54: 28–34.

63 Mucida, D., Park, Y., Kim, G. et al. (2007). Reciprocal TH 17 and regulatory T cell differentiation mediated by retinoic acid. *Science* 317: 256–260.

64 Xia, T., Lai, W., Han, M. et al. (2017). Dietary ZnO nanoparticles alter intestinal microbiota and inflammation response in weaned piglets. *Oncotarget* 8: 64878–64891.

13

Understanding the Role of Microbiota in Cancer

Parneet Kaur[1], Lisa F. M Lee Nen That[2], Saurabh Kulshreshtha[1], and Jessica Pandohee[3]

[1] Faculty of Applied Sciences and Biotechnology, Shoolini University of Biotechnology and Management Sciences, Solan, India
[2] School of Science, RMIT University, Victoria, Australia
[3] Telethon Kids Institute, Nedlands, Western Australia, Australia

13.1 Introduction

Cancer is one of the most fatal diseases in the twenty-first century. The most common cancers account for nearly 2.3 million cases (breast cancer), 2.2 million cases (lung cancer), 1.9 million cases (colon and rectum cancer), 1.4 million cases (prostate cancer), and 1.2 million cases (skin, non-melanoma cancer). Several clinical trials in order to understand the mechanism of actions of the initiation and development of cancers in humans, as well as the drug delivery and efficacy in treating and curing cancers have enabled lives of patients to be extended. With the discovery of the gut microbiota, it has become increasingly evident that the microbiota in general have the ability to provide several health benefits to its hosts. For instance, the microbiota play an essential role in maintenance of human health and the gastrointestinal tract, and influence the organs such as brain, liver, and pancreas.

While the microbiota also have the ability to prevent cancer, the microbiota may occasionally contain tumour-associated microbes that cause a range of benign and malignant cancers. Moreover, the existence of specialised microbiota has been shown to increase the effectiveness of the anti-cancer therapy with the help of chemotherapeutic drugs and immunomodulatory oligonucleotides [1], although the alteration in gut microbiota may lead to the resistance towards chemotherapy drugs. The tumour growth is suppressed with an intact microbiota in function [2]. The gut microbiota consists of trillions of bacteria along with fungi, archaea, and viruses and alterations of these may lead to various pathological conditions [3]. Therefore, understanding the role of such a complex interaction between the microbiota and its host is a challenging task. The role of cancer-causing microbes in humans and its interactions with the healthy microbiota is rapidly being unravelled. In this chapter, a detailed discussion on how the gut microbiota affects cancers and how the disease can be prevented and perhaps cured is discussed.

The Gut Microbiota in Health and Disease, First Edition. Edited by Nimmy Srivastava, Salam A. Ibrahim, Jayeeta Chattopadhyay, and Mohamed H. Arbab.
© 2023 John Wiley & Sons Ltd. Published 2023 by John Wiley & Sons Ltd.

13.2 Role of Microbiota in Cancers

13.2.1 Gastric Cancer

The influence of microbiota on cancer risk is multifactorial, impacting the metabolism of the host, functioning of the immune system, and cellular proliferation [4]. One of the leading causes of death worldwide is gastric cancer, and it is the fifth most common type of cancer. The causative agent of gastric cancer is the infection by *Helicobacter pylori*. The infection caused by *Helicobacter pylori* leads to inflammation of the gastric mucosa and causes destruction of glands of the stomach by secreting hydrochloric acid, which leads to atrophic gastritis. This Class I carcinogen play an important role in initiating steps of gastric carcinogenesis by causing increased inflammation and changes in the function of gastric mucosa, resulting in lifelong infection [5, 6].

In a recent study, the gastric microbiota was shown to consist of proteobacteria, firmicutes, Bacteroidetes, actinobacteria, fusobacteria, and specific fungal consortium (mycobiome) [7–9]. It was also shown that in gastric cancer, there is an increase in microbial community, metabolic pathways, amino acid and nitrate metabolism, membrane transport, and carbohydrate digestion and absorption as compared with the healthy gastric tissues [5]. In a recent study, samples of Korean patients with gastric cancer were analysed and *Helicobacter pylori*, *Propionibacterium acnes*, and *Prevotellacopri* showed an impact in the cancer development, whereas *Lactococcus lactis* is a protective factor [10]. For the effective treatment of gastric cancer, it is essential to eliminate the *Helicobacter pylori* and other microbiota, which are harmful to human health

13.2.2 Colorectal Cancer

Ten percent of all new cancer cases occurring globally are colorectal cancer. The gut microbiota consist of a large population of microorganisms that interact with host intestinal cells and affect the immunity and metabolome in the gastrointestinal tract [11]. The precursor for colorectal cancer is Colorectal adenomas [12]. In recent studies several gut microbial communities in patients were analysed and there was an increase in the abundance of Fusobacterium and altered microbial taxonomies [13]. The process of colorectal cancer is an intricate process, which is affected by both genetic and environmental factors; these factors include inflammation, immune regulation, metabolism of dietary components, and genotoxin production.

Microbiota are also used as a biomarker for the presence of the severity of the disease. In a recent study, *Streptococcus bovis* was found in the tissues, this is associated with high risk of colorectal cancer [14]. There are certain fecal markers which detect early colorectal cancer so that it may be treated at an early stage [11]. Moreover, the stool samples of the colorectal cancer patients contain *Bacteriodes fragilis*, *Enterococcus*, *Shigella*, *Klebssiella*, *Streptococcus*, and *Peptostreptococcus* [15]. One study found that the tumour is associated with the structure of gut microbiota, and the results proved that dysbiosis in the gut is one of the reasons that colorectal cancer evolves [16].

Several models, such as driver-passenger and keystone models are optimised for the study of the development of colorectal cancer. In the driver-passenger hypothesis, the role of various bacteria in the development of colorectal cancer were studied [17]. In this model, the microbes were classified into two different groups and demonstrated that the driver micro-organisms caused DNA damage and started the progression of the colorectal cancer, but these organisms are not always present as a marker [17]. In the second hypothesis, the key-stone pathogen is described as a microorganism that supports the disease-associated dysbiosis microbiota, and these microorganisms have a low abundance in the ecosystem [18]. Colorectal cancer may be prevented by adopting a healthy lifestyle and dietary patterns.

13.2.3 Liver Cancer

Liver cancer is the third leading cause of the death by cancer. The microbiota of the gut colonise immediately after birth and play a critical role in the health of the host by assisting digestion, production of vitamins, generation of bile acids, and modulating both local and systemic immunity [19–22]. The factors such as diet, lifestyle of an individual, age, medication, and illness affect the microbiota of the gut, which further impact the development of the disease [23]. The liver is directly exposed to gut microbiota and metabolites via the portal vein [24]. Liver cancer is impacted by gut microbiota by modulating various factors such as bile acids, immune checkpoint inhibitors, and toll-like receptors [25].

Non-alcoholic fatty liver syndrome (NAFLD) is one of the chronic liver diseases which include steatosis, non-alcoholic steatohepatitis (NASH), fibrosis, and cirrhosis [23]. In a recent study, it was found that gut dysbiosis has a key function in the development of NASH via regulation of inflammation, resistance of insulin, metabolism of choline, and bile acid production [26–28]. In another recent study, the patients suffering from NASH had significantly lower levels of Bacteroidetes [29], whereas non-obese patients with NAFLD had increased numbers of Bacteroidetes and lower abundance of Firmicutes [30].

In healthy conditions, the entry of bacterial products from the gut is prevented from leaking into the portal circulation by the intestinal barrier. The immune cells of the liver clear the microbial products and bacteria passing through the gut barrier. The gut microbiota reduces inflammation, improves insulin sensitivity, and activates the innate immune system via toll-like receptors which causes inflammation, liver damage, and liver diseases [31]. Liver cirrhosis is the end-stage of chronic liver disease and is characterised by fibrosis and portal hypertension, and may lead to hepatic failure and cancer [30]. The interaction between microbiota and bile acids plays an important role in the liver cirrhosis [32]. In a study, it was revealed that in fecal samples of cirrhotic patients, there is an increase in Protobacteria and Fusobacteria and a decrease in Bacteroidetes [33]. One study found that probiotics and fecal microbiome transplantation may be used in cancer treatment as an adjuvant strategy to increase the efficacy of chemotherapy and immunotherapy [34].

13.2.4 Pancreatic Cancer

Pancreatic ductal adenocarcinoma (PDAC) is a highly lethal disease. The human microbiota protects from diseases by supporting nutrition, hormonal homeostasis, modulation of inflammation, detoxifying compounds, and providing bacterial metabolites that have metabolic effects [35]. It is also found that the microbes are related with PDAC susceptibility, initiation, and progression. The mechanisms by which microbiota affects PDAC are [36]; (i) the microbes activate the inflammatory responses and lead to molecular alterations, which promotes the activation or the suppression of the immune system. Further, the gut bacteria increase their anti-tumour effect by the activation of the specific immune cells. (ii) The specific strains of gut bacteria and intrapancreatic bacteria induces a tolerogenic immunosuppressive microenvironment that favours progression in cancer and resistance to immunotherapies.

Previous studies have provided a link between pancreatic cancer and periodontal pathogen *P. gingivalis* [37], which is a biomarker for the risk of death due to colorectal and pancreatic cancer [38]. The major microorganisms that include *P. gingivalis, FusobacteriumI Aggregatibacter* species, *Prevotella* species, and *Capnocytophaga* species have a role in the commencement of pancreatic cancer [39]. In a recent study, the potential roles of intratumoral microorganisms in anticancer therapeutics such as pancreatic cancer was being studied [40], where it was determined that gut microorganisms have no direct role with pancreatic tissues. In a study by, Mitsuhashi et al. it was discovered that a number of Fusobacterium species were higher in infected patients with pancreatic cancer than the number of non-cancerous cells [41]. A recent technique for therapeutics for cancer is the microbiota transplantation and use of microbial markers. Fecal microbiota transplantation (FMT) will enhance anti-cancer immunity of the host cells and improve ineffectiveness and resistance in cancer patients [25]. New strategies such as probiotics, faecal microbiota transplantation (FMT), dietary changes, and antibiotics increase the efficiency of the current therapeutics and reduce toxicity [25].

13.3 Mechanism in which Microbiota Kill Cancer Cells

Cancer is considered as the major health problem with an increased rate of death. For the management of cancer, gut microbiota and TME (Tumour Microenvironment) play an important role. Gut microbiota play an essential role in functional development and maintenance of the host immune system [42, 43]. The multiple gut microbiota establish a symbiotic relationship with the immune system of the host and promote the host homeostasis, while also causing or worsening the creation and growth of the cancer [38]. The alteration of gut microbiota may lead to a feasible strategy for the anticancer therapy [44].

The metabolites of the gut flora enter human cells and symbiotically react with each other to promote variety of tumour inhibitory effects, inhibiting inflammation by maintaining the integrity of epithelial barrier and intestinal tract [45]. For the clearance of the tumour, the gut microbiota interact with immune cells which slow the metastasis of cancer cells and inhibit chronic inflammation [46]. The biomolecules produced from the intestinal microbes, such as SCFAs and inosine, affect the shape of TME and the cancer process [46].

For the effective treatment of cancer, gut microbes stimulate the body to produce CD47, which is a signal molecule that communicates with the immune system to produce a good effect of tumour immunotherapy by blocking CD47 [47, 48]. Further, CD47 interacts with the signal regulatory protein (SIRP), which are present on macrophages and dendritic cells [48]. In a recent study, it was found that CD8+T-cells are essential for anti-CD47 mediated tumour regression [49]. The anaerobes present in the gut such as *Bifidobacterium* are widely used in treating gastrointestinal disease [50, 51]. The interaction between the host system and the intestinal flora prevents tissue damaging inflammatory responses [52]. The microbiota controls the systemic and the innate immunity. For the proliferation of the cancer cells, the genetic mutations and alterations within the tissues are required [53, 54]. In a recent study, the gut microbiota was shown to affect the response to both immune and chemotherapy by regulating different myeloid cells, which function in the tumour microenvironment [52].

13.4 Microbiota that Promote Health Post Cancer Treatment

The microbial communities have evolved into diverse array of specialised lineage to adapt to different habitats, which have moulded the evolution of modern life. Gut microbes are crucial microorganisms with specialised functions in immune responses to cancer treatment and therapy. In recent years, treatments such as chemotherapy and radiotherapy are used. Currently, a new technology of using intestinal microbiota for increasing the efficacy and reduction of the toxicity of the current chemotherapeutic drugs is popular, and it improves the sensitivity to immunotherapy [55]. Immunotherapy is one of the most used technologies for treatment of cancer; in this treatment, the tumour cells are identified and killed. The interaction of T cell receptors and MHC molecules is controlled by series of immune checkpoints, which send signals for the activation and inhibition of T-cells [55].

In a recent study, it was revealed that the efficacy of the checkpoint inhibitors is affected by the gut microbiota of the patient, and it was perceived that the disparities are present in responses by the interaction between the immune checkpoint inhibitors and gut microbiota [56, 57]. Another approach for treating cancer is the ionising radiation therapy; in this technology, immunogenic tumour cell death may be induced by local irradiation, systemic immunity, and inflammation are promoted [58]. Ionising radiation therapy also causes certain side effects such as genomic instability, bystander effect on nearby cells, and immune and inflammatory reactivity [59]. This method also alters the composition of how microbiota break the intestinal barriers and causes apoptosis in intestinal crypts [60].

Cellular mutation caused by irradiation is another source of cancer, therefore being able to mitigate and restore the original cell status is crucial in preventing cancer. One clinical trial was named the 'Gut Microbiome and Gastrointestinal Toxicities as Determinants of Response to Neoadjuvant Chemo for Advanced Breast Cancer,' and the major objective was to prove that the normal gut bacteria help the body to fight cancer [55]. The gut microbiota is implicated in many aspects of drug metabolism, pharmacokinetics, anticancer effect, and toxicity [61]. In a study, it was discovered that the gut microbes such as *Bifidobacterium*, *Lactobacillus*, and *Streptococcus* are protective against pelvic radiation-induced gut toxicity and reduce the incidence of severe diarrhea [62, 63]. In the future, the goal of the researchers will be to discover a bacterial species or combination of species that reduces the toxicity and promotes anti-cancer therapy [64].

13.5 Conclusion

Cancer is a terrifying and indiscriminating disease. Research in last fifty years has demonstrated that there are factors such as environmental, genetic, and ageing that may increase the risks for developing cancer. At a molecular level, a significant amount of work remains to be done to provide a more comprehensive understanding of the commencement of tumours and how they develop into malignant and deadly cells. This chapter has focused on explaining the mechanism in which the gut microbiota are supressing or causing cancer. Further functions of the microbiota in assisting recovery post-cancer therapy are also discussed.

References

1 Perez-Chanona, E. and Trinchieri, G. (2016). The role of microbiota in cancer therapy. *Curr. Opin. Immuno.* 39: 75–81.

2 Cheng, W.Y., Wu, C.-Y., and Yu, J. (2020). The role of gut microbiota in cancer treatment: friend or foe? *Gut* 69 (10): 1867–1876.

3 Smet, A., Kupcinskas, J., Link, A. et al. (2022). The role of microbiota in gastrointestinal cancer and cancer treatment: chance or curse? *Cell. Mol. Gastroent. Hepatol.* 13 (3): 857–874.

4 Louis, P., Hold, G.L., and Flint, H.J. (2014). The gut microbiota, bacterial metabolites and colorectal cancer. *Nat. Rev. Micro.* 12 (10): 661–672.

5 Ferreira, R.M., Pereira-Marques, J., Pinto-Ribeiro, I. et al. (2018). Gastric microbial community profiling reveals a dysbiotic cancer-associated microbiota. *Gut* 67 (2): 226–236.

6 Teal, E., Dua-Awereh, M., Hirshorn, S.T. et al. (2020). Role of metaplasia during gastric regeneration. *Am. J. Physio.-Cell Physio.* 319 (6): C947–C954.

7 Aviles-Jimenez, F., Vazquez-Jimenez, F., Medrano-Guzman, R. et al. (2014). Stomach microbiota composition varies between patients with non-atrophic gastritis and patients with intestinal type of gastric cancer. *Sci. Rep.* 4: 4202.

8 Engstrand, L. and Lindberg, M. (2013). Helicobacter pylori and the gastric microbiota. *Best Prac. Res. Clin. Gastroent.* 27 (1): 39–45.

9 Hansen, A.B.R., Johannesen, T.B., Spiegelhauer, M.R. et al. (2020). Distinct composition and distribution of the gastric microbiota observed between dyspeptic and gastric cancer patients evaluated from gastric biopsies. *Microbio. Heal. Dis.* 2: e340.

10 Gunathilake, M.N., Lee, J., Choi, I.J. et al. (2019). Association between the relative abundance of gastric microbiota and the risk of gastric cancer: a case-control study. *Sci. Rep.* 9: 13589.

11 Wong, S.H. and Yu, J. (2019). Gut microbiota in colorectal cancer: mechanisms of action and clinical applications. *Nat. Rev. Gastroent. Hepatol.* 16 (11): 690–704.

12 Strum, W.B. (2016). Colorectal adenomas. *NEJ. Med.* 374 (11): 1065–1075.

13 McCoy, A.N., Araújo-Pérez, F., Azcárate-Peril, A. et al. (2013). Fusobacterium is associated with colorectal adenomas. *PLoS One* 8 (1): e53653.

14 Gupta, A., Madani, R. and Mukhtar, H. (2010). Streptococcus bovis endocarditis, a silent sign for colonic tumour. *Colorec. Dis.* 12 (3): 164–171.

15 Wang, T., Cai, G., Qiu, Y. et al. (2012). Structural segregation of gut microbiota between colorectal cancer patients and healthy volunteers. *ISME J.* 6 (2): 320–329.

16 Genua, F., Raghunathan, V., Jenab, M. et al. (2021). The role of gut barrier dysfunction and microbiome dysbiosis in colorectal cancer development. *Front. Oncol.* 11: 626349.

17 Zintzaras, E. (2012). Is there evidence to claim or deny association between variants of the multidrug resistance gene (MDR1 or ABCB1) and inflammatory bowel disease? *Inflam. Bowel Dis.* 18 (3): 562–572.

18 Hajishengallis, G., Darveau, R.P. and Curtis, M.A. (2012). The keystone-pathogen hypothesis. *Nat. Rev. Microbio.* 10 (10): 717–725.

19 Pennisi, E. (2013). Cancer therapies use a little help from microbial friends. *Science* 342 (6161): 921–921.

20 Wan, M.L.Y. and El-Nezami, H. (2018). Targeting gut microbiota in hepatocellular carcinoma: probiotics as a novel therapy. *Hepatobil. Surg. Nutr.* 7 (1): 11–20.

21 Ma, J., Zhou, Q. and Li, H. (2017). Gut microbiota and nonalcoholic fatty liver disease: insights on mechanisms and therapy. *Nutrients* 9 (10): 1124.

22 Zamparelli, M.S., Rocco, A., Compare, D. et al. (2017). The gut microbiota: a new potential driving force in liver cirrhosis and hepatocellular carcinoma. *Unit. Euro. Gastroent. J.* 5 (7): 944–953.

23 Henao-Mejia, J., Elinav, E., Jin, C. et al. (2012). Inflammasome-mediated dysbiosis regulates progression of NAFLD and obesity. *Nature* 482 (7384): 179–185.

24 Tripathi, A., Debelius, J., Brenner, D.A. et al. (2018). The gut–liver axis and the intersection with the microbiome. *Nat. Rev. Gastroent. Hepatol.* 15 (7): 397–411.

25 Zhang, C., Yang, M. and Ericsson, A.C. (2020). The potential gut microbiota-mediated treatment options for liver cancer. *Front. Oncol.* 10: 524205.

26 Boursier, J., Mueller, O., Barret, M. et al. (2016). The severity of nonalcoholic fatty liver disease is associated with gut dysbiosis and shift in the metabolic function of the gut microbiota. *Hepatology* 63 (3): 764–775.

27 Quigley, E.M. and Monsour, H.P. (2015). The gut microbiota and nonalcoholic fatty liver disease. *Sem. Liver Dis.* 35 (3): 262–269.

28 Miura, K. and Ohnishi, H. (2014). Role of gut microbiota and Toll-like receptors in nonalcoholic fatty liver disease. *W. J. Gastroent.* 20 (23): 7381–7391.

29 Mouzaki, M., Comelli, E.M., Arendt, B.M. et al. (2013). Intestinal microbiota in patients with nonalcoholic fatty liver disease. *Hepatology* 58 (1): 120–127.

30 Wang, B., Jiang, X., Cao, M. et al. (2016). Altered fecal microbiota correlates with liver biochemistry in nonobese patients with non-alcoholic fatty liver disease. *Sci. Rep.* 6: 32002.

31 Wang, L. and Wan, Y.-J.Y. (2019). The role of gut microbiota in liver disease development and treatment. *Liver Res.* 3 (1): 3–18.

32 Ridlon, J.M., Kang, D.J., Hylemon, P.B. et al. (2014). Bile acids and the gut microbiome. *Cur. Opin. Gastroent.* 30 (3): 332–338.

33 Chen, Y., Ji, F., Guo, J. et al. (2016). Dysbiosis of small intestinal microbiota in liver cirrhosis and its association with etiology. *Sci. Rep.* 6: 34055.

34 Vivarelli, S., Salemi, R., Candido, S. et al. (2019). Gut microbiota and cancer: from pathogenesis to therapy. *Cancers (Basel)* 11 (1): 38.

35 The Human Microbiome Project Consortium. (2012). Structure, function and diversity of the healthy human microbiome. *Nature* 486 (7402): 207–214.

36 Wei, M.-Y., Shi, S., Liang, C. et al. (2019). The microbiota and microbiome in pancreatic cancer: more influential than expected. *Molec. Cancer* 18: 97.

37 Michaud, D.S., Izard, J., Wilhelm-Benartzi, C.S. et al. (2013). Plasma antibodies to oral bacteria and risk of pancreatic cancer in a large European prospective cohort study. *Gut* 62 (12): 1764–1770.

38 Michaud, D.S., Joshipura, K., Giovannucci, E. et al. (2007). A prospective study of periodontal disease and pancreatic cancer in US male health professionals. *J. Nat. Cancer Inst.* 99 (2): 171–175.

39 Karpiński, T.M. (2019). The microbiota and pancreatic cancer. *Gastroent. Clin. N. Am.* 48 (3): 447–464.

40 Thomas, H. (2017). Intra-tumour bacteria promote gemcitabine resistance in pancreatic adenocarcinoma. *Nat. Rev. Gastroent. Hepat.* 14: 632.

41 Mitsuhashi, K., Nosho, K., Sukawa, Y. et al. (2015). Association of Fusobacterium species in pancreatic cancer tissues with molecular features and prognosis. *Oncotarget* 6 (9): 7209–7220.

42 Khan, M.A.W., Ologun, G., Arora, R. et al. (2020). Gut microbiome modulates response to cancer immunotherapy. *Diges. Dis. Sci.* 65: 885–896.

43 Garcia-Carbonell, R., Yao, S.-J., Das, S. et al. (2019). Dysregulation of intestinal epithelial cell RIPK pathways promotes chronic inflammation in the IBD Gut. *Front. Immuno.* 10: 1094.

44 Ling, Z., Shao, L., Liu, X. et al. (2019). Regulatory T cells and plasmacytoid dendritic cells within the tumor microenvironment in gastric cancer are correlated with gastric microbiota dysbiosis: a preliminary study. *Front. Immun.* 10: 533.

45 van der Veeken, J., Glasner, A., Zhong, Y. et al. (2020). The transcription factor Foxp3 shapes regulatory T cell identity by tuning the activity of trans-acting intermediaries. *Immunity* 53 (5): 971–984.

46 Qiu, Q., Lin, Y., Ma, Y. et al. (2021). Exploring the emerging role of the gut microbiota and tumor microenvironment in cancer immunotherapy. *Front. Immu.* 11: 612202.

47 Liu, X., Pu, Y., Cron, K. et al. (2015). CD47 blockade triggers T cell–mediated destruction of immunogenic tumors. *Nat. Med.* 21 (10): 1209–1215.

48 Barclay, A.N. and Van den Berg, T.K. (2014). The interaction between signal regulatory protein alpha (SIRPα) and CD47: structure, function, and therapeutic target. *Ann. Rev. Immuno.* 32: 25–50.

49 Xu, M.M., Pu, Y., Han, D. et al. (2017). Dendritic cells but not macrophages sense tumor mitochondrial DNA for cross-priming through signal regulatory protein alpha signaling. *Immunity* 47 (2): 363–373.

50 Furrie, E., Macfarlane, S., Kennedy, A. et al. (2005). Synbiotic therapy (Bifidobacterium longum/Synergy 1) initiates resolution of inflammation in patients with active ulcerative colitis: a randomised controlled pilot trial. *Gut* 54 (2): 242–249.

51 Zhou, S., Gravekamp, C., Bermudes, D. et al. (2018). Tumour-targeting bacteria engineered to fight cancer. *Nat. Rev. Cancer* 18 (12): 727–743.

52 Akanbong, E.A., Şenol, A., Sudağıdan, M. et al. (2021). Unraveling microbiome: the role of microbiota in patients' response to oncological treatment and its influence on host-biochemistry. *Int. J. Veter. Anim. Res. (IJVAR)* 4 (2): 69–77.

53 Hanahan, D. and Weinberg, R.A. (2000). The hallmarks of cancer. *Cell* 100 (1): 57–70.

54 Vogelstein, B., Papadopoulos, N., Velculescu, V.E. et al. (2013). Cancer genome landscapes. *Science* 339 (6127): 1546–1558.

55 Ma, W., Mao, Q., Xia, W. et al. (2019). Gut microbiota shapes the efficiency of cancer therapy. *Front. Microbio.* 10: 1050.

56 Sivan, A., Corrales, L., Hubert, N. et al. (2015). Commensal Bifidobacterium promotes antitumor immunity and facilitates anti-PD-L1 efficacy. *Science* 350 (6264): 1084–1089.

57 Vétizou, M., Pitt, J.M., Daillère, R., et al. (2015). Anticancer immunotherapy by CTLA-4 blockade relies on the gut microbiota. *Science* 350 (6264): 1079–1084.

58 Kroemer, G., Galluzzi, L., Kepp, O. et al. (2013). Immunogenic cell death in cancer therapy. *Ann. Rev.f Immuno.* 31: 51–72.

59 Azzam, E.I. and Little, J.B. (2004). The radiation-induced bystander effect: evidence and significance. *Hum. Experim. Toxico.* 23 (2): 61–65.

60 Barker, H.E., Paget, J.T.E., Khan, A.A. et al. (2015). The tumour microenvironment after radiotherapy: mechanisms of resistance and recurrence. *Nat. Rev. Cancer* 15 (7): 409–425.

61 Spanogiannopoulos, P., Bess, E.N., Carmody, R.N. et al. (2016). The microbial pharmacists within us: a metagenomic view of xenobiotic metabolism. *Nat. Rev. Microbio.* 14 (5): 273–287.

62 Touchefeu, Y., Montassier, E., Nieman, K. et al. (2014). Systematic review: the role of the gut microbiota in chemotherapy-or radiation-induced gastrointestinal mucositis–current evidence and potential clinical applications. *Aliment. Pharmaco. Therap.* 40 (5): 409–421.

63 Delia, P., Sansotta, G., Donato, V. et al. (2007). Use of probiotics for prevention of radiation-induced diarrhea. *World J. Gastroenter.* 13 (6): 912–915.

64 Roy, S. and Trinchieri, G. (2017). Microbiota: a key orchestrator of cancer therapy. *Nat. Rev. Cancer* 17 (5): 271–285.

14

Impact of Gut Microbiota on Mental Health in Humans

Sagnik Nag[1], Ankita Saini[2], Richismita Hazra[3], and Jutishna Bora[4]

[1] Department of Biotechnology, School of Biosciences & Technology, Vellore Institute of Technology (VIT), Tiruvalam Rd, Tamil Nadu, India
[2] Department of Microbiology, University of Delhi (South Campus), Benito Juarez Road, New Delhi, India
[3] Amity Institute of Biotechnology, Amity University Kolkata, West Bengal, India
[4] Amity Institute of Biotechnology, Amity University Jharkhand, Ranchi, India

14.1 Introduction

14.1.1 Importance of Gut Microbiota

Microbiota refers to the myriad of microorganisms interacting and colonising in a specific location including bacteria, archaea, and eukarya. They are believed to have co-evolved with the host over thousands of decades to bring about a remarkable impact on the host during homeostatic conditions as well as diseased conditions [1]. Approximately more than 10^{14} microorganisms inhabit our GI tract, encompassing ~10× the excess bacterial cells than the total number of human cells [2]. The density and composition of the microbiota are influenced by chemical factors, nutritional factors, and immunological gradients along the gut. Owing to its huge genomic composition and metabolic complement, the gut microbiota benefits the host in a broad spectrum of ways. Maintenance of the integrity of the mucosal barrier, provision of nutrients, and protection against pathogens are a few of the crucial roles played by the microbes present within the gut. Microorganisms have a symbiotic relationship when it comes to association with humans. It has been found that the microbiota of the gut is closely linked with brain systems mainly that control stress regulators. Gut microbiota in every individual is shaped from early childhood, depending upon gestational factors and external factors such as use of antibiotics. Each individual gut microbiota is specific and performs functions such as immunomodulation, nutrient metabolism, defense against pathogens, and others unique to that individual [3].

Diet is considered to play a pivotal role in shaping the gut microbiota across the lifetime. Gut microbes are believed to have acclimatisation properties to certain types of lifestyles due to the relatively smaller number of biochemical niches present in the gut than in other microbial-rich environments. The host benefits from the microbiota through a variety of physiological activities including the improvement of gut integrity, energy harvest, shielding against pathogens, and regulating host immunity. Dysbiosis, a condition resulting from the altered microbial condition, has the potential for disrupting these mechanisms. Apart from its role in various systems in the body, the gut microbes play a crucial role in mental health and overall well-being of an individual [4] (see Figure 14.1).

14.1.2 The Microbiota–Gut–Brain Axis

The Gut–Brain axis (GBA) is a bidirectional process in which the gastrointestinal tract and Central Nervous System (CNS) interact with each other by neurohumoral communication [5]. GBA is responsible for maintaining the homeostasis of the body. It has been demonstrated that microbiota impact GBA by the cells of intestine and enteric nervous system (ENS) alongside CNS by metabolic pathways. A minor disturbance in this axis will result in dysfunction throughout the circuit. The primary components of the gut–brain axis are the intestinal microbes through which communication is mediated between the gut and the CNS via bloodstream, as demonstrated by a study [6].

There are multifaceted ways through which the gut microbiota establishes a strong relationship with the brain axis. The modulatory pathways and approaches play an imperative role in healthy physiological functioning of the human body. Some of them can be elaborated as follows.

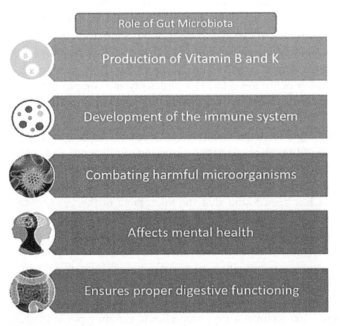

Figure 14.1 Importance of gut microbiota in human health. *Source:* (for image in Combating harmful microorganisms: Lotus_studio/Adobe Stock).

- **Gut to brain (bottom up modulation):** There are molecules produced by microbes, e.g., secondary bile acids and Tryptophan metabolites, which interact with enteroendocrine cells (EEC) and may either reach the brain directly or reach the vagus nerve efferents [7]. Microbiota may produce neuroactive compounds such as dopamine and norepinephrine. EEC present in gut epithelia have 20 molecules for their signal transduction. It has been shown in the experiments that microbial metabolites, such as bile acids, regulate hunger [5].

- **Enterochromaffin signaling:** ECC cells of the GI tract produce 5-HT, which is responsible for GI motility. Microbiota of GI secrete fluids, which are helpful in this modulation. Many experiments on germ-free mice showed a 2-fold decrease in 5-HT levels, indicating the important role microbiota play [8].

- **Neuroimmune Signaling:** Gut microbiota influence the development of microglia cells of the CNS. Studies on GF mice having immature microglia showed a weakened response when attacked by pathogens [9].

- **Direct Neural Signaling:** Gut peptides and dietary compounds are recognised by vagal receptors, which pass on signals to CNS. Toll-like receptors 3 and 7 directly recognise viral RNA; while receptor 4 recognises lipopolysaccharides, which are expressed in ENS [9].

- **Microbial Metabolites:** Some metabolites produced by microbes are helpful in direct activation of neurons. If the concentrations of bile acids are low, it is helpful in expression of receptors such as FXR and TGR 5 [10].

- **Brain to Gut:** Stress affects the gut microbiome. The Autonomic Nervous System (ANS) regulates secretion of mucus, gastric acid, epithelial fluids, and antimicrobial peptides [5]. It has also been observed in this study that the children born from parents undergoing stress have altered microbiomes with increased chances of inflammation.

- **GI Motility:** The assessment of intestinal transit time by Bristol Stool Scale indicates correlation with microbial richness and composition. Stress may cause leaky gut either by modulation of epithelial permeability or alteration in intestinal mucosal layers. These alterations lead to increased translocation of gut microbes. Brain injury in mice during experiments resulted in altered mucoprotein and goblet cell production [11].

- **Direct Modulation by Neurotransmitters:** Many sequences in gut microbiota are identical to the human genome for binding sites of melatonin. It has been found that melatonin concentration in the gut of rats and pigs was a 10-fold serum concentration [12]. It has also been noted that epinephrine and norepinephrine increase the virulence of enteric pathogens or microbes via activation of quorum sensing mechanisms.

There is a well-established communication among microbiota, gut, and brain with experiments conducted on gut microbiota for neuropsychiatric disorders. It has been observed that patients with IBS are invariably the ones suffering from anxiety. In an experiment on Rhesus monkeys where anxiety was created, it was found that the population of Lactobacillus decreased considerably. Microbes release metabolites, which trigger inflammation in CNS leading to pain, depression, autism, and stroke. This proves that there is a correlation between CNS and the gut microbiota [13], as seen in Figure 14.2.

The co-existing bilateral relationship between the brain and the gut imperatively affects the basic physiology of the human body. The diseases of the gut are linked with alterations within the GBA due to genetic and epigenetic factors. The treatment of such diseases adversely/positively (rarely) affect intestinal microbiota. A possible cause of

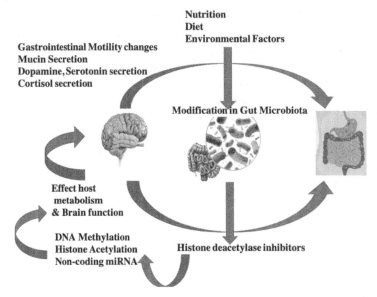

Figure 14.2 Experimental evidence showing the role of microbiota in influencing GBA. *Source:* (for image in modification in Gut Microbiota: Freshidea / Adobe Stock); (for image in effct host metabolism & Brain function: Science RF / Adobe Stock).

depression is the inflammation caused by disruption of GI barriers. In vivo studies have shown the direct role of altered gut microbes and metabolites in the progression of neurodevelopmental diseases [14]. The Blood–Brain Barrier (BBB) is important to prevent neuroinflammation. Gut dysfunctions and inflammation sometime result in autism spectrum disorders (ASD) through compromising the BBB and immunological abnormalities [15].

14.2 Gut Dysbiosis and Mental Health Disorders

With the advent of technology, relative studies in linking the cross-talk between the enteric nervous system and cognitive axis of the brain has emerged progressively. Permutation in this interplay delineates the rationale behind the pathophysiology of several psychiatric disorders such as anxiety, mood, cognition, and psychiatric beht colonisers (gut dysbiosis) being intertwined with development of mental health disorder [16].

Additionally, diet, antibiotic medications, genetics, and age anchor the dynamicity of the GBA and progression of a number of mental health disorders. Changes in gut microbiota derived from high-energy diets has proven to be an influencing factor for paradigm shift in anxiety, memory, or cognitive changes [17].

There is a continuous parallel between gut dysbiosis and pathogenesis of psychiatry disorders. Metabolites released after altered gut microbiota disturb the healthy functioning of the gut microbiota, and hence leading to several neuro-psychotic disorders [18] (see Figure 14.3).

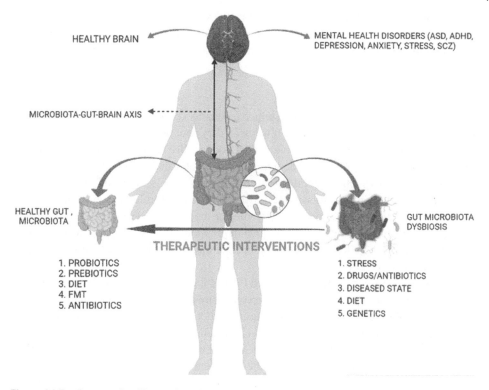

Figure 14.3 Comparative illustration of healthy gut microbiota and dysbiosis conditions under the intervention of GBA.

14.2.1 Neurodevelopmental Disorders

Neurodevelopmental disorders (NDDs) are onset of symptoms, particularly at an early stage of life, leading to impairment of CNS functioning. Brain malfunctioning induces sensory-motor disorders, disability of language-learning, mental retardation, and Autism. Altered GI in patients with autism have been linked with degree of pathology and the gut microbiota [19]. Autism patients with higher GI disturbance index are more often striken with multiple symptoms, such as acid reflux, abdominal discomfort, diarrhea, and constipation (sometimes both) than in patients with lower GI disturbance index [20].

Increased growth of some enteric bacteria, particularly from genera *Bacteroides* and *Clostridium* with diminishing growth of healthy bacteria (*Bifidobacterium*), have been reported in children with autism spectrum disorder (ASD). Heterogeneity of gut microbiota was found to be disturbed in patients with ASD, resulting in impairment of CNS functioning. Therefore, any perturbation of healthy gut microbiota results in detrimental effects on neurochemicals such as serotonin, dopamine, and short chain fatty acids (SCFAs), and thus leads to neurodevelopmental disorders [21].

Bifidobacteria, a significant bacterial genus of the gut microbiota, play a pivotal role in polysaccharide digestion, host-body pathogen exclusion, production of vitamins (B-group), and antimicrobial agents. Consequently, treatment with Bifidobacteria was proven to be of paramount importance in treating patients with mental health disorders such as depression and anxiety [22]. Individuals with ASD showed improvement and reduction in GI perturbations with Fecal Microbial Transplantation (FMT) treatment along with antibiotics administration, a bowel cleanse, and stomach-acid suppressants [23].

14.2.2 Mood Disorders

Mood disorder is a mental condition in which a person experiences long periods of extreme happiness, extreme sadness, or both. It is affected by genetics as well as the environment. Mood disorders alter behavior and may affect your ability to deal with routine activities. The common mood disorders are depression and bipolar disorder. Urbanisation leads to bad lifestyle choices such mechanistic routine, increased noise, reduced diet quality, and pollution. Recent scientific experiments have proven a direct influence on the influence of the mood with a correlation of the right types of food and healthy nutrition along with changes in gut microbiome that can induce depression. As a result, the gut microbiome becomes altered, which leads to the occurrence of more psychiatric problems, depression, and mood disorders [24].

Influence of a Western diet, i.e., processed foods which are very low in fibre content, high in saturated fats and sugars have resulted in compromised epithelial permeability referred to as 'leaky gut.' The gut microbiome flourishes on a diet rich in fibre, unsaturated fatty acids, and polyphenols, and these substances are metabolised by gut microbes into anti-inflammatory metabolites such as SCFAs. The polyphenols interact with gut microbiota and produce many bioactive metabolites, which modulate the risk factors of depression [25]. It has been observed that non-consumption of probiotics increases the chances of depression and may decrease the alertness of the brain. In addition to that role, they also influence the hypothalamic–pituitary–adrenal axis (HPA), affecting a person's the mood [26, 27].

I) Depression: Grief is the major symptom of clinical depression and occurs as a response to any traumatic event that happened in the past. The various types of depression are:
  i) Postpartum depression, which occurs post-delivery;
  ii) Dysthymia, a chronic form that can last up to two years;
  iii) Seasonal Affective Disorder (SAD), mainly in response to a certain season of the year and most common beginning in Autumn and continuing until Spring; and
  iv) Psychotic depression, which is a severe depression combined with hallucinations and/or delusions [28].
II) Bipolar Disorders: Mood swings are a common symptom and may range from depression to mania. There are four types:
  i) Bipolar I: This is the most severe form and may require hospitalisation;
  ii) Bipolar II: Experience of hypomania which is less severe and no need for hospitalisation;
  iii) *Cyclothymia* disorder: A milder form in which mood swings occur from mild or moderate to high; or from mild or moderate to low;
  iv) Substance abuse disorder: A person is unable to control the use of any drug or medication and becomes addicted [28].

Mounting evidence has shown that gut microbiome may influence functions of the brain by neuroimmune and neuro-endocrine pathways. SCFA-producing bacteria were reduced and the genera involved in lipid metabolism were increased in patients with depression

[29]. In bipolar disorders (BD) and major depressive disorder (MDD), populations of *Enterobacteriaceae* and *Actinobacteria* were increased, while *Faecalibacterium* spp. tended to be reduced. Butyrate/lactate producing bacterial population was low in children diagnosed with ASD [29]. Schizophrenia was accompanied by increased populations of Proteobacteria, causing dysbiosis of gut as reported by [30], see Table 14.1.

The improvement in patients' health after consuming psychotropic drugs also influences the diversity of microbiota in the gut. This results in weight gain, metabolic disturbance, and inflammatory activities in patients. Most of the psychotropic drugs target neurotransmitters and alter the concentrations of serotonin, dopamine, and noradrenaline. The latter being produced by gut microbiota, may have effects on them as well in the form of constipation and diarrhea. Some antidepressants have antimicrobial effects. Experimental evidence has shown that antipsychotics may have inhibitory effects on the growth of gut microorganisms, indicating that these behave as antibiotics [36].

Studies have shown that in schizophrenic patients, chronic treatment with risperidone was associated with weight gain and a lower ratio of *Bacteroidetes* to *Firmicutes* [37]. In general, antidepressants have a role in increasing the beta diversity of gut bacteria and in turn reduce their richness.

14.2.3 Depression Disorders

Depressive disorder, or depression, is usuallly an enfeebling psychiatric disorder characterised by low emotional disposition, loss of confidence, and apathy. This mental illness is

Table 14.1 Gut microbiome studies in humans for mood disorders.

Mood Disorders	Bacteria Involved	Increased/Decreased Population	Reference
MDD	*Actinobacteria*	Increased	[31]
	Bacteroidetes	Decreased	
	a. *Proteobacteria & Bacteroidetes*	Decreased	[32]
	b. *Actinobacteria & Fimicutes*	Increased	
BD	*Flavonifractor*	Increased	[33]
BD	a. *Actinobacteria & Coriobacteria*	Increased	[34]
	b. *Ruminococcaceae & Faecalibacterium*	Decreased	
a. BD	*Proteobacteria, Ruminococcus, Veillonella, & Lanchnospira*	Increased	[35]
	Bacteroides	Decreased	
b. BDM	a. *Enterobacteriaceae, Ruminococcus, Megamonas, & Bifidobacterium adolescentis*	Increased	
	b. *Bacteroides*	Decreased	
c. BDD	*Selenomonadales, Lachnospira, Eubacrerium, & Plebelus*	Increased	

Notes: MDD: Major depressive disorder; BD: Bipolar Disorder; BDD: Bipolar disorder with depressive episode; BDM: Bipolar disorder with manic episodes.

caused by multiple factors and is a major contributor to the global disease burden. It correlates with disruptions in the HPA axis, thereby causing inflammatory responses. It brings about anhedonia, altered appetite, lack of concentration, guilt feeling, sleep disturbances, psychomotor agitation, and suicidal ideation [38].

Various studies of depression disorder on animal models have been conducted, among which some preclinical and clinical studies have provided shreds of evidence suggesting that alterations in the gut microbiota, short-chain fatty acids derived from microorganisms, D-amino acids, and metabolites have major roles in the pathophysiology of depression through the brain–gut–microbiota axis. Alterations in the composition of the gut microbiome trigger the production of microbial lipopolysaccharides, which activates inflammatory responses. Certain signals are sent to the vagus nerve by Cytokines, thereby linking the HPA axis and affecting behavioral change. Some evidence shows a direct link between gastrointestinal tract inflammation and neuroinflammation, which affects the kynurenine pathway [39].

Subjects diagnosed with mental disorders including depression have been found to demonstrate gut microbiome dysbiosis. The composition and variability of bacteria between healthy and MDD patients displayed remarkable disparity. Mostly *Firmicutes*, *Bacteroides*, and *Actinobacteria* were found in the gut of depressed subjects. The use of supplemental probiotics has proven to be a potential practice to address depression-associated issues. The Mediterranean diet is highly associated with the improvement of mental health, unlike foods with an elevated fat content that not only lead to obesity, but also cause inflammation of body systems. *Bifidobacterium* and *Lactobacillus* strains have been investigated to improve depressive symptoms overall. According to a recent study, butyrate-producing gut microbes including *Faecalibacterium* and *Coprococcus*, when present in high amounts in humans, improve the quality of living, while subjects with lower amounts of these species are more likely to have depressive disorders [40].

14.2.4 Alcohol Use Disorder (AUD)

AUD refers to a blend of mental impairment that includes alcohol dependence, alcohol abuse, and alcohol addiction. It has significant adverse effects on the lifespan and quality of living. Individuals with AUD are mostly diagnosed with anxiety, depression, and cognitive impairments. Alcoholism or alcohol addiction is a brain disorder that is associated with the brain reward circuit and is characterised by relapse and remission. Alcoholism, when combined with psychiatric comorbidities, makes the recovery process more complex [41].

The human intestine is bounded by enterocytes, goblet cells, and various antimicrobial substances, which affect the microbiome in the mucus layer, and a few other immune cells in the *lamina propria*. Although the exact relation between alcohol and leaky gut has not been identified yet, scientists suggest that intestinal dysbiosis, immune activation, and inflammation may have roles to play in this regard. Studies have suggested that alcohol impairs the intestinal barrier, causes modifications to the intestinal permeability, and alters the composition of the gut microbiota [42]. Alcohol addiction has a close relation with absorption impairment in the duodenum, which leads to impaired thiamine storage in the liver. Among patients diagnosed with AUD, the most common reason for death is alcoholic liver disease. Among alcoholics, GI alterations bring about nutritional deficiencies including deficits in vitamin A, thiamine, and niacin. Alcohol consumption disrupts the gut barrier function, a phenomenon known as leaky gut. Alcoholism or alcohol addiction is a complex disorder, throughout the development of which subjects acquire a multitude of cognitive alterations. These alterations and dysfunctions affect emotional processing, memory, and executive functioning [43].

14.3 Psychiatric Medication and the Microbiome

The rationale behind the regulation of psychiatric disorders is the fair interplay between the microbes and action of the brain; a tab for potential psychiatric medications. Psychiatry or psychotropic medications are believed to show a differential impact on the gut microbiota composition. The amount and type of medications taken could have a solid influence on the composition of gut microbes. Thus, the pliability of the gut microbiota could be regarded as a potential target for the therapeutic approach [44].

Psychotropic drugs address the treatment of mental health disorders by debilitating the symptoms of auditory hallucinations, excessive mood swings, behavioral patterns, etc. The complex regime of medications include treatment with antidepressants, anti-anxiety medications, stimulants, antipsychotics, and mood stabilisers. Selective serotonin reuptake inhibitors (SSRIs) are classified as antidepressants which include escitalopram and fluvoxamine, they exhibit antimicrobial effects and potency in depression, anxiety, panic disorder, post-traumatic stress, obsessive-compulsive disorder (OCD), migraine, and other conditions [44]. Anti-anxiety agents, or anxiolytics, like diazepam and lorazepam treat anxiety disorders, sleep disorders, panic attacks and stress. Antipsychotics such as aripiprazole and clozapine, and mood stabilisers such as carbamazepine and lithium, are effective in schizophrenia, psychosis associated with depression, and mania [45].

The relativity of the complexity of gut microbiota and drug pharmacokinetics (fate of xenobiotics) potentially strikes the immunity and the metabolism of the body [46]. Drug pharmacokinetics demonstrate a significant effect on microbial diversity. Antipsychotics such as aripiprazole are believed to increase the load of species belonging to *Clostridium*, *Peptoclostridium*, *Intestinibacter*, and *Christenellaceae*. However, antidepressants such as escitalopram and fluvoxamine exhibit antimicrobial activity against *Leishmania rhamnosus* and *E. coli* [44].

The scope of pharmacokinetics with effects of dynamic microbiome on the drug absorption and metabolism give us strong implications on futuristic therapeutic interventions, pharmacological drug action, and biotransformations [47].

14.4 Probiotic Treatments for Mental Health Disorders

Probiotics are living microorganisms known to heighten the welfare of gut health when consumed in a requisite amount. Consumption of probiotics is both strain- and disease-specific with an impact on both enteric system and CNS (see Table 14.2). Several preclinical studies have exemplified the treatment with probiotics in improving various mental health-related disorders such as mood, anxiety, and cognitive diseases by altering neurochemical operations [48].

Table 14.2 Enlisted probiotic strains showing therapeutic potential in relieving symptoms or in treatment of various mental disorders.

Probiotic Strains	Mental Health Disorders	Symptom Relief	References
Bifidobacterium longum; *Lactobacillus helveticus*	Depression and anxiety	Reduced psychological distress	[50]
Bifidobacterium longum 1714	Psychological distress	Reduced stress and improved memory	[51]
Bifidobacterium bifidum W23 *Bifidobacterium lactis W52, Lactobacillus acidophilus W37, Lactobacillus brevis W63* *Lactobacillus caseiW56* *Lactococcus lactis W19* *Lactococcus lactis W58* *Lactobacillus salivarius W24*	Mood disorders	Reduced rumination and aggressive thoughts	[52]
Bifidobacterium bifidum *Lactobacillus acidophilus Lactobacillus casei* *Lactobacillus fermentum*	Alzheimer's disease	Revived cognitive and metabolic status	[53]
Bifidobacterium bifidum *Lactobacillus acidophilus, Lactobacillus fermentum*	Parkinson's disease	Downregulate cytokines and up regulate growth factor, peroxisome proliferator	[54]
Lactobacillus plantarum *Lactobacillus acidophilus Lactobacillus rhamnosus*	Autism spectrum disorder (ASD) in children	Improved autism and gastrointestinal (GI) symptoms	[55]

The term "Psychobiotics" often comes into play when referring to the treatment of psychiatric disorders with probiotics. Psychobiotics are broad-spectrum bacteria which regulate the neuroimmune axis and neuroendocrine stress-response systems along with different hormonal pathways [49].

Lactobacillus and *Bifidobacterium* species probiotic combinations have shown a significant abatement in various mental health disorders. A blend of diet (macro- and micronutrients) along with the probiotics induces complementary health benefits to gut–brain axis.

With regard to neurochemical transmission, probiotics may prevent stress-induced adrenocorticotropic hormone (ACTH), corticosterone, adrenaline, and noradrenaline elevations. Probiotic use also upgrades brain plasticity, memory, and neuronal health. Regulation of neurotransmitters under the influence of probiotics consumption suggested overall positive results on enteric and central nervous systems [56].

Probiotics elevate the levels of gamma-aminobutyric acid (GABA) in the body, induce improved memory, and reduce anxiety- and depressive-like behaviors. Accordingly, probiotics may be used as a complementary treatment for some mental health disorders by contracting with certain symptoms such as mood, anxiety, and cognitive disorders [47].

14.5   Future Therapeutic Approach

Gut microbiota is known to help the body's vital functions such as metabolic pathways, vitamin production, and regulation of the immune system. In general, most of the neuro-psychiatric drugs act against commensal microbes [57]. Success in treating the symptoms of BD or failure to respond to the drug is all dependent upon how the gut microbiome and medication interact with each other.

Today is the age of microbial revolution where many lifestyle diseases are treated by manipulation of the microbes in our bodies. It has been demonstrated that more than 90% of *Clostridioides difficile*-associated disease (CDAD) was cured using bacterial transplant. Bacterial transplant is currently widely used for the treatment of IBS, hepatic encephalopathy, and steatosis. Obesity, autoimmune diseases, and diseases of the nervous system are also significantly improved with the introduction of good bacteria [58].

Fecal matter transplant (FMT) is a popular technique used for treatment of psychiatric disorders. The dysbiosis of gut microbiome is treated by administering fecal matter from healthy individuals. It has been shown that the incoming microbes will face competition from existing microorganisms, but will eventually show tolerance to the friendly bacteria [59]. Studies were conducted on GF mice where anxiety and IBS symptoms were assessed by FMT. Stool banks have become popular recently, which provide donors with highly screened fecal matter rich in beneficial bacteria. Capsule FMT has further simplified the process of delivering good bacteria to the donor.

MDD and anxiety disorders are currently being treated with antidepressants. Due to many side effects faced by the patients, there emerges the need for alternative techniques such as FMT for curing mental disorders. The mechanism of action of FMT is still unclear and only based on hypothetical approaches. Meyyppan et al. have listed some of the limitations in studying and standardising FMT; the main among them being the sample size and randomisation of the controlled trials. One of the approaches identifies serotonin imbalance as the main cause of depression and 90% production of serotonin is by EC cells of gut [60].

Dietary fibres [DFs] are complex carbohydrates having varied physicochemical properties. Fructo- and galacto-oligosaccharides are also DFs, and they tolerate digestion by host enzymes and aid in fermentation processes in the large intestine. DFs are responsible for the formation of SCFAs by gut microbiota, which promotes health and well-being. The role of probiotics in restoration of microbial population, and a possible role in treatment of depression and other mood disorders have been elucidated [61]. It has been noticed that infants whose mothers were on probiotics prior to delivery were better adapted to metabolic and immunological diseases. However, they still believe that there is insufficient data with regard to use of probiotics and their appreciable benefit or harm to pregnant women. Pre- and probiotics may contribute immensely in the mitigation of global issues affecting the society in the form of disease and pandemics. The only caution to be observed is that the administered probiotic must promote homeostasis. Recently, the role of probiotics in absorbing heavy metals from food growing in contaminated regions is also examined [62].

It can be concluded that a bidirectional brain-to-gut axis (BGA) imparts a major influence on the mental health of individuals, and probiotics have proved to be beneficial for mental health. Few limitations hindering the study include the majority of trials done on animals/rats, the small size of the sample, and presence of the third variable, i.e., confounding factor. Overcoming these gaps in the future may make treatment for chronic mental disorders easy by modifications of BGA.

14.6 Conclusion

The dynamic bidirectional communication between the gut and brain executes the strong effect on mental health and brain homeostasis. As outlined, the synergistic communication along GBA has an influential association with some neuropsychiatric disorders. The potential functionality of the gut microbiota has been proven to show an unmediated relationship with the diet, which is ultimately associated with psychopathological outcomes. Moreover, probiotics have been proven to be constructive in treating mental health disorders. Furthermore, comorbidities such as a western diet, lifestyle, alcohol, and obesity may have an overall impact on the beneficial effects of psychobiotics. In particular, smoking and alcohol use could influence the human microbiome following down-regulation of brain functions. The degree of complexity of the recovery process is directly proportional to the stage of psychiatric condition.

The increasing evidence and contemporary outlook suggests that patients with psychiatric disorders such as depression, anxiety, bipolar disorder, schizophrenia, ADHD, and ASD have a notable distinctive composition of their gut microbiota. Albeit, much remains to discover regarding brain functioning the the areas of nutrition, gut health, and drug pharmacokinetics as far as comprehensive psychiatric care is concerned. Despite this, the proposal of psychotropic medication is considered persuasive with regard to the futuristic approach.

References

1 Andoh, A. (2016). Physiological role of gut microbiota for maintaining human health. *Digestion* 93 (3): 176–81.

2 Fan, Y. and Pedersen, O. (2021 January). Gut microbiota in human metabolic health and disease. *Nat. Rev. Microbiol.* 19 (1): 55–71.

3 Rinninella, E., Raoul, P., Cintoni, M. et al. (2019 January). What is the healthy gut microbiota composition? A changing ecosystem across age, environment, diet, and diseases. *Microorganisms* 7 (1).

4 Lucas, G. (2018 November). Gut thinking: the gut microbiome and mental health beyond the head. *Microb. Ecol. Health Dis.* 29 (2): 1548250.

5 Martin, C.R., Osadchiy, V., Kalani, A. et al. (2018). The brain–gut–microbiome axis. *Cell Mol. Gastroent. Hepatol.* 6 (2): 133–48.

6 Skonieczna-Żydecka, K., Marlicz, W., Misera, A. et al. (2018 December). Microbiome: the missing link in the gut–brain axis: focus on its role in gastrointestinal and mental health. *J. Clin. Med.* 7 (12).

7 Schächtle, M.A. and Rosshart, S.P. (2021). The microbiota–gut–brain axis in health and disease and its implications for translational research. *Front. Cell Neurosci.* 15: 698172.

8 Reigstad, C.S., Salmonson, C.E., Rainey, J.F. III et al. (2015 April). Gut microbes promote colonic serotonin production through an effect of short-chain fatty acids on enterochromaffin cells. *FASEB J. Off. Publ. Fed. Am Soc. Exp. Biol.* 29 (4): 1395–1403.

9 Jacobson, A., Yang, D., Vella, M. et al. (2021 May). The intestinal neuro-immune axis: crosstalk between neurons, immune cells, and microbes. *Mucosal Immunol.* 14 (3): 555–65.

10 Huang, C., Wang, J., Hu, W. et al. (2016 September). Identification of functional farnesoid X receptors in brain neurons. *FEBS Lett.* 590 (18): 3233–3242.

11 Khlevner, J., Park, Y., and Margolis, K.G. (2018 December). Brain–gut axis: clinical implications. *Gastroenterol. Clin. North Am.* 47 (4): 727–39.

12 Strandwitz, P. (2018 August). Neurotransmitter modulation by the gut microbiota. *Brain Res.* 1693 (Pt B): 128–133.

13 Chong, P.P., Chin, V.K., Looi, C.Y. et al. (2019). The microbiome and irritable bowel syndrome: a review on the pathophysiology, current research and future therapy. *Front. Microbiol.* 10: 1136.

14 Eshraghi, R.S., Davies, C., Iyengar, R. et al. (2020 December). Gut-induced inflammation during development may compromise the blood–brain barrier and predispose to autism spectrum disorder. *J. Clin. Med.* 10 (1).

15 Muller, P.A., Schneeberger, M., Matheis, F. et al. (2020 July). Microbiota modulate sympathetic neurons via a gut-brain circuit. *Nature* 583 (7816): 441–446.

16 Cryan, J.F. and Dinan, T.G. (2012 October). Mind-altering microorganisms: the impact of the gut microbiota on brain and behavior. *Nat. Rev. Neurosci.* 13 (10): 701–712.

17 Rogers, G.B., Keating, D.J., Young, R.L. et al. (2016 June). From gut dysbiosis to altered brain function and mental illness: mechanisms and pathways. *Mol. Psych.* 21 (6): 738–748.

18 Fond, G., Boukouaci, W., Chevalier, G. et al. (2015 February). The "psychomicrobiotic": Targeting microbiota in major psychiatric disorders: a systematic review. *Pathol. Biol. (Paris)* 63 (1): 35–42.

19 Mulle, J.G., Sharp, W.G., and Cubells, J.F. (2013 February). The gut microbiome: a new frontier in autism research. *Curr. Psych. Rep.* 15 (2): 337.

20 Chaidez, V., Hansen, R.L., and Hertz-Picciotto, I. (2014 May). Gastrointestinal problems in children with autism, developmental delays or typical development. *J. Autism Dev. Disord.* 44 (5): 1117–1127.

21 Krajmalnik-Brown, R., Lozupone, C., Kang, D.W. et al. (2015 March). Gut bacteria in children with autism spectrum disorders: challenges and promise of studying how a complex community influences a complex disease. *Microb. Ecol. Health Dis.* 26: 26914.

22 Desbonnet, L., Garrett, L., Clarke, G. et al. (2008 December). The probiotic *Bifidobacteria infantis*: an assessment of potential antidepressant properties in the rat. *J. Psychiatr. Res.* 43 (2): 164–174.

23 Kang, D.W., Adams, J.B., Coleman, D.M. et al. (2019 April). Long-term benefit of Microbiota Transfer Therapy on autism symptoms and gut microbiota. *Sci. Rep.* 9 (1): 5821.

24 Bleys, D., Luyten, P., Soenens, B. et al. (2018 January). Gene–environment interactions between stress and 5-HTTLPR in depression: a meta-analytic update. *J. Affect. Disord.* 226: 339–345.

25 Panossian, A. (2017 August). Understanding adaptogenic activity: specificity of the pharmacological action of adaptogens and other phytochemicals. *Ann. N.Y. Acad. Sci.* 1401 (1): 49–64.

26 Knuesel, T., and Mohajeri, M.H. (2022). The role of the gut microbiota in the development and progression of major depressive and bipolar disorder. *Nutrients* 14 (1). doi.org/mdpi. com/2072-6643/14/1/37.

27 Martins, L.B., Braga Tibães, J.R., Sanches, M. et al. (2021 March). Nutrition-based interventions for mood disorders. *Expert. Rev. Neurother.* 21 (3): 303–315.

28 Rakofsky, J., and Rapaport, M. (2018 June). Mood disorders. *Contin. Life. Learn. Neurol.* 24 (3): 804–827.

29 Huang, T.-T., Lai, J.-B., Du, Y.-L. et al. (2019). Current understanding of gut microbiota in mood disorders: an update of human studies. *Front. Genet.* 10: 98.

30 Zhang, M., Ma, W., Zhang, J. et al. (2018 September). Analysis of gut microbiota profiles and microbe–disease associations in children with autism spectrum disorders in China. *Sci. Rep.* 8 (1): 13981.

31 Shen, Y., Xu, J., Li, Z. et al. (2018 July). Analysis of gut microbiota diversity and auxiliary diagnosis as a biomarker in patients with schizophrenia: a cross-sectional study. *Schizophr. Res.* 197: 470–477.

32 Chen, Z., Li, J., Gui, S. et al. (2018 March). Comparative metaproteomics analysis shows altered fecal microbiota signatures in patients with major depressive disorder. *Neuroreport* 29 (5): 417–425.

33 Chen, J.-J., Zheng, P., Liu, Y.-Y. et al. (2018). Sex differences in gut microbiota in patients with major depressive disorder. *Neuropsychiatr. Dis. Treat.* 14: 647–655.

34 Coello, K., Hansen, T.H., Sørensen, N. et al. (2019 January). Gut microbiota composition in patients with newly diagnosed bipolar disorder and their unaffected first-degree relatives. *Brain Behav. Immun.* 75: 112–118.

35 Painold, A., Mörkl, S., Kashofer, K. et al. (2019 February). A step ahead: exploring the gut microbiota in inpatients with bipolar disorder during a depressive episode. *Bipolar Disord.* 21 (1): 40–49.

36 Guo, L., Ji, C., Ma, Q. et al. (2018). The diversity and the abundance of gut microbiome in patients with bipolar disorder. *Chin. J. Psych.* 51: 98–104.

37 Maier, L., Pruteanu, M., Kuhn, M. et al. (2018 March). Extensive impact of non-antibiotic drugs on human gut bacteria. *Nature* 55 (7698): 623–628.

38 Kunugi, H. (2021). Gut microbiota and pathophysiology of depressive disorder. *Ann. Nutr. Metab.* 77 (2): 11–20.

39 Limbana, T., Khan, F., and Eskander, N. (2020 August). Gut microbiome and depression: how microbes affect the way we think. *Cureus* 12 (8).

40 De Filippis, F., Pasolli, E., and Ercolini, D. (2020 July). The food-gut axis: lactic acid bacteria and their link to food, the gut microbiome and human health. *FEMS Microbiol. Rev.* 44 (4): 454–489.

41 Wang, S.C., Chen, Y.C., Chen, S.J. et al. (2020 January). Alcohol addiction, gut microbiota, and alcoholism treatment: a review. *Int. J. Mol. Sci.* 21 (17): 6413.

42 Dubinkina, V.B., Tyakht, A.V., Odintsova, V.Y. et al. (2017 December). Links of gut microbiota composition with alcohol dependence syndrome and alcoholic liver disease. *Microbiome* 5 (1): 1–4.

43 Vassallo, G., Mirijello, A., Ferrulli, A. et al. (2015 May). Alcohol and gut microbiota: the possible role of gut microbiota modulation in the treatment of alcoholic liver disease. *Alim. Pharmacol. Ther.* 41 (10): 917–927.

44 Cussotto, S., Strain, C.R., Fouhy, F. et al. (2019 May). Differential effects of psychotropic drugs on microbiome composition and gastrointestinal function. *Psychopharmacology (Berl)* 236 (5): 1671–1685.

45 Gardner, D.M., Baldessarini, R.J., and Waraich, P. (2005 June). Modern antipsychotic drugs: a critical overview. *CMAJ* 172 (13): 1703–1711.

46 Maier, L., Pruteanu, M., Kuhn, M. et al. (2018 March). Extensive impact of non-antibiotic drugs on human gut bacteria. *Nature* 555 (7698): 623–628.

47 Clarke, G., Sandhu, K.V., Griffin, B.T. et al. (2019 April). Gut reactions: breaking down xenobiotic–microbiome interactions. *Pharmacol. Rev.* 71 (2): 198–224.

48 Dinan, T.G., Stanton, C., and Cryan, J.F. (2013 November). Psychobiotics: a novel class of psychotropic. *Biol. Psych.* 74 (10): 720–726.

49 Sarkar, A., Lehto, S.M., Harty, S. et al. (2016 November). Psychobiotics and the manipulation of bacteria–gut–brain signals. *Trends Neurosci.* 39 (11): 763–781.

50 Messaoudi, M., Lalonde, R., Violle, N. et al. (2011 March). Assessment of psychotropic-like properties of a probiotic formulation (*Lactobacillus helveticus* R0052 and *Bifidobacterium longum* R0175) in rats and human subjects. *Br. J. Nutr.* 105 (5): 755–764.

51 Allen, A.P., Hutch, W., Borre, Y.E. et al. (2016 November). *Bifidobacterium longum* 1714 as a translational psychobiotic: modulation of stress, electrophysiology and neurocognition in healthy volunteers. *Transl. Psych.* 6 (11): e939.

52 Steenbergen, L., Sellaro, R., van Hemert, S. et al. (2015 August). A randomized controlled trial to test the effect of multispecies probiotics on cognitive reactivity to sad mood. *Brain Behav. Immun.* 48: 258–264.

53 Akbari, E., Asemi, Z., Daneshvar Kakhaki, R. et al. (2016 November). Effect of probiotic supplementation on cognitive function and metabolic status in Alzheimer's disease: a randomized, double-blind and controlled trial. *Front. Aging Neurosci.* 8: 256.

54 Tamtaji, O.R., Taghizadeh, M., Daneshvar Kakhaki, R. et al. (2019 June). Clinical and metabolic response to probiotic administration in people with Parkinson's disease: a randomized, double-blind, placebo-controlled trial. *Clin. Nutr.* 38 (3): 1031–1035.

55 Shaaban, S.Y., El Gendy, Y.G., Mehanna, N.S. et al. (2018 November). The role of probiotics in children with autism spectrum disorder: a prospective, open-label study. *Nutr. Neurosci.* 21 (9): 676–681.

56 Wallace, C.J.K. and Milev, R. (2017 February). The effects of probiotics on depressive symptoms in humans: a systematic review. *Ann. Gen. Psychiatry* 16: 14.

57 Bahr, S.M., Tyler, B.C., Wooldridge, N. et al. (2015 October). Use of the second-generation antipsychotic, risperidone, and secondary weight gain are associated with an altered gut microbiota in children. *Transl. Psychiatry* 5 (10): e652–e652.

58 Olesen, S.W., Panchal, P., Chen, J. et al. (2020 March). Global disparities in faecal microbiota transplantation research. *Lancet Gastroenterol. Hepatol.* 5 (3): 241.

59 Lau, A.W.Y., Tan, L.T.-H., Ab Mutalib, N.-S. et al. (2021 February). The chemistry of gut microbiome in health and diseases. *Prog. Microbes. Mol. Biol.* 4 (1). doi.org/journals. hh-publisher.com/index.php/pmmb/article/view/379.

60 Chinna Meyyappan, A., Forth, E., Wallace, C.J.K. et al. (2020 June). Effect of fecal microbiota transplant on symptoms of psychiatric disorders: a systematic review. *BMC Psych.* 20 (1): 299.

61 Clapp, M., Aurora, N., Herrera, L. et al. (2017 September). Gut microbiota's effect on mental health: the gut–brain axis. *Clin. Pract.* 7 (4): 987.

62 Grev, J., Berg, M., and Soll, R. (2018 December). Maternal probiotic supplementation for prevention of morbidity and mortality in preterm infants. *Cochrane Database Syst. Rev.* 12 (12): CD012519.

15

Interaction between Gut Microbiota and Central and Enteric Nervous Systems: The Gut–Brain Axis Concept

Mohamed Hussein Arbab

Associate Professor of Medical Microbiology, Omdurman Ahlia University, Sudan

15.1 Introduction

The immune system is a built-in defence system that exists in complex organisms to protect the host from health threats such as tissue injury, pathogen infection, and tumorigenesis. During immune defence, the biological process of inflammation is responsible for initiating an immune response. This involves the production and secretion of inflammatory cytokines and chemokines, which together with the expression of cell surface receptors, form signaling cascades that integrate both innate and adaptive immune cells into the immune response. It was originally thought that the cells in the immune system were solely responsible for facilitating inflammation and immune responses; however, there are clear regulatory links with the nervous system that show the immune system is not autonomous, but functions in close association with the nervous system. It is now clear that these two systems are intimately connected and reciprocally influence the function of each other, and this constitutes the neuroimmune network [1]. Anatomically, nerves and immune cells are connected throughout the human body. Mechanistically, nerve cells and immune cells produce soluble factors that communicate through their cognate receptors to regulate immune processes such as inflammation. Indeed, the central nervous system (CNS) has been suggested to be a virtual secondary lymphoid organ that is involved in the regulation of immune responses throughout the human body [2]. Communication between neurons and immune cells in the regulation of inflammation contributes not only to cellular defence, but also to inflammatory-associated pathology. As a result of restrictive entry of immune cells into the brain, brain cells other than neurons, such as microglia and astrocytes, also act as a first line of defence to control inflammation and immune responses in both CNS and peripheral tissues [3–10]. In addition to communication between different cells within the organism, interspecies communication between the microbiota and host brain cells, neurons, and immune cells occurs, may have an impact on health and disease. In this chapter, we briefly summarise the involvement of neurons and immune cells in the regulation of inflammation, as well

The Gut Microbiota in Health and Disease, First Edition. Edited by Nimmy Srivastava, Salam A. Ibrahim, Jayeeta Chattopadhyay, and Mohamed H. Arbab.
© 2023 John Wiley & Sons Ltd. Published 2023 by John Wiley & Sons Ltd.

as the involvement of microbiota in the development of the nerve and immune systems. We then focus on recent findings on the contribution of microbiota in the regulation of cellular defence.

The family of pathogen-associated molecular patterns (PAMPs) that are derived from microbes, and damage-associated molecular patterns (DAMPs) derived from host cells, are the main categories of 'danger' molecules that initiate innate immune responses and inflammation [11]. Upon pathogen invasion or tissue damage, these molecules are released and detected by pattern recognition receptors (PRRs) that are expressed by innate surveillance immune cells. Toll-like receptors (TLRs) are a class of PRRs that sense the presence of conserved microbial molecular patterns for early immune recognition of a pathogen. The binding of PAMPs or DAMPs to TLRs on innate immune cells such as macrophages initiates infectious or non-infectious acute inflammatory responses, respectively. These events result in intracellular cascades such as the Nuclear factor-kappaB (NF-κB) pathway to initiate the transcription of both pro- and anti-inflammatory cytokines [12]. This leads to subsequent activation and recruitment of adaptive lymphocytes to the site of inflammation, where cytokines such as IFN-γ, IL-10, or TGF-β are released to clear the infection and/or to settle down inflammation and initiate tissue repair. When acute inflammation fails to settle, it may progress to prolonged, low-level inflammation resulting in chronic conditions such as autoimmune diseases and cancer. Therefore, the level and process of inflammation are tightly regulated to avoid inflammation-associated pathology.

15.2 The Neuronal Communications

The nervous system regulates numerous physiological responses including movement, digestion, body temperature, stress, and secretion of various enzymes and hormones. All these responses are regulated by communication between neurons of different parts of the nervous system with the central nervous system (CNS) in the brain and the peripheral nervous system (PNS), which connects the CNS to every part of the body through the spinal cord. Neurons communicate with each other to send messages to and from the brain and spinal cord to various parts of the body by both electrical and chemical signals involving a range of soluble molecules, which interact with cell surface receptors [13]. The signaling process initiates as dendrites, which receive external stimuli, followed by the cell body generating an electrical signal (action potential) that propagates along the axon to the nerve terminal. This results in the release of chemical signaling molecules as neuronal messengers, such as neurotransmitters [14], to regulate the responses of target cells such as neurons, muscles, and immune cells. Cells of the nervous system participate in immune surveillance and cellular defence at different levels and regions via both neural and non-neural communicating pathways [15]. These include the blood–brain barrier (BBB) pathway [16], the neuroendocrine pathways [17], and the microbiota–gut–brain (MGB) axis [18], in which soluble molecules such as neurotransmitters, hormones, and cytokines are the main communication tools [1, 19].

15.3 Neuroimmune Regulation of Inflammation and Cellular Defence

Research in the area of neuroimmunology has revealed that neurological signaling utilising soluble molecules is involved in the communication between neurons and immune cells, which regulates inflammation and immune responses. Neurons have been found to express various cytokine and chemokine receptors such as the IL-6 receptor and CXCR4 that allow them to receive proinflammatory stimuli from immune cells [20–22]. Treatment with TNF-α and IL-1β has been shown to evoke a neural response in mouse vagus nerve cells in a dose-dependent manner [23]. Indeed, these proinflammatory cytokines were found to be more effective than LPS, norepinephrine, and nerve growth factor for activating primary neurons in cultures [24]. In addition to immune cells, human and mouse neurons express TLRs [25, 26] that enable them to directly detect danger signals [27, 28]. Expression of TLR-7 by mouse airway neurons was also found to be increased after stimulation with neuropeptide substance P, and contributes to airway inflammation and immune defence [29]. Activation of sensory neurons through either cytokine or PAMPs/DAMPs leads to the production of neuronal signaling molecules, including neurotransmitters (reviewed in Pinho-Ribeiro et al. [30]. In addition, neurons are also capable of producing cytokines to regulate inflammation; this has been observed where stimulation of P2X purinoceptor 7 receptors (P2X7Rs) on the neural membrane trigger the release of multiple cytokines by mouse neurons and provide neuroprotection [31]. Similar to neurons, many subsets of immune cells have been found to express receptors for various neurotransmitters as well as being capable of producing neurotransmitters upon activation [32, 33]. Serotonin, which is a multi-functional neurotransmitter, has been found to drive both proinflammatory [34] and anti-inflammatory [35, 36] responses through serotonin receptors expressed on mouse immune cells such as T cells. Gamma-aminobutyric acid (GABA), which is a neurotransmitter in the brain and pancreatic islets, has been found to inhibit the release of inflammatory cytokines by human peripheral blood mononuclear cells (PBMC) and CD4+T cells by blocking calcium signaling and NF-κB activity [37, 38]. Treatment with GABA or GABAergic drugs in mouse bone marrow-derived macrophages (BMDM) inhibited the production of proinflammatory cytokines TNF-α and IL-6, but enhanced antimicrobial responses of BMDM through intracellular calcium release and autophagy [39]. Recent studies by two independent groups have both reported that mouse T cell-derived acetylcholine promotes immune infiltration and the production of proinflammatory cytokines at the site of pathogen invasion to clear the infection [40, 41]. Therefore, signaling through neurotransmitters and their receptors may lead to either pro- or anti-inflammatory responses, depending on the local stimuli and the target cells they are acting on (reviewed in Hodo et al. [42]). Overall, cells of the immune and nervous systems communicate with each other through a common language using soluble molecules and cell surface receptors. Such signaling processes allows the integration of neurological and immunological signals to detect pathogen invasion, regulate inflammation, and orchestrate tissue homeostasis [33, 43, 44].

15.3.1 Involvement of Microbiota in the Development of the Nervous and Immune Systems and Modulation of Inflammation

It was originally considered that the fetal and perinatal immune systems develop in a relatively sterile environment where microbial and maternal immune cells have restricted entry. However, the human placenta and amniotic fluid have been found to harbour a unique microbiome, which shares features of microbiota detected in the infant meconium, and might contribute to the initiation of microbiota colonisation in the gut [45, 46]. In addition, a recent human study discovered the presence of several types of bacteria in the fetal gut, skin, placenta, and lungs in the second trimester of gestation [47]. These bacteria were found to be able to induce activation of memory T cells isolated from the fetal mesenteric lymph node, suggesting their contribution in priming the fetal immune cells during early human development [47]. It is now clear that microbial encounters occur in at least three stages of early mammalian life: in utero (during pregnancy); microbes acquired at the time of delivery; and microbes established postnatally by the acquisition of maternal and environmental bacteria [48–50]. Early life exposure to microbiota imprint long-lasting changes in the offspring's nervous and immune systems that affect the health and risk of diseases throughout life [51–55]. The enteric nervous system (ENS), which is part of the autonomic nervous system (ANS), is a unique nervous system that largely functions independently from but does communicate with the CNS. Innervation of the gut by the network of ENS provides a unique opportunity for gut microbiota to form a multidirectional communication axis with the local neurons, immune cells, and brain cells [56]. This forms the microbiota–gut–brain (MGB) axis, which drives a variety of processes including intestinal barrier function, blood–brain barrier (BBB) function, and neuroimmune crosstalk to regulate not only brain health [57] but also the development and function of the host defence systems (reviewed in Bistoletti et al. [18] and others [58–60]).

15.3.2 The Importance of Microbiota for the Development of the Nervous and Immune Systems

The importance of microbiota in the development and health of the brain and CNS has been clearly shown in mice lacking gut microbiota, where development of anxiolytic-like behaviour and neurodegenerative disease was observed [61–63]. Compared to specific pathogen-free mice, germ-free mice were found to have altered expression of genes involved in signaling mechanisms that affect motor control and anxiety behaviour [64]. Mice transplanted with gut microbiota from patients with neurobehavioral disorders also showed altered brain structure and anxious behaviour [65]. Studies in obese and non-obese individuals also found that alterations in microbial composition affect brain microstructure and cognitive function [66]. Maternal probiotic administration of mice with *Lactobacillus acidophilus* and *Bifidobacterium infantis* has been shown to promote neuronal and oligodendrocyte progenitor cell development in the offspring [67]. At the molecular level, the microbiota have been found to not only regulate the production, transportation, and functioning of neurotransmitters, but are also capable of producing neurotransmitters to regulate the development of the brain and CNS [68, 69]. *Bifidobacteria*, which are a group of commensal bacteria in the gut, have been found to harbour the gene and enzymatic machinery to generate neurotransmitters such as GABA and tyrosine [70]. Altering the composition of the gut microbiota with a high-sugar and high-fat diet altered neurotransmitter metabolism and affected brain function [71]. Although the precise molecular mechanisms of microbiota interaction with host cells are largely unknown, there is growing evidence that the microbiota interact with host cells and affect their development and function through microbial-derived soluble molecules (reviewed in Silva et al. [72] and Wall et al. [73]). Short-chain fatty acids (SCFAs) are one of the most studied metabolites produced by the gut microbiota through fermentation of dietary fibre and indigestible polysaccharides. Microbial-derived SCFAs have been found to promote the production of serotonin by host cells [74]. This contributes to the maintenance of the neuroanatomy and maturation of the ENS [75]. Mice fed with a diet containing a low level of SCFAs during gestation have been found to have impaired neurocognitive functions of the offspring [76]. Germ-free mice and mice deficient for SCFA receptors have both been found to display global defects in the maturation and function of microglial cells, leading to impaired cellular defence in the CNS [77]. In another mouse study, microbial metabolites other than SCFAs derived from spore-forming gut bacteria were also found to serve as signaling molecules to regulate the biosynthesis of serotonin, contributing to gastrointestinal motility and platelet function [78]. To endow a newborn with the ability to mount an immune response against pathogen invasion after birth, mammalian immunity starts to develop during the prenatal period of life and continues to evolve throughout the lifetime of the individual [79]. Maternal microbiota and early life microbiota exposure during birth and through breast milk have been found to influence the lineage development and the education of the hematopoietic cells, as well as functional responses of immune cells in the newborn [49, 80]. The effects of microbiota on immune cells have also been found to occur via their metabolites. Mucosal-associated invariant T cells (MAIT) are gut resident innate immune cells that play an important role in gut inflammation and defence against pathogen infection. Bacterial riboflavin-derived antigen, 5-OP-RU, was found to be able to travel from mucosal surfaces to the thymus and be taken up by the major histocompatibility complex class I-related protein (MR1) to promote the generation of MAIT [81, 82]. Consequently, early life exposure to microbial riboflavin may regulate the development of and also interact with MAIT cells, to promote gut immunity and homeostasis [83]. The SCFA butyrate, a major gut metabolite, has also been found to facilitate either the differentiation of T regulatory cells or effector T helper-1 cells under various conditions, suggesting that the influence of gut microbiota on the differentiation of immune cells is subjected to the local environment [84].

The microbiota have been found to induce neural expression of AhR, which enable the neurons to sense and respond to the luminal environment by upregulating neuron-specific effector mechanisms [85].

References

1 Dantzer, R. (2018). Neuroimmune interactions: from the brain to the immune system and vice versa. *Physiol. Rev.* 98: 477–504.

2 Negi, N. and Das, B.K. (2018). CNS: not an immunoprivileged site anymore but a virtual secondary lymphoid organ. *Int. Rev. Immunol.* 37: 57–68.

3 Xu, S., Lu, J., Shao, A.J. et al. (2020). Glial cells: role of the immune response in ischemic stroke. *Front. Immunol.* 11: 294.

4 Williams, K. Jr., Ulvestad, E., Cragg, L. et al. (1993). Induction of primary T cell responses by human glial cells. *J. Neurosci. Res.* 36: 382–390.

5 Antel, J.P., Becher, B., Ludwin, S.K. et al. (2020). Glial cells as regulators of neuroimmune interactions in the central nervous system. *J. Immunol.* 204: 251–255.

6 Chhatbar, C. and Prinz, M. (2021). The roles of microglia in viral encephalitis: from sensome to therapeutic targeting. *Cell. Mol. Immunol.* 18: 250–258.

7 Wyatt-Johnson, S.K. and Brutkiewicz, R.R. (2020). The complexity of microglial interactions with innate and adaptive immune cells in Alzheimer's disease. *Front. Aging Neurosci.* 12: 592359.

8 Olson, J.K. and Miller, S.D. (2004). Microglia initiate central nervous system innate and adaptive immune responses through multiple TLRs. *J. Immunol.* 173: 3916–3924.

9 Ibiza, S., Garćia-Cassani, B., Ribeiro, H. et al. (2016). Glial-cell-derived neuroregulators control type 3 innate lymphoid cells and gut defence. *Nature* 535: 440–443.

10 Paape, M.J., Shafer-Weaver, K., Capuco, A.V. et al. (2000). Immune surveillance of mammary tissue by phagocytic cells. *Adv. Exp. Med. Biol.* 480: 259–277.

11 Ramadan, A., Land, W.G., and Paczesny, S. (2017). Editorial: danger signals triggering immune response and inflammation. *Front. Immunol.* 8: 979.

12 Mueller, C. (2012). Danger-associated molecular patterns and inflammatory bowel disease: is there a connection? *Dig. Dis.* 30 (Supp. 3): 40–46.

13 Lovinger, D.M. (2008). Communication networks in the brain: neurons, receptors, neurotransmitters, and alcohol. *Alcohol Res. Health* 31: 196–214.

14 Franco, R., Pacheco, R., Lluis, C. et al. (2007). The emergence of neurotransmitters as immune modulators. *Trends Immunol.* 28: 400–407.

15 Eskandari, F., Webster, J.I., and Sternberg, E.M. (2003). Neural immune pathways and their connection to inflammatory diseases. *Arthritis Res. Ther.* 5: 251–265.

16 Marchetti, L. and Engelhardt, B. (2020). Immune cell trafficking across the blood–brain barrier in the absence and presence of neuroinflammation. *Vasc. Biol.* 2: H1–H18.

17 Savino, W., Silva, P.O., and Besedovsky, H. (2009). Network of bidirectional interactions between the neuroendocrine and immune systems. *Ann. NY Acad. Sci.* 1153: xi.

18 Bistoletti, M., Bosi, A., Banfi, D. et al. (2020). The microbiota–gut–brain axis: focus on the fundamental communication pathways. *Prog. Mol. Biol. Transl. Sci.* 176: 43–110.

19 Thyaga Rajan, S. and Priyanka, H.P. (2012). Bidirectional communication between the neuroendocrine system and the immune system: relevance to health and diseases. *Ann. Neurosci.* 19: 40–46.

20 Sawada, M., Itoh, Y., Suzumura, A. et al. (1993). Expression of cytokine receptors in cultured neuronal and glial cells. *Neurosci. Lett.* 160: 131–134.

21 Tran, P.B., Banisadr, G., Ren, D. et al. (2007). Chemokine receptor expression by neural progenitor cells in neurogenic regions of mouse brain. *J. Comp. Neurol.* 500: 1007–1033.

22 Salvador, A.F., de Lima, K.A., and Kipnis, J. (2021). Neuromodulation by the immune system: a focus on cytokines. *Nat. Rev. Immunol.* 21: 526–541.

23 Zanos, T.P., Silverman, H.A., Levy, T. et al. (2018). Identification of cytokine-specific sensory neural signals by decoding murine vagus nerve activity. *Proc. Natl. Acad. Sci. USA* 115: e4843–e4852.

24 Listwak, S.J., Rathore, P., and Herkenham, M. (2013). Minimal NF-jB activity in neurons. *Neuroscience* 250: 282–299.

25 Frederiksen, H.R., Haukedal, H., and Freude, K. (2019). Cell type specific expression of toll-like receptors inhuman brains and implications in Alzheimer's disease. *Bio. Med. Res. Int.* 1–18.

26 Kaul, D., Habbel, P., Derkow, K. et al. (2012). Expression of Toll-like receptors in the developing brain. *PLoS One* 7: e37767.

27 Donnelly, C.R., Chen, O., and Ji, R.R. (2020). How do sensory neurons sense danger signals? *Trends Neurosci.* 43: 822–838.

28 Park, C.K., Xu, Z.Z., Berta, T. et al. (2014). Extracellular micro RNAs activate nociceptor neurons to elicit pain via TLR7 and TRPA1. *Neuron* 82: 47–54.

29 Larsson, O., Tengroth, L., Xu, Y.et al. (2018). SubstanceP represents a novel first-line defense mechanism in the nose. *J. All. Clin. Immunol.* 141: 128–136, e123.

30 Pinho-Ribeiro, F.A., Verri, W.A. Jr, and Chiu, I.M. (2017). Nociceptor sensory neuron-immune interactions in pain and inflammation. *Trends Immunol.* 38: 5–19.

31 Lim, J.C., Lu, W., Beckel, J.M. et al. (2016). Neuronal release of cytokine IL-3 triggered by mechanosensitive auto-stimulation of the P2X7 receptor is neuroprotective. *Front. Cell. Neurosci.* 10: 270.

32 Rosenberg,K.M. and Singh, N.J. (2019). Mouse T cells express a neurotransmitter-receptor signature that is quantitatively modulated in a subset- and activation-dependent manner. *Brain Behav. Immun.* 80: 275–285.

33 Kerage, D., Sloan, E.K., Mattarollo, S.R. et al. (2019). Interaction of neurotransmitters and neurochemicals with lymphocytes. *J. Neuroimmuno.* 332: 99–111.

34 Wan, M., Ding, L., Wang, D. et al. (2020). Serotonin: a potent immune cell modulator in autoimmune diseases. *Front .Immuno.* 11: 186.

35 Domínguez-Soto, Á., Usategui, A., Casas-Engel, M.L. et al. (2017). Serotonin drives the acquisition of a profibrotic and anti-inflammatory gene profile through the 5-HT7R-PKA signaling axis. *Sci. Rep.* 7: 14761.

36 Nau, F. Jr., Yu, B., Martin, D. et al. (2013). Serotonin 5-HT2A receptor activation blocks TNF-a mediated inflammation in vivo. *PLoS One* 8: e75426.

37 Datusalia, A.K. and Sharma, S.S. (2016). NF-jB inhibition resolves cognitive deficits in experimental type 2 diabetes mellitus through CREB and Glutamate/GABA neurotransmitters pathway. *Curr. Neurovasc. Res.* 13: 22–32.

38 Bhandage, A.K., Jin, Z., Korol, S.V. et al. (2018). GABA regulates release of inflammatory cytokines from peripheral blood mononuclear cells and CD4+ T cells and is immunosuppressive in Type 1 diabetes. *E. Bio. Medicine.* 30: 283–294.

39 Kim, J.K., Kim, Y.S., Lee, H.M. et al. (2018). GABAergic signaling linked to autophagy enhances host protection against intracellular bacterial infections. *Nat. Commun.* 9: 4184.

40 Cox, M.A., Duncan, G.S., Lin, G.H.Y. et al. (2019). Cholineacetyl transferase-expressing T cells are required to control chronic viral infection. *Science* 363: 639–644.

41 Ramirez, V.T., Godinez, D.R., Brust-Mascher, I. et al. (2019). T-cell derived acetylcholine aids host defenses during enteric bacterial infection with Citrobacterrodentium. *PLoS Pathog.* 15: e1007719.

42 Hodo, T.W., de Aquino, M.T.P., Shimamoto, A. et al. (2020). Critical neurotransmitters in the neuroimmune network. *Front. Immunol.* 11: 1869.

43 Qiu, Y., Peng, Y., and Wang, J. (1996). Immunoregulatory role of neurotransmitters. *Adv. Neuroimmuno.* 6: 223–231.

44 Levite, M. (2008). Neurotransmitters activate T-cells and elicit crucial functions via neurotransmitter receptors. *Curr. Opin. Pharmacol.* 8: 460–471.

45 Aagaard, K., Ma, J., Antony, K.M. et al. (2014). The placenta harbors a unique microbiome. *Sci. Transl. Med.* 6: 237ra265.

46 Collado, M.C., Rautava, S., Aakko, J. et al. (2016). Human gut colonisation may be initiated in utero by distinct microbial communities in the placenta and amniotic fluid. *Sci. Rep.* 6: 23129.

47 Mishra, A., Lai, G.C., Yao, L.J. et al. (2021). Microbial exposure during early human development primes fetal immune cells. *Cell* 184: 3394–3409, e20.

48 Younge, N., McCann, J.R., Ballard, J. et al. (2019). Fetal exposure to the maternal microbiota in humans and mice. *JCI Insight* 4: e127806.

49 Kalbermatter, C., Fernandez Trigo, N., Christensen, S. et al. (2021). Maternal microbiota, early life colonization and breast milk drive immune development in the newborn. *Front. Immunol.* 12: 683022.

50 Pronovost, G.N. and Hsiao, E.Y. (2019). Perinatal interactions between the microbiome, immunity, and neuro development. *Immunity* 50: 18–36.

51 Jain, N. (2020). The early life education of the immune system: moms, microbes and (missed) opportunities. *Gut Micro.* 12: 1824564.

52 Sampson, T.R. and Mazmanian, S.K. (2015). Control of brain development, function, and behavior by the microbiome. *Cell. Host. Micro.* 17: 565–576.

53 Zheng, D., Liwinski, T., and Elinav, E. (2020). Interaction between microbiota and immunity in health and disease. *Cell. Res.* 30: 492–506.

54 Ma, Q., Xing, C., Long, W. et al. (2019). Impact of microbiota on central nervous system and neurological diseases: the gut-brain axis. *J. Neuroinflam.* 16: 53.

55 Al Nabhani, Z. and Eberl, G. (2020). Imprinting of the immune system by the microbiota early in life. *Mucosal Immunol.* 13: 183–189.

56 Furness, J.B., Callaghan, B.P., Rivera, L.R. et al. (2014). The enteric nervous system and gastrointestinal innervation: integrated local and central control. *Adv. Exp. Med. Biol.* 817: 39–71.

57 Rao, M. and Gershon, M.D. (2016). The bowel and beyond: the enteric nervous system in neurological disorders. *Nat. Rev. Gastroenterol. Hepatol.* 13: 517–528.

58 Muller, P.A., Matheis, F., Schneeberger, M. et al. (2020). Microbiota-modulated CART+ enteric neurons autonomously regulate blood glucose. *Science* 370: 314–321.

59 O'Connor, K.M., Lucking, E.F., Cryan, J.F. et al. (2020). Bugs, breathing and blood pressure: microbiota–gut–brain axis signalling in cardiorespiratory control in health and disease. *J. Physiol.* 598: 4159–4179.

60 Schächtle, M.A. and Rosshart, S.P. (2021). Themicrobiota–gut–brain axis in health and disease and its implications for translational research. *Front. Cell. Neurosci.* 15: 698172.

61 Pan, J.X., Deng, F.L., Zeng, B.H. et al. (2019). Absence of gut microbiota during early life affects anxiolytic behaviors and monoamine neurotransmitters system in the hippocampal of mice. *J. Neurol. Sci.* 400: 160–168.

62 Luczynski, P., McVey Neufeld, K.A., Oriach, C.S. et al. (2016). Growing up in a bubble: using germ-free animals to assess the influence of the gut microbiota on brain and behavior. *Int. J. Neuropsychol.* 19: pyw020.

63 Huang, F. and Wu, X. (2021). Brain neurotransmitter modulation by gut microbiota in anxiety and depression. *Front. Cell. Dev. Biol.* 9: 649103.

64 Diaz Heijtz, R., Wang, S., Anuar, F. et al. (2011). Normal gut microbiota modulates brain development and behavior. *Proc. Natl. Acad. Sci. USA* 108: 3047–3052.

65 Tengeler, A.C., Dam, S.A., Wiesmann, M. et al. (2020). Gut microbiota from persons with attention-deficit/hyperactivity disorder affects the brain in mice. *Microbiome* 8: 44.

66 Fernandez-Real, J.M., Serino, M., Blasco, G. et al. (2015). Gut microbiota interacts with brain microstructure and function. *J. Clin. Endocrinol. Metab.* 100: 4505–4513.

67 Lu, J., Lu, L., Yu, Y. et al. (2020). Maternal administration of probiotics promotes brain development and protects offspring's brain from postnatal inflammatory insults in C57/BL6J mice. *Sci. Rep.* 10: 8178.

68 Strandwitz, P. (2018). Neurotransmitter modulation by the gut microbiota. *Brain Res.* 1693: 128–133.

69 Chen, Y., Xu, J., and Chen, Y. (2021). Regulation of neurotransmitters by the gut microbiota and effects on cognition in neurological disorders. *Nutrients* 13: 2099.

70 Luck, B., Horvath, T.D., Engevik, K.A. et al. (2021). Neurotransmitter profiles are altered in the gut and brain of mice mono-associated with *Bifidobacterium dentium*. *Biomolecules* 11: 1091.

71 Guo, Y., Zhu, X., Zeng, M. et al. (2021). A diet high in sugar andfat influences neurotransmitter metabolism and the affects brain function by altering the gut microbiota. *Transl. Psych.* 11: 328.

72 Silva, Y.P., Bernardi, A., and Frozza, R.L. (2020). The role of short-chainfatty acids from gut microbiota in gut–brain communication. *Front. Endocrinol. (Lausanne)* 11: 25.

73 Wall, R., Cryan, J.F., Ross, R.P. et al. (2014). Bacterial neuroactive compounds produced by psychobiotics. *Adv. Exp. Med. Biol.* 817: 221–239.

74 Reigstad, C.S., Salmonson, C.E., Rainey, J.F. III et al. (2015). Gut microbes promote colonic serotonin production through an effect of short-chain fatty acids on enterochromaffin cells. *FASEB J.* 29: 1395–1403.

75 DeVadder, F., Grasset, E., Mannerås Holm, L. et al. (2018). Gut microbiota regulates maturation of the adult enteric nervous system via enteric serotonin networks. *Proc. Natl. Acad. Sci. USA* 115: 6458–6463.

76 Yu, L., Zhong, X., He, Y. et al. (2020). Butyrate, but not propionate, reverses maternal diet-induced neurocognitive deficits in offspring. *Pharmacol. Res.* 160: 105082.

77 Kim, Y., Park, J., and Choi, Y.K. (2019). The role of astrocytes in the central nervous system focused on BK channel and heme oxygenase metabolites: a review. *Antioxi. (Basel)* 8: 121.

78 Heithoff, B.P., George, K.K., Phares, A.N. et al. (2021). Astrocytes are necessary for blood–brain barrier maintenance in the adult mouse brain. *Glia* 69: 436–472.

79 Kirischuk, S., Héja, L., Kardos, J. et al. (2016). Astrocyte sodium signaling and the regulation of neurotransmission. *Glia* 64: 1655–1666.

80 Li, K., Li, J., Zheng, J. et al. (2019). Reactive astrocytes in neurodegenerative diseases. *Aging Dis.* 10: 664–675.

81 Sanmarco, L.M., Wheeler, M.A., Gutiérrez-Vázquez, C. et al. (2021). Gut-licensed IFNc+ NK cells drive LAMP1+TRAIL+ anti-inflammatory astrocytes. *Nature* 590: 473–479.

82 Logsdon, A.F., Erickson, M.A., Rhea, E.M. et al. (2018). Gut reactions: how the blood–brain barrier connects the microbiome and the brain. *Exp. Biol. Med. (Maywood)* 243: 159–165.

83 Guarnieri, T., Abruzzo, P.M., and Bolotta, A. (2020). More than a cell biosensor: aryl hydrocarbon receptor at the intersection of physiology and inflammation. *Am. J. Physiol. Cell. Physiol.* 318: C1078–C1082.

84 Pernomian, L., Duarte-Silva, M., and de Barros Cardoso, C.R. (2020). The aryl hydrocarbon receptor (AHR) as a potential target for the control of intestinal inflammation: insights from an immune and bacteria sensor receptor. *Clin. Rev. Allergy Immunol.* 59: 382–390.

85 Nehmar, R., Fauconnier, L., Alves-Filho, J. et al. (2021 May). Aryl hydrocarbon receptor (AhR)-dependent Il-22 expression by type 3 innate lymphoid cells control of acute joint inflammation. *J. Cell. Mol. Med.* 25 (10): 4721–4731.

16

Immune-Modulation and Gut Microbiome

Sarah Adjei-Fremah[1], Mulumebet Worku[2], and Salam Ibrahim[3]

[1] *Department of Biological Sciences, Winston-Salem State University, Winston-Salem North Carolina, USA*
[2] *Department of Animal Sciences, North Carolina Agricultural and Technical State University, Greensboro, North Carolina, USA*
[3] *Department of Family and Consumer Sciences, North Carolina Agricultural and Technical State University, Greensboro, North Carolina, USA*

16.1　Introduction

The gut microbiota is composed of complex and dynamic microbial communities including bacteria, archaea, viruses, protozoa, and fungi, and the collective genome of all microbial communities makes up the gut microbiome [1]. The gut microbial diversity classification consists of four predominant phyla; *Firmicutes*, *Bacteroides*, *Proteobacteria*, and *Actinobacteria*, comprising 90% of microbiota in humans. The most abundant, *Firmicutes* phylum (60–80%), consists of 200 different microbial genera including *Lactobacillus*, *Clostridium*, *Enterococcus*, and *Ruminicoccus*. The *Actinobacteria* phylum consists of the *Bifidobacteria* genera [2]. Comparatively, the human microbiome has over three million genes, while different animal species have uniquely diverse microbiomes of equal or greater complexity compared to human microbiome [3]. Interestingly, studies have shown microbiome sharing between humans and animals in close contact. Kraemer et al. [4] reported microbiome sharing between humans and livestock (pigs) and sharing between children and nearby cattle [5]. The diverse communities in the gut microbiome function to support immunity; both local and systemic. Research findings over the past decade have indicated that the gut microbiome plays a key function in human physiological processes and maintenance of homeostasis and health. As in humans, animal gut microbiomes function in gut development, utilisation, and digestion of feed, and immunity [6]. In this chapter, we will discuss the mechanisms of immune modulation by the gut microbiome, factors (diet, probiotic, etc.) that trigger gut dysbiosis, and their resulting immune response.

16.2   Dysbiosis of the Gut Microbiome

Alteration in the gut microbiota composition, known as dysbiosis, results in reduction of microbial diversity and loss of beneficial microbial populations. Disturbance in the gut microbiome population and function is caused by several factors including nutritional (diet), age, antibiotics, genetics, and other environmental factors [7]. The gut microbiome and its associated metabolites function to maintain host wellness. Therefore, gut dysbiosis impairs the normal function of the gut by affecting intestinal permeability, digestion, and metabolism [8]. In addition, dysbiosis of microbiome can disrupt host homeostasis due to the essential role of microbes in immune modulation, activation of both innate and adaptive immune systems [9].

16.3   Gut Dysbiosis and Diseases

Dysbiosis has been unfavorably associated with the pathogenesis and progression of many human diseases including inflammatory bowel disease (IBD) [10], metabolic diseases such as obesity, non-alcoholic fatty liver (NAFLD) [11, 12], asthma [13], colorectal carcinoma [14], and cardiovascular disease [15]. Table 16.1 presents selected diseases and their associated dysbiotic characteristics. The effect of gut dysbiosis and association with diseases is well-established and extensively reviewed in previous publications [16, 17]. In this chapter, we will focus specifically on two selected diseases; IBD and NAFLD.

Table 16.1   Selected gut-microbiome associated diseases.

Disease	Gut Dysbiosis Characteristics	Immune Modulation	Reference
Inflammatory Bowel Disease	Reduce Bacteroidetes and Firmicutes (*Faecalibacterium prausnitzii* and *Roseburia* spp.) Increase *Enterobacteriaceae* and *Ruminococcus* spp.	Reduce pro-inflammatory cytokines (IL-12, IFN-γ) Increase anti-inflammatory IL-10	[20, 21]
Non-alcoholic fatty liver disease	Significant increase of *E. coli* Lower *Firmicutes* and *Bacteroides* Higher levels of *Prevotella*	Inflammation through influx of TLR4 and TLR9 agonists Enhance expression of hepatic TNF-α	[27, 29, 30]
Irritable Bowel Syndrome	Increase in *Escherichia coli* Decrease in *Bifidobacteria* Decrease *Firmicutes* and increase *Proteobacteria*	Increase number of immune cells such as mast cells and lymphocytes Increase cytokines (IL-6, TNF-α, and IL-1β)	[31, 32]
Acute kidney injury	Increase *Enterobacteriacea* Decrease *Lactobacilli* and *Ruminococaaeae*	Reduce Th17, Th1 response Increase T cell and macrophages	[33, 34]

Adapted from [19, 17].

16.3.1 Inflammatory Bowel Disease

Inflammatory bowel disease is a chronic, intestinal, immune-mediated disease that affects the digestive system. Multifactorial causes of IBD are environmental and genetic factors, which have an effect on microbial composition in the gut. Two main types of IBD exist; Crohn's disease (CD), which occurs throughout the GIT, and ulcerative colitis (UC), which affects the large intestine [18]. The exact pathogenesis of IBD is not elucidated, but crosstalk between microbe and host factors such as immunity, inflammation regulation, microbes' recognition, and host defense regulation contribute to IBD development and progression [19]. Research suggests a two-way relationship between IBD and gut dysbiosis. First, microbial imbalance leads to the development of IBD, secondly, it serves as a further consequence of inflammation in the gut. The IBD condition has been linked to reduced *Bacteroidetes* and *Firmicutes* [20]. Sokol et al. [21] showed these bacteria had anti-inflammatory function in decreasing pro-inflammatory cytokines (IL-12, IFN-γ) and promoting anti-inflammatory IL-10. Gastrointestinal immunity is essential in maintaining intestinal homeostasis. A key indication in IBD is prolonged immune response to microbial-derived antigenic materials [22]. Studies reported a spectrum of highly specific antibodies used for the diagnosis of CD, including anti-*Saccharomices cerevisiae* (ASCA), anti-chitobiosid, and anti-outer membrane porin C (anti-OmpC). Contrary to CD, antibodies associated with UC are anti-neutrophil cytoplasmic autoantibodies (pANCA) and antibodies against goblet cells (GAB) [23]. Because IBD is linked with intestinal mucosa proinflammatory immune response, most current therapeutic treatment includes anti-inflammatory antibodies that target proinflammatory cytokines such as TNF-α, IL-12, and IL-23 [24].

16.3.2 Non-alcoholic Fatty Liver Disease

Non-alcoholic fatty liver disease (NAFLD) is a chronic liver disease characterised by fat accumulation, which may progress further to non-alcoholic steatohepatitis (NASH), fibrosis, cirrhosis, and hepatocellular carcinoma [25]. Although the pathogenesis of NAFLD is yet to be understood, the gut microbiota has been implicated in NAFLD through interaction of the gut–liver axis [26]. A greater proportion of blood transported from the intestines to the liver exposes the liver to bacterial cell wall components, such as lipopolysaccharides (LPS), peptidoglycans, and other gut microbiome metabolites (ammonia and acetaldehyde) [27]. Both human and animal studies have shown association between gut dysbiosis and disease progression and severity in NAFLD patients. Boursier et al. [28] identified association between *Bacteroides* abundance and NASH, and *Ruminococcus* spp. was significantly linked to fibrosis. Another study in mice reported alterations in gut microbiome were linked with increased expression of proinflammatory TNF-α [29]. Furthermore, analysis of patients' fecal microbiome identified 20% more *Bacteroidetes* and 24% less *Firmicutes* in NAFLD patients than healthy control. Various research findings have expanded our understanding and highlighted the role of intestinal dysbiosis and subsequent immune modulation in the development and disease progression of NAFLD [27].

16.4 Gut Microbiome-Mediated Immune Modulation

The gut microbiome may affect human health and homeostasis through mechanisms such as defense against pathogens. The gut microbiota resides and multiplies on the intestinal surface creating a conducive environment to protect against invading pathogens [19]. There is a bidirectional communication between gut microbiome and host immune system. The gut microbiome is an effective stimulator of immune response and promotes both innate and adaptive immunity [35]. The immune signals triggered by the gut microbiome serve as a powerful modulator of gut commensals and offers protection against invading opportunistic pathogens [36]. Therefore, disruption of the gut barrier function promotes the gut's permeability to commensal microbes and microbial metabolites, resulting in an atypical response to immunity including inflammation, allergy, and autoimmune issues [19, 37]. Figure 16.1 presents a summary of the gut microbiome, gut dysbiosis factors, diseases, and immune modulations. These disorders are mediated by molecular imitation and dysregulation of T cell response. An important role of the gut microbiome is to regulate the gastrointestinal T-lymphocytes balance (i.e., regulatory T cell/T helper type 17 ratio). A balance and tight regulation of the Treg/TH17 ratio is crucial to prevent abnormal immune-inflammatory response and maintain intestinal homeostasis [19, 38]. Studies have shown that commensal microbes such as *Bifidobacterium infantis* and *Bacteroides fragilis* are able to stimulate growth of FOXP3 and IL-10 Treg cells, which are

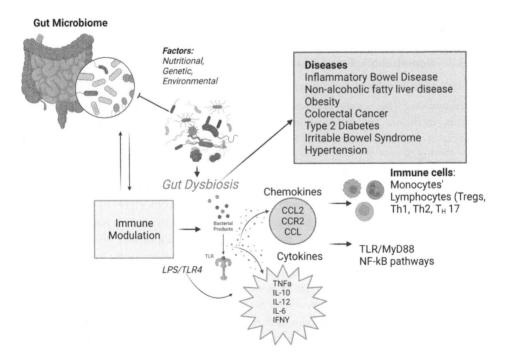

Figure 16.1 A schematic of the gut microbiome, dysbiosis, associated diseases, and immune modulation mediators.

able to suppress inflammation and strengthen gut barrier function [39]. Additionally, the microbial metabolite short chain fatty acids provide protection to the gut barrier against pro-inflammatory cytokines [40].

16.4.1 Innate Immunity

The gut microbiome plays a crucial role in the development of host innate immunity on both local and systemic levels [41]. As the first line of defense, the innate immunity is triggered when pathogen-associated molecule patterns (PAMPs) are recognised by pattern recognition receptors (PRR). Within the PRR family, toll-like receptors (TLRs) can recognise cell surface PAMPs of various microbes and stimulate an immune response. The TLR and PAMP interaction is vital in microbiota-mediated immune modulation [42]. The immune response activates signaling pathways known as TLR/MyD88, NF-kB, and Galectins pathways. Gut microbiome and metabolites such as LPS and PGN interact with different TLRs. LPS, a cell wall component of gram-negative bacteria binds to TLR4 [43], and animal studies have shown LPS stimulate TLR4 expression [44–47]. Gronbach and others [48] showed higher LPS expression in mice microbiota stimulated gut inflammation. Their results suggested a TLR4 pathway mediated suppression of regulatory T-lymphocyte and/ or activation of effector helper-T (T_H1/T_H17) through host TLR4 signaling pathway. A study by Asiamah et al. [49] reported different microbial PAMPS including lipopolysaccharide, peptidoglycan, and viral RNA polyinosinic–polycytidylic acid binding to their associated TLRs mediated secretion of different cytokines [49], but changes in microbial species was not reported. TLR5 recognition of the bacterial flagellin activated innate immune and changed colonic microbial species [50].

16.4.2 Adaptive Immunity

The adaptive immunity mediates responses to microbes through protection against microbial invasion and promoting symbiotic relationships of beneficial gut microbial organisms. To stimulate dysfunctional responses of the adaptive immune system, bacterial proteins may cross-react with human antigens [51]. Host adaptive immune system deficiency would lead to changes in microbiome such as increased levels of bacterial flagellin [52]. Other studies have found immunoglobulin A (IgA) and T-cell-mediated responses to alter gut microbiome composition and diversity [53]. Alteration in microbial composition such as increase in *Escherichia coli*, and decrease in *Bifidobacteria* in IBS, trigger immune response, which increased the number of immune cells such as mast cells and lymphocytes [20–21]. Yang [34] observed increased *Enterobacteriacea* and decreased *Lactobacilli* in the gut, subsequent increase in T-cell and macrophages, and reduced Th17 and Th1 response.

16.5 Gut Microbiome Modulators

Gut dysbiosis occurs due to several factors including diet, probiotics, and others (genetic, environmental factors, antibiotic, age) as shown in Figure 16.1. Therefore, changes in dietary eating habits, food/feed component modification, and use of probiotic or prebiotic supplements may modulate the gut microbiome and enhance the effectiveness of immune response and overall health and well-being of animals and humans [54], as presented in Table 16.2.

16.5.1 Diet

Diet is one of the most important factors that influence the microbiome. Studies have shown that changes in diet (plant and animal-based diet) alter the microbiome composition [55]. Dietary component and essential food nutrients including carbohydrates, proteins, fats, short chain fatty acids (SCFA), and micronutrients (vitamins and minerals) may alter the gut microbiome [56]. Studies in humans and animals have shown influence of diet on the diversity of gut microbiota [57]. Human studies have focused on the three main macronutrients; carbohydrates, proteins, and fats. Foods with high fibre content increased population of *Bacteroidetes* and lactic acid bacteria *Ruminococcus* spp. [58]. Murphy et al. [59] reported that high fat diet decreased *Firmicutes*.

16.5.2 Diet, Gut Microbiome, and Immunity

Diet alters the gut microbiome, which in turn modulates the immune system. Diet directly affects immunity by altering immune cells, and indirectly induces alterations in the gut

Table 16.2 Gut microbiome modulators, effect on microbiome profiles, and immune modulation outcomes.

Factors/modulators	Experimental type	Gut Microbiome/Immune modulation signature	References
High-fibre diet	Human	Increased microbiome function, cytokine response score was unchanged	[68]
High-fermented food diet	Human	Increased microbiome diversity, decreased inflammatory signals and activity	[68]
Probiotics (*Lactobacillus casei*)	Mouse	Increased innate immunity markers CD-206 and TLR2	[76]
Multi-strain probiotics (*Lactobacillus acidophilus, Sachharomycescerevisae, Enterococcus faecium*)	Animal (Cow, Goat)	Increased expression of innate and adaptive immune response (TLR4) Cytokines (IL-10, IL-8)	[45, 80–81]
Probiotic (*Bifidobacterium pseudocatenulatum* CECT 7765)	Mouse	Decrease serum cholesterol, triglyceride, leptin, interleukin (IL)-6, and monocyte chemotactic protein-1	[73]
Prebiotic (Arabinoxylan)	Mouse	Increased *Bacteroides-Prevotella* spp.	[73]
Prebiotic (fructans)	Animal	Increase *Bacteroides* and *Bifidiobacterium* spp.	[74]
Pectin and pectin oligosaccharide (Prebiotics)	Human	Promote *Eubacterium eligens*, which strongly promote IL-10	[79]

microbial population and non-immune tissues [60]. Inside the host gut, a diet's first site of interaction is the gastrointestinal epithelium, which serves as barrier connecting the host and microbiome through a tight junction; this mechanism was demonstrated in a study [61]. Mice fed high-fat diet had decreased expression of tight junction proteins linked to elevated intestinal permeability and translocation of bacterial products [62]. Similar findings were reported by Wastyk et al. [63], where they demonstrated different diets targeted the microbiome and modulated immune status in humans. Their study findings highlighted that high-fibre diet increased gut microbiome-encoded glycan degrading carbohydrate active enzymes, and a high-fermented food diet promoted microbiome diversity and reduced markers of inflammation. Worku et al. [64] also reported that diet may modulate innate immunity response makers in goats. A microarray analysis found plant polyphenol extract impacted immune markers such as CD40, toll-like receptors [65], and Galectins [66] in dairy cows. Natural herbs and spices essential oils have shown antimicrobial activity against pathogens such as *E. coli*, *Listeria monocytogenes*, and *Staphylococcus aureus* [67]. Additionally, mice fed high-fat diet had increased expression of chemokines *CCL*, *CCL2*, and *CCR2*, which resulted in penetration of proinflammatory monocytes and lymphocytes into intestinal tissues [68]. Comparatively, a study in germ-free mice (i.e., with no microbiome), showed decreased TNF-α expression. Consumption of dietary fats affects gastrointestinal barriers and may directly induce production of immune cells including macrophages, monocytes, and T cells to promote permeability of the gut and systemic proinflammatory response [69].

16.5.3 Short-Chain Fatty Acids

Metabolic fermented products such as short-chain fatty acids (SCFAs) serve as an essential source of energy for intestinal epithelial cells and thus reinforce the mucosal barrier [70]. Other metabolites such as propionate and butyrate have anti-inflammatory and anti-carcinogenic effects due to the ability to restrict the function of histone deacetylase in immune cells [71].

16.6 Prebiotics

Prebiotics are selective fermented ingredients which cause alteration in gastrointestinal microbial composition and function. Prebiotics are beneficial in strengthening gut mucosal barrier, promote mucosal immunity, decrease the pH and SCFA, and inhibit growth of pathogens [72]. Administration of prebiotics in diet may alter the gut microbial composition. In a study on mice, the addition of prebiotic wheat Arabinoxylan (10%) increased *Bacteroides-Prevotella* spp. and *Roseburia* spp. [73] Supplementation of diet with fructans increased *Bacteroides* and the beneficial microbe *Bifidiobacterium* spp. population [74].

16.7 Probiotics

Probiotics are widely recognised as live non-pathogenic microbes with health benefits, which are due to their immunomodulatory activity in the gut. Microbial species commonly used as probiotics include *Bifidobacteria* and *Lactobacillus* [75]. Probiotics are used as additive agents to reverse dysbiotic gut condition, and they may induce secretion of cytokines and IgA in the intestinal mucosa [76]. Oral administration of *Lactobacillus casei* probiotic bacterium in Bald/c mice increased innate immunity markers CD-206 and TLR2 [77]. Administration of *Bifidobacterium pseudocatenulatum* decreased serum glucose levels leptin, IL-6, and monocyte chemotactic protein-1 in obese mice [78]. Similar studies have highlighted the benefit of probiotic supplements in reducing metabolic and immunological dysfunction related to obesity, NAFLD, and other gut dysbiosis associated diseases [79].

16.8 Galectins, Gut Microbiome, and Immune Modulation

Complex lectin glycan interactions that are part of the innate immune system regulate gut homeostasis and combat pathogenesis. Cell mediated immunity such as the formation of neutrophils extracellular traps (NETosis) is induced by gut microbes and involves neutrophil accumulation, activation, and functions [82, 83]. Members of the gut microbiome may induce and circumvent NETosis. Microbial surface glycans are recognised by host cell lectins such as galectins. Glycan and lectin interactions positively and negatively regulate microbial attachment, invasion, survival, pathogenesis, and the host's immune response. Innate immune factors are essential to homeostasis and contribute to its regulation. Pathogenesis in the gut such as IBD is associated with neutrophil accumulation and activation such as NETosis [83]. Galectins are a group of animal lectins with functional roles in immunity, inflammation, and development [84]. Several galectins can bind to microbial glycans, and function in microbial infection and immune response.

Galectins may detect microbial infection, antimicrobial activity, inhibit inflammation, and induce apoptosis. With respect to the gut microbiome, Galectin-4 is expressed in gastrointestinal tissues [85], where they bind to induce peripheral and muscosal lamina propria T cells at CD3 epitope. Serum galectin levels are biomarkers in diseases such as IBD [86]. Galectin-9 is induced by dietary synbiotics and is involved in suppression of allergic symptoms in mice and humans [87]. Galectin-3 interacts with commensal organisms and products such as LPS to regulate inflammation, bacterial clearance, and healing [88]. Studies show that Gal-3 plays a role in maintaining the balance between oral microbiota and the host immune response and diseases pathogenesis. Therapeutic effects of Galectin-3 are being studied and used for targeted delivery. Galectins may serve as biomarkers of gut health and immune activation [87, 89], and as possible therapeutic targets [84] and as regulators for effective dietary immunomodulation against microbial products such as LPS [45, 89] and their receptors [89].

16.9 Conclusion

In summary, this chapter provides an overview of the immune modulation by gut microbiomes, factors such as diet, probiotic, and host factors that trigger gut dysbiosis, and the resulting immune response. This information may allow for better understanding of the research progress and for development of targeted therapeutic interventions against diseases associated with gut dysbiosis.

References

1 Belizário, J.E. and Faintuch, J. (2018). Microbiome and gut dysbiosis. In: *Metabolic Interaction in Infection*, (ed. R. Silvestre and E. Torrado) 459–476. Springer, Cham.

2 Shreiner, A.B., Kao, J.Y., and Young, V.B. (2015 January). The gut microbiome in health and in disease. *Cur. Opin. Gastroenterol.* 31 (1): 69.

3 Fernandes, G.R., Tap, J., Bruls, T. et al. (2011). Enterotypes of the human gut microbiome. *Nature* 473 (7346): 174180.

4 Kraemer, J.G., Ramette, A., Aebi, S. et al. (2018 March). Influence of pig farming on the human nasal microbiota: key role of airborne microbial communities. *App. Environ. Microbio.* 84 (6): e0247017.

5 Mosites, E., Sammons, M., Otiang, E. et al. (2017 February). Microbiome sharing between children, livestock and household surfaces in western Kenya. *PLoS One* 12 (2): e0171017.

6 Bauer, E., Williams, B.A., Smidt, H. et al. (2006 March). Influence of the gastrointestinal microbiota on development of the immune system in young animals. *Cur. Issu. Intest. Microbial.* 7 (2): 35–52.

7 Odamaki, T., Kato, K., Sugahara, H. et al. (2016 December). Age-related changes in gut microbiota composition from newborn to centenarian: a cross-sectional study. *BMC Microbiol.* 16 (1): 1–2.

8 Rothschild, D., Weissbrod, O., Barkan, E. et al. (2018 March). Environment dominates over host genetics in shaping human gut microbiota. *Nature* 555 (7695): 210–215.

9 Dixit, K., Chaudhari, D., Dhotre, D. et al. (2021 August). Restoration of dysbiotic human gut microbiome for homeostasis. *Life Sci.* 278: 119622.

10 Carding, S., Verbeke, K., Vipond, D.T. et al. (2015 December). Dysbiosis of the gut microbiota in disease. *Microb. Ecol. Heal. Dis.* 26 (1): 26191.

11 Putignani, L., Del Chierico, F., Vernocchi, P. et al. (2016 February). Dysbiotrack Study Group. Gut microbiota dysbiosis as risk and premorbid factors of IBD and IBS along the childhood–adulthood transition. *Inflamm. Bowel Dis.* 22 (2): 487–504.

12 Li, X., Watanabe, K., and Kimura, I. (2017 December). Gut microbiota dysbiosis drives and implies novel therapeutic strategies for diabetes mellitus and related metabolic diseases. *Front. Immunol.* 8: 1882.

13 Hufnagl, K., Pali-Schöll, I., Roth-Walter, F. et al. (2020 February). Dysbiosis of the gut and lung microbiome has a role in asthma. *Semin. Immunopathol.* 42 (1): 75–93. Springer Berlin Heidelberg.

14 Schwabe, R.F. and Jobin, C. (2013 November). The microbiome and cancer. *Nat. Rev. Cancer* 13 (11): 800–812.

15 Estruch, R., Ros, E., Salas-Salvadó, J. et al. (2018 June). Primary prevention of cardiovascular disease with a Mediterranean diet supplemented with extra-virgin olive oil or nuts. *N.E. J. Med.* 378 (25): e34.

16 Gomaa, E.Z. (2020 December). Human gut microbiota/microbiome in health and diseases: a review. *Antonie Van Leeuwenhoek* 113 (12): 2019–2040.

17 Scotti, E., Boué, S., Sasso, G.L. et al. (2017 November). Exploring the microbiome in health and disease: implications for toxicology. *Toxicol. Res. App.* 1: 2397847317741884.

18 Schirmer, M., Franzosa, E.A., Lloyd-Price, J. et al. (2018 March). Dynamics of metatranscription in the inflammatory bowel disease gut microbiome. *Nat. Microbiol.* 3 (3): 337–346.

19 Kho, Z.Y. and Lal, S.K. (2018). The human gut microbiome: a potential controller of wellness and disease. *Front. Microbiol.* 9: 1835.

20 Lane, E.R., Zisman, T.L., and Suskind, D.L. (2017). The microbiota in inflammatory bowel disease: current and therapeutic insights. *J. Inflamm. Res.* 10: 63.

21 Sokol, H., Pigneur, B., Watterlot, L. et al. (2008 October). *Faecalibacterium prausnitzii* is an anti-inflammatory commensal bacterium identified by gut microbiota analysis of Crohn disease patients. *Proc. Nat. Acad. Sci.* 105 (43): 16731–16736.

22 Fakhoury, H.M., Kvietys, P.R., Al Kattan, W. et al. (2020 June). Vitamin D and intestinal homeostasis: barrier, microbiota, and immune modulation. *J. Ster. Biochem. Molec. Bio.* 200: 105663.

23 Tesija Kuna, A. (2013 February). Serological markers of inflammatory bowel disease. *Biochemia. Medica.* 23 (1): 28–42.

24 Christensen, K.R., Steenholdt, C., Buhl, S.S. et al. (2015). Systematic information to health-care professionals about vaccination guidelines improves adherence in patients with inflammatory bowel disease in anti-TNFα therapy. *Off. J. Am. Coll. Gastroent. ACG* 110 (11): 1526–1532.

25 Safari, Z. and Gérard, P. (2019 April). The links between the gut microbiome and non-alcoholic fatty liver disease (NAFLD). *Cell. Molec. Life Sci.* 76 (8): 1541–1558.

26 Compare, D., Coccoli, P., Rocco, A. et al. (2012 June). Gut–liver axis: the impact of gut microbiota on non-alcoholic fatty liver disease. *Nut. Metab. Cardio. Dis.* 22 (6): 471–476.

27 Safari, Z. and Gérard, P. (2019 April). The links between the gut microbiome and non-alcoholic fatty liver disease (NAFLD). *Cell Mole. Life Sci.* 76 (8): 1541–1558.

28 Boursier, J., Mueller, O., Barret, M. et al. (2016 March). The severity of nonalcoholic fatty liver disease is associated with gut dysbiosis and shift in the metabolic function of the gut microbiota. *Hepatology* 63 (3): 764–775.

29 Henao-Mejia, J., Elinav, E., Jin, C. et al. (2012 February). Inflammasome-mediated dysbiosis regulates progression of NAFLD and obesity. *Nature* 482 (7384): 179–185.

30 Wang, B., Jiang, X., Cao, M. et al. (2016 August). Altered fecal microbiota correlates with liver biochemistry in nonobese patients with non-alcoholic fatty liver disease. *Sci. Rep.* 6 (1): 1–11.

31 Pittayanon, R., Lau, J.T., Yuan, Y. et al. (2019 July). Gut microbiota in patients with irritable bowel syndrome—a systematic review. *Gastroenterology* 157 (1): 97–108.

32 Lazaridis, N. and Germanidis, G. (2018 March). Current insights into the innate immune system dysfunction in irritable bowel syndrome. *Ann. Gastroent.* 31 (2): 171.

33 Chen, T., Li, R., and Chen, P. (2021). Gut microbiota and chemical-induced acute liver injury. *Front. Physiol.* 12: 753.

34 Yang, L., Bian, X., Wu, W. et al. (2020 November). Protective effect of Lactobacillus salivarius Li01 on thioacetamide-induced acute liver injury and hyperammonaemia. *Microb. Biotech.* 13 (6): 1860–1876.

35 Pickard, J.M., Zeng, M.Y., Caruso, R. et al. (2017 September). Gut microbiota: role in pathogen colonization, immune responses, and inflammatory disease. *Immuno. Rev.* 279 (1): 70–89.

36 Negi, S., Das, D.K., Pahari, S. et al. (2019 October). Potential role of gut microbiota in induction and regulation of innate immune memory. *Front. Immunol.* 10: 2441.

37 Al Bander, Z., Nitert, M.D., Mousa, A. et al. (2020 January). The gut microbiota and inflammation: an overview. *Int. J. Environ. Res. Pub. Heal.* 17 (20): 7618.

38 Lawley, T.D. and Walker, A.W. (2013 January). Intestinal colonization resistance. *Immunology* 138 (1): 1–11.

39 Chen, T., Kim, C.Y., Kaur, A. et al. (2017). Dietary fibre-based SCFA mixtures promote both protection and repair of intestinal epithelial barrier function in a Caco-2 cell model. *Food Funct.* 8 (3): 1166–1173.

40 Peng, L., He, Z., Chen, W. et al. (2007 January). Effects of butyrate on intestinal barrier function in a Caco-2 cell monolayer model of intestinal barrier. *Ped. Res.* 61 (1): 37–41.

41 Khosravi, A., Yáñez, A., Price, J.G. et al. (2014 March). Gut microbiota promote hematopoiesis to control bacterial infection. *Cell Host Micro.* 15 (3): 374–381.

42 Rakoff-Nahoum, S., Paglino, J., Eslami-Varzaneh, F. et al. (2004 July). Recognition of commensal microflora by toll-like receptors is required for intestinal homeostasis. *Cell* 118 (2): 229–241.

43 Anitha, M., Vijay-Kumar, M., Sitaraman, S.V. et al. (2012 October). Gut microbial products regulate murine gastrointestinal motility via Toll-like receptor 4 signaling. *Gastroenterology* 143 (4): 1006–1016.

44 Adjei-Fremah, S., Ekwemalor, K., Asiamah, E.K. et al. (2018 January). Effect of probiotic supplementation on growth and global gene expression in dairy cows. *J. App. Anim. Res.* 46 (1): 257–263.

45 Adjei-Fremah, S., Ekwemalor, K., Asiamah, E. et al. (2016 December). Transcriptional profiling of the effect of lipopolysaccharide (LPS) pretreatment in blood from probiotics-treated dairy cows. *Genom. Data* 10: 15–18.

46 Adjei-Fremah, S., Ekwemalor, K., Worku, M. et al. (2018 July). Probiotics and ruminant health. *Rijeka: InTech.* 1.

47 Ekwemalor, K., Adjei-Fremah, S., Asiamah, E. et al. (2016 October). 0167 Exposure of bovine blood to pathogen associated and non-pathogen associated molecular patterns results in transcriptional activation. *J. Anim. Sci.* 94 (sup. 5): 81.

48 Gronbach, K., Flade, I., Holst, O. et al. (2014 March). Endotoxicity of lipopolysaccharide as a determinant of T-cell-mediated colitis induction in mice. *Gastroenterology* 146 (3): 765–775.

49 Asiamah, E.K., Ekwemalor, K., Adjei-Fremah, S. et al. (2019 September). Natural and synthetic pathogen associated molecular patterns modulate galectin expression in cow blood. *J. Anim. Sci. Tech.* 61 (5): 245.

50 Vijay-Kumar, M., Aitken, J.D., Carvalho, F.A. et al. (2010 April). Metabolic syndrome and altered gut microbiota in mice lacking Toll-like receptor 5. *Science* 328 (5975): 228–231.

51 Galland, L. (2014 December). The gut microbiome and the brain. *J. Medici. Food* 17 (12): 1261–1272.

52 Cullender, T.C., Chassaing, B., Janzon, A. et al. (2013 November). Innate and adaptive immunity interact to quench microbiome flagellar motility in the gut. *Cell Host Micro.* 14 (5): 571–581.

53 Suzuki, K. and Fagarasan, S. (2008 November). How host-bacterial interactions lead to IgA synthesis in the gut. *Trends Immunol.* 29 (11): 523–531.

54 Graf, D., Di Cagno, R., Fåk, F. et al. (2015 December). Contribution of diet to the composition of the human gut microbiota. *Microb. Eco. Health Dis.* 26 (1): 26164.

55 Kashtanova, D.A., Popenko, A.S., Tkacheva, O.N. et al. (2016 June). Association between the gut microbiota and diet: fetal life, early childhood, and further life. *Nutrition* 32 (6): 620–627.

56 Maslowski, K.M. and Mackay, C.R. (2011 January). Diet, gut microbiota and immune responses. *Nature Immunol.* 12 (1): 5–9.

57 Scott, K.P., Gratz, S.W., Sheridan, P.O. et al. (2013 March). The influence of diet on the gut microbiota. *Pharma. Res.* 69 (1): 52–60.

58 Kim, C.H., Park, J., and Kim, M. (2014 December). Gut microbiota-derived short-chain fatty acids, T cells, and inflammation. *Immune Net.* 14 (6): 277–288.

59 Murphy, E.F., Cotter, P.D., Healy, S. et al. (2010 December). Composition and energy harvesting capacity of the gut microbiota: Relationship to diet, obesity and time in mouse models. *Gut* 59 (12): 1635–1642.

60 Burr, A.H., Bhattacharjee, A., and Hand, T.W. (2020 September). Nutritional modulation of the microbiome and immune response. *J. Immunol.* 205 (6): 1479–1487.

61 Okumura, R. and Takeda, K. (2017 May). Roles of intestinal epithelial cells in the maintenance of gut homeostasis. *Experi. Molec. Med.* 49 (5): e338.

62 Cani, P.D., Bibiloni, R., Knauf, C. et al. (2008 June). Changes in gut microbiota control metabolic endotoxemia-induced inflammation in high-fat diet-induced obesity and diabetes in mice. *Diabetes* 57 (6): 1470–1481.

63 Wastyk, H.C., Fragiadakis, G.K., Perelman, D. et al. (2021 August). Gut-microbiota-targeted diets modulate human immune status. *Cell* 184 (16): 4137–4153.

64 Worku, M., Abdalla, A., Adjei-Fremah, S. et al. (2016). The impact of diet on expression of genes involved in innate immunity in goat blood. *J. Agri. Sci.* 8 (3): 1.

65 Adjei-Fremah, S., Jackai, L.E., Schimmel, K. et al. (2018 January). Microarray analysis of the effect of Cowpea (*Vigna unguiculata*) phenolic extract in bovine peripheral blood. *J. App. Ani. Res.* 46 (1): 100–106.

66 Adjei-Fremah, S. and Worku, M. (2021 February). Cowpea polyphenol extract regulates galectin gene expression in bovine blood. *Ani. Biotech.* 32 (1): 1–2.

67 Tajkarimi, M.M., Ibrahim, S.A., and Cliver, D.O. (2010 September). Antimicrobial herb and spice compounds in food. *Food Con.* 21 (9): 1199–1218.

68 Kawano, Y., Nakae, J., Watanabe, N. et al. (2016 August). Colonic pro-inflammatory macrophages cause insulin resistance in an intestinal Ccl2/Ccr2-dependent manner. *Cell Metab.* 24 (2): 295–310.

69 Yoshida, H., Miura, S., Kishikawa, H. et al. (2001 November). Fatty acids enhance GRO/CINC-1 and interleukin-6 production in rat intestinal epithelial cells. *J. Nutri.* 131 (11): 2943–2950.

70 Wei, Y., Chang, L., Ishima, T. et al. (2021 February). Abnormalities of the composition of the gut microbiota and short-chain fatty acids in mice after splenectomy. *Brain Behav. Imm. Health* 11: 100198.

71 Lin, H.V., Frassetto, A., Kowalik, E.J. Jr et al. (2012 April). Butyrate and propionate protect against diet-induced obesity and regulate gut hormones via free fatty acid receptor 3-independent mechanisms. *PloS One* 7 (4): e35240.

72 Simpson, H.L. and Campbell, B.J. (2015 July). Dietary fibre–microbiota interactions. *Aliment. Pharma. Therapeut.* 42 (2): 158–179.

73 Neyrinck, A.M., Possemiers, S., Druart, C. et al. (2011 June). Prebiotic effects of wheat arabinoxylan related to the increase in bifidobacteria, *Roseburia* sp. and *Bacteroides/Prevotella* in diet-induced obese mice. *PloS One* 6 (6): e20944.

74 Moschen, A.R., Wieser, V., and Tilg, H. (2012 October). Dietary factors: major regulators of the gut's microbiota. *Gut Liv.* 6 (4): 411.

75 Ohashi, Y. and Ushida, K. (2009). Health-beneficial effects of probiotics: its mode of action. *Ani. Sci. J.* 80 (4): 361–371.

76 Azad, M., Kalam, A., Sarker, M. et al. (2018 October). Immunomodulatory effects of probiotics on cytokine profiles. *BioMed Res. Int.* 2018: 1–10.

77 Galdeano, C.M. and Perdigon, G. (2006 February). The probiotic bacterium *Lactobacillus casei* induces activation of the gut mucosal immune system through innate immunity. *Clin.Vacc. Immunol.* 13 (2): 219–226.

78 Cano, P.G., Santacruz, A., Trejo, F.M. et al. (2013 November). Bifidobacterium CECT 7765 improves metabolic and immunological alterations associated with obesity in high-fat diet-fed mice. *Obesity* 21 (11): 2310–2321.

79 Chung, W.S., Meijerink, M., Zeuner, B. et al. (2017 November). Prebiotic potential of pectin and pectic oligosaccharides to promote anti-inflammatory commensal bacteria in the human colon. *FEMS Microbio. Ecol.* 93 (11): fix127.

80 Ekwemalor, K., Asiamah, E., Osei, B. et al. (2017). Evaluation of the effect of probiotic administration on gene expression in goat blood. *J. Mol. Bio. Res.* 7 (1): 88.

81 Adjei-Fremah, S., Ekwemalor, K., Asiamah, E.K. et al. (2018 January). Effect of probiotic supplementation on growth and global gene expression in dairy cows. *J. App. Ani. Res.* 46 (1): 257–263.

82 Chen, K., Shao, L.H., Wang, F. et al. (2021 October). Netting gut disease: neutrophil extracellular trap in intestinal pathology. *Oxi. Med. Cell. Longev* 2021: 1–10.

83 Worku, M., Rehrah, D., Ismail, H.D. et al. (2021 January). A review of the Neutrophil Extracellular Traps (NETs) from cow, sheep and goat models. *Int. J. Mol. Sci.* 22 (15): 8046.

84 Klyosov, A.A., Witczak, Z.J., Platt, D. (eds.). (2008). *Galectins*. John Wiley & Sons.

85 Paclik, D., Danese, S., Berndt, U. et al. (2008). Galectin-4 controls intestinal inflammation by selective regulation of peripheral and mucosal T cell apoptosis and cell cycle. *PloS One* 3 (7): e2629.

86 Yu, T.B., Dodd, S., Yu, L.G. et al. (2020 January). Serum galectins as potential biomarkers of inflammatory bowel diseases. *PloS One* 15 (1): e0227306.

87 de Kivit, S., Saeland, E., Kraneveld, A.D. et al. (2012 March). Galectin-9 induced by dietary synbiotics is involved in suppression of allergic symptoms in mice and humans. *Allergy* 67 (3): 343–352.

88 Ray, S. and Maunsell, J.H. (2011 April). Different origins of gamma rhythm and high-gamma activity in macaque visual cortex. *PLoS Bio.* 9 (4): e1000610.

89 Ekwemalor, K., Asiamah, E., and Worku, M. (2016 January). Effect of a mushroom (*Coriolus versicolor*) based probiotic on the expression of toll-like receptors and signal transduction in goat neutrophils. *J. Mol. Bio. Res.* 6 (1): 71.

17

Current Molecular Technologies for Assaying the Gut Microbiota: Next-generation DNA Sequencing

Harshit Sajal[1], Yuvaraj Sivamani[2], and Sumitha Elayaperumal[1]

[1] *Department of Biotechnology and Bioinformatics, JSS Academy of Higher Education and Research, Mysore, Karnataka, India*
[2] *Department of Pharmaceutical Chemistry, Cauvery College of Pharmacy, Mysuru, Karnataka, India*

17.1 Introduction and Overview

The trillions of microbes that are colonised in the human intestine significantly influence human metabolism and health [1]. Numerous significant discoveries linking the bacterial taxa present in the human gastrointestinal tract to illnesses from the cardiovascular, neurologic, respiratory, psychiatric, autoimmune, metabolic, gastrointestinal, hepatic, and oncologic spectra have been realised as a result of growing scientific interest in and understanding of the human gut microbiota [2, 3]. In contrast to the host's constitutive resources, the gut microbiota serves the human host in a variety of capacities, including those related to nutrition, immunity, and physiology [4]. Indigenous species of bacteria are essential for the growth and health of newborns [5]; therefore, the gut microbiota is regarded as an organ of the human body with unique roles and complexity [6]. Research on the gut microbiota has been limited as a result of the difficulty in growing many of these gastrointestinal microbial species in a laboratory environment [7]. Culture-independent next-generation sequencing (NGS) methodologies allowed for massively parallel detection, fast and cost-effective exploration, and quantification of the genes and genomes of single cells and complex communities of microorganisms. NGS may directly sequence microbial DNA or RNA in samples of feces, blood, or tissue, for instance. The two most prevalent NGS technologies are currently amplicon sequencing and shotgun metagenomic sequencing. Since the transcriptome has been determined, RNA sequencing adds a new step to the definition of microbiota function, making it a legitimate and, in some respects, a superior method for microbial characterisation [8]. The primary form of information regarding the microbiota in the human gut came from feces analysis; this easily available metabolic waste has significance since its microbial composition has been determined to have potential in disease diagnostics, disease prognosis, and therapeutic intervention. The most widely used NGS method for determining the taxonomic and phylogenetic composition of bacterial communities is 16S rRNA gene amplicon analysis [9]. However, the fecal bacterial population's identified composition may be affected by the experiment design and methodology, including the collection and storage technique and the DNA extraction method [10]. Unfortunately, these high-throughput gene/genome-focused approaches do not provide much in the way of mechanistic understanding of how the gut microbiota interacts with the host and with one another, and the role of these interactions in the host metabolic system. Making the transition from gene/genome-centric analysis to mechanism-centric approaches by combining omics and experimental data with current system-level understanding will be a vital next step in gut microbiome investigations [11]. Our understanding of the pathophysiological pathways has advanced significantly because of recent NGS advancements and the widespread use of bioinformatics, genomics, and mathematical databases. In particular, by exploiting the Human Microbiome Project (HMP) [12].

17.2 Research on the Gut Microbiome Using Next-generation Sequencing

Which bacteria species are present in a specific sample is a crucial query in studies on the gut microbiota. NGS analysis may answer questions regarding intraspecies and distribution of the population, the relative abundance of the microbes present, functional profiles, and more. DNA sequencing technology was invented in 1975 and is based on a DNA polymerase that incorporates a selectively labelled chain-terminating ddNTP during in vitro DNA replication [13]. However, high-throughput research has typically been costly, time-consuming, and arduous. NGS has gradually replaced the more traditional Sanger sequencing method in sequencing equipment. The foundation of NGS technologies is massively parallel sequencing, which has been thoroughly reviewed [14]. Thermo Fisher Scientific, Roche, Pacific Bioscience, Illumina, and other companies' sequencers have been successfully employed to investigate complex biological material. Amplicon and shotgun sequencing are two types of NGS that may be used to study microbiomes (which include transcriptomics and metagenomics), however, RNA sequencing adds a step to the definition of microbiota function and is considered a superior tool for microbial characterisation. Figure 17.1 outlines the gene/genome-centric approach for studying the gut microbiota using NGS techniques such as Amplicon and Shotgun sequencing.

17.2.1 Amplicon Sequencing

The most widely utilised method for describing gut microbiome diversity is amplicon-based profiling. A part of the sample DNA is amplified using polymerase chain reaction (PCR), and the resultant product is sequenced. The most typical PCR target is the bacterial 16S ribosomal RNA (rRNA) gene. As a result, 16S rRNA sequencing and analysis are frequently used to refer to amplicon sequencing. In 1985, Lane [15] described the classification of uncultured bacteria using the 16S rRNA gene. The highly conserved and widely distributed 16S rRNA gene marker is a taxonomically useful gene marker for bacteria and archaea. This 1500 bp long gene is divided into nine conserved sections and nine hypervariable regions (V1–V9) that differ between bacterial species and genera [16]. To bind the conserved sections while amplifying an interfering variable region, the forward and reverse

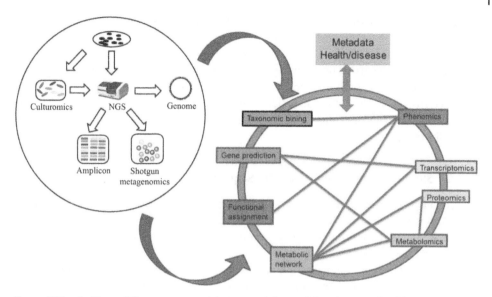

Figure 17.1 Outlines of the genome-centric approach for studying the gut microbiota.

primers of PCR were created. In 16S amplicon NGS investigations, regions V1–V5 are most frequently read to identify bacterial taxa to reduce the volume, duration, and expense of sequencing [17]. It is crucial to keep in mind that no single region is completely isolated from all bacteria, and various conclusions may come from sequencing sections that are purposefully produced at high levels [18]. The results may be skewed by the amplification of some overlapping regions, leading to an over- or under-representation of taxa, but it may also help to recognise separate species within a genus. In microbiota communities, full 16S rRNA gene sequencing by NGS may provide species and strain characterisation [19].

Following PCR amplification of the desired region of interest, the amplicons are sequenced and data cleansing is performed. The process of cleaning data involves several steps, such as (i) adaptor and primer sequence trimming; (ii) removing base and sequences of poor quality from reads; and (iii) eliminating matched sequences from the control collection, including the Illumina PhiX control, chimera sequences, human contamination reads, chloroplast, and mitochondrial contaminants. Following analysis, the sequencing data is often grouped into operational taxonomic units (OTUs). Distance-based OTU or sequence clusters are initially built without a reference database. OTUs are used to characterise genus and phylum with sequence similarities of 95% and 80%, respectively, but a species is often defined by an OTU sequence identity of more than 97% (or with only 3% dissimilarity) [20]. Computational alignment in the sense of 16S rRNA sequence databases such as SILVA, the Ribosomal Database Project (RDP), or Greengenes is used to resolve taxonomic identification. Then, the downstream analysis uses the discovered taxa and OTUs. A less used alternative analytical technique for amplicon sequencing, which produces amplicon sequence variants, is exact nucleotide matching amplicon sequence variant (ASV).The accuracy of reference databases affects how ASV taxon designations are made. Because the majority of bacterial cells have multiple copies of the rRNA gene, which usually have distinct nucleotide sequences, ASVs may divide single genomes into many

groups [21]. Although there are proponents of both strategies (OTUs vs. ASVs), it is important to remember that both are computational techniques for predicting taxonomy [21, 22].

On Illumina and Thermo platforms, 16S rRNA-based studies of different bacterial
populations may be carried out utilising the Ion Torrent (IT) and MiSeq Personal Genome
Machine (PGM) benchtop sequencers. Although both the IT and Illumina systems
sequence DNA by looking for nucleotide additions during DNA synthesis, their different
operating approaches may affect how well they perform and consequently affect the data
they collect [23].

17.2.2 Shotgun Metagenomic and RNA Sequencing

Shotgun metagenomic sequencing and RNA sequencing, in contrast to amplicon sequencing, investigate the entire DNA or RNA in a given sample, as this provides a more comprehensive method for simultaneously examining the taxonomic diversity and functional
potential of the gut microbiome.

Following extraction, fragmentation of DNA is carried out to perform shotgun metagenomic sequencing. Sample identification and sequencing of DNA are facilitated by the
ligation of the barcodes and adapters to the end of each segment. Once the output of the data
is derived, data cleansing is carried out before aligning to the reference database including
GenBank and Reference Sequence (RefSeq), to explore probable taxa and functions. These
enormous databases hold all genomes that are available to the general public. Additionally,
smaller pathogen-specific databases such as the Eukaryotic Pathogen Database (EuPathDB)
and the Pathosystems Resource Integration Center (PATRIC) are used [24]. The shotgun
metagenomic sequencing method is comparable to the RNA sequencing method. The key
step after the fragmentation of RNA includes the conversion of RNA fragments to complementary DNA (cDNA) in the presence of the reverse transcriptase enzyme. Following this,
the cDNA is sequenced using the DNA sequencing process [25].

The summary of a metagenomics workflow is shown in Figure 17.2 [26]. Step 1 includes
the experimental technique and research design, this step is important in metagenomics,
which is commonly underestimated. Computational pre-processing is Step 2, computational
quality control (QC) that eliminate basic sequence biases or artifacts, including quality trimming, eliminating duplicate sequences, and adaptor sequences (using, for example, FastQC,
Picard tools, or Trimmomatic121). Data are subsampled to standardise read numbers and to
remove non-target DNA sequences when comparing the variety of taxa or functions. Step 3 is
sequence analysis. Depending on the experiment's objective, the ideal strategy is to combine
'read-based' and 'assembly-based' approaches. Both strategies have benefits and drawbacks.
Step 4 is to analyse and interpret the data so a multivariate statistical approach may be carried
forward. Step 5 is validation; follow-up analyses are required because conclusions derived
from highly dimensional biological data may be skewed by study-driven biases.

17.2.3 Comparisons between NGS Methods

By using shotgun metagenomic analysis, RNA sequencing, and 16S rRNA, the microorganisms in a microbiome may be identified; however, the latter two also identify members
of other domains such as fungus, parasites, and viruses. RNA viruses are only examined

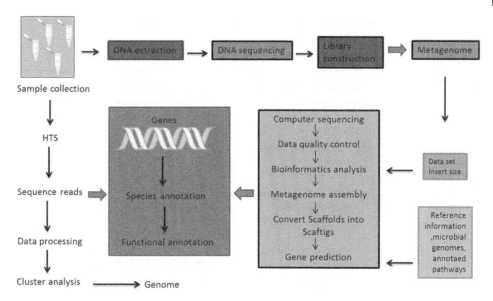

Figure 17.2 A summary of a metagenomics workflow.

by RNA sequencing. Shotgun metagenomic analysis may detect changes at the strain level while 16S rRNA sequencing has low resolution and sensitivity for species-level changes. Genus- and species-level advancements have been made thanks to sequencing [27]. A functional profile cannot be quickly determined from the data from 16S rRNA sequencing since it only analyses sequences from one significant gene. The functional profiles of bacteria are predicted using methods such as PICRUSt2 or PICRUSt (Phylogenetic Investigations of Communities by Reconstruction of Unobserved States), Tax4Fun, or Tax4Fun2. Depending on the 16S primers used for amplification, the functional potentials identified using shotgun metagenomics vary. In contrast, both RNA sequencing and Shotgun metagenomics sequence every piece of microbial DNA and RNA, thereby enabling the exploration of the functional potential of various microbes. The result of these analyses will help us to understand which genes are transcribed under various pathological conditions.

When employing an NGS technique, host contamination, bias, false positives, and post-sequencing computational requirements are additional considerations. In comparison with other NGS approaches, 16S rRNA sequencing has a lower risk of host contamination because the gene being amplified and read (16S rRNA gene) is specific to bacteria. The probability of false positives increases with decreasing sample biomass, but it decreases with 16S rRNA sequencing, thanks to extensive reference databases and computational error correcting techniques. On the other hand, because of primer-dependent PCR amplification bias and differences in the variable areas, the bias risk connected with 16S rRNA sequencing is greater [19]. Table 17.1 represents comparisons of popular microbiome sequencing techniques.

The final consideration is cost, which is unquestionably one of the most crucial aspects in determining the initial sort of NGS to carry out. The quantity and depth of sequencing play a role in the cost disparities between the techniques. The sequencing depth is the number of times a specific nucleotide base appears in a sample's sequencing. NGS-based metagenomic

Table 17.1 Comparisons of popular microbiome sequencing techniques.

Methods

	Amplicon(16S, 18S, ITS)	Shotgun metagenomics	RNA sequencing
What is sequenced?	DNA coding for the 16S, 18S ribosomal subunit or ITS	Host and microbial DNA	Host and microbial RNA
What is the taxonomic resolution?	Phylum-genus, sometimes species	Species-strains	Species-strains
What is the taxonomic coverage?	Bacteria, archaea (16S); eukaryotes (18S)	Bacteria, archaea, eukaryotes, DNA viruses	Bacteria, archaea, eukaryotes, DNA and RNA viruses
Are appropriate reference databases available?	Over 3 million 16S gene sequences from humans and environmental sources are available	Over 100000 genomes with a bias toward human microbiomes	Over 100000 genomes with a bias toward human microbiomes
Does host contamination occur?	Limited	Yes, but can be mitigated by the host DNA/RNA depletion methods	Yes, but can be mitigated by the host DNA/RNA depletion methods
Can sequencing data yield a functional profile?	Not directly, but the functional profile may be predicted computationally	Yes, with appropriate computational expertise	Yes, with appropriate computational expertise
What is the minimum input for detection?	10 copies	1 ng	1 ng
What is the potential for false positives?	Lower due to extensive reference databases and error correction tools	Higher due to host DNA contamination of draft genomes	Higher due to host RNA/DNA contamination of draft genomes
What is the potential for bias?	Medium to high due to dependence on primers, targeted variable region, and PCR amplification	Lower due to the untargeted nature of the methodology	Lower due to the untargeted nature of the methodology
What level of computational skills is required?	Beginner–intermediate	Intermediate–advanced	Intermediate–advanced

Source: [24] / American Society for Clinical Investigation / CC BY 4.0.

sequencing methods have an advantage over the conventional sequencing approaches in that they are able to detect the presence of microbial communities in low abundance. Since shotgun metagenomics and RNA sequencing analyses often require quite a bit more sequence data than 16S rRNA sequencing, those researches are more expensive.

17.3   Collection, Storage, and DNA Extraction Methodology

The majority of information on the microbiota makeup of the human gastrointestinal system comes from next-generation sequencing studies of human feces. Its microbial composition has been found to offer the potential for disease diagnosis, disease prediction, and therapeutic intervention because it contains remnants of food DNA, human DNA, and various inhibitors that impede PCR amplification and NGS methods. Feces rank among the most challenging biological materials for isolating bacterial DNA. The identified fecal bacterial population's makeup may, however, be affected by the experimental design and methodology, including the collection and storage strategy, as well as the DNA extraction method. Examining the numerous methods for bacterial DNA extraction from feces and optimising protocols and techniques that would offer enough quantity, purity, and integrity of the DNA are essential to obtaining high-quality samples for further research. The workflow overview of various NGS methods is shown in Figure 17.3.

17.3.1   Sample Collection and Storage

Procedures for collecting samples are one of the first and most important steps in ensuring the stability and integrity of the collected data. As recommended by current collecting techniques, fresh feces should be used immediately or quickly frozen at −80°F or −20°C. Freezing at specific temperatures preserves specific microbial community composition in fecal samples; thus, microbial diversity and composition also depend on the storage temperature. Nucleic acid stabilising chemicals and preservative buffers, such as TE-buffer or RNAlater, were found to have a negative impact on DNA quantity and quality, by modifying microbial diversity, and changing the proportions of particular taxa [27]. Numerous studies have shown that factors such as the amount of freeze–thaw cycles a sample endures, and the time between sample collection and freezing may affect the microbial community profiles that are discovered [28]. Few commercially systems are currently available for stabilising and collecting waste, such as OMNIgene; GUT is also used to preserve the sample microbiota makeup after freezing, with only slight changes to fresh stool samples [10].

17.3.2   DNA Extraction and Quantification

The composition of the subsequent sequencing data may be impacted by the DNA extraction technique. The extraction process must be efficient for a variety of microbial taxa to yield appropriate sequencing results; otherwise DNA from bacteria that are easier to lyse may predominate in the sequencing results. Bead beating, or mechanical lysis, is often regarded as a superior method of extracting DNA to chemical lysis. Nevertheless, the effectiveness of methods based on bead beating varies. Vigorous extraction procedures, such as bead beating, may lead to the generation of shorter DNA fragments and loss of target sequence, which may be overcome by using fragment size-selection methods.

Contamination may occur during the processing of the sample, including laboratory supplies or kits leading to variable degrees of microbial contamination. Metagenomics data sets derived from low-biomass samples, such as skin swabs, are especially prone to this issue since there is less 'genuine' signal to compete with low levels of contamination [29]. Contamination may also come from the PhiX control DNA, which is frequently employed in Illumina-based sequencing techniques, as well as human or host DNA. Another possible risk factor is a crossover from prior sequencing runs. The three most widely used DNA extraction kits, MP, MO BIO, and QI kits, were able to successfully extract bacterial DNA when using feces samples [30].

Quantity and quality of DNA is determined by using spectrophotometric, Nanodrop, and benchtop fluorometers based on the readouts of the fluorescence and absorbance, respectively. The purity of the nucleic acid (DNA) is determined by the nanodrop, where the absorbance ratio A260/A280, and concentration of DNA may also be determined by using a fluorometer. The absorbance ratio at A260/A280 and DNA concentration values are listed as mean SEM values (multiple samples per group).

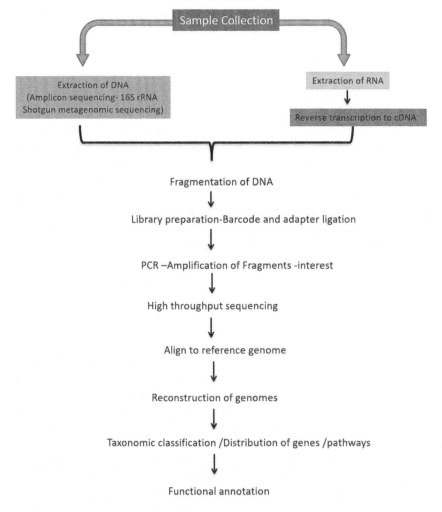

Figure 17.3 Overview of different NGS mythologies. Adapted from [24].

17.4   DNA Sequencing and Post-processing

There are three processes within an outline of the key steps; RNA sequencing, shotgun metagenomic sequencing, and 16S rRNA gene sequencing [24]. With RNA sequencing, PCR is employed to amplify random cDNA fragments generated by RNA reverse transcription or bacterial 16S rRNA gene variable sections (16S rRNA amplicon sequencing). To eliminate the introduction of PCR-related experimental bias, DNA-based shotgun metagenomic sequencing without PCR amplification should be performed. However, in samples with low DNA concentrations, PCR amplification of the DNA library is utilised on occasion, the traditional Illumina-based sequencing chemistry. Complex taxonomic and functional analyses of NGS data frequently make use of freely available technologies.

17.5   Metabolic Modelling of the Human Gut Microbiome

The shortcomings of the genomic sequencing-based approach were overcome by NGS. This approach has enabled the exploration of the mechanisms of the microbiome on human health, which has paved the way to understanding the gut microbiome. To unveil the role of gut microbiomes in human health it is highly essential to quantify the metabolic interactions between the gut microbes and the host. In this case, addressing the systems-level interactions between gut microorganisms and metabolism will be effective with a modelling-based approach.

The study of microbial metabolism and human health typically uses genome-scale metabolic models (GEMs) and sophisticated systems biology techniques. GEMs are computational models of genome-scale biological metabolism. The first GEM, which was developed in 1999, focused on the bacteria *Haemophilus influenzae*. Even though the modelled organisms only have a limited amount of evolutionary knowledge, more than 120 GEMs have now been reconstructed. There have been various evaluations regarding GEM reconstruction and computer analysis of the recovered GEMs. The underlying framework for metabolic reconstructions is, to put it briefly, gene–protein-reaction links that transcend the genotype–phenotype map and connect known genes to functional categories. These relationships are produced using relevant orthologous data and genomic annotations [11].

References

1 Bäckhed, F., Ley, R.E., Sonnenburg, J.L. et al. (2005). Host-bacterial mutualism in the human intestine. *Science* 307 (5717): 1915–1920.

2 Matijašić, M., Meštrović, T., Perić, M. et al. (2016). Modulating composition and metabolic activity of the gut microbiota in IBD patients. *Int. J. Mol. Sci.* 17 (4): 578. https://doi.org/10.3390/IJMS17040578.

3 Lynch, S.V. and Pedersen, O. (2016). The human intestinal microbiome in health and disease. *N. Engl. J. Med.* 375 (24): 2369–2379.

4 Guarner, F. and Malagelada, J.R. (2003). Gut flora in health and disease. *Lancet* 361 (3556): 512–519.

5 Jost, T., Lacroix, C., Braegger, C.P. et al. (2012). New insights in gut microbiota establishment in healthy breast fed neonates. *PLoS One* 7 (8): e44595.

6 O'Hara, A.M. and Shanahan, F. (2006). The gut flora as a forgotten organ. *EMBO Rep.* 7 (7): 688–693.

7 Lagier, J.C., Million, M., Hugon, P. et al. (2012). Human gut microbiota: repertoire and variations. *Front. Cell. Infect. Microbiol.* 2: 136.

8 Cottier, F., Srinivasan, K.G., Yurieva, M. et al. (2018). Advantages of meta-total RNA sequencing (MeTRS) over shotgun metagenomics and amplicon-based sequencing in the profiling of complex microbial communities. *NPJ Bio. Microb.* 4 (1): 1–7.

9 Claesson, M.J. and O'Toole, P.W. (2010). Evaluating the latest high-throughput molecular techniques for the exploration of microbial gut communities. *Gut Micro.* 1 (4): 277–278.

10 Panek, M., Čipčić Paljetak, H., Barešić, A. et al. (2018). Methodology challenges in studying human gut microbiota effects of collection, storage, DNA extraction and next generation sequencing technologies. *Sci. Rep.* 8 (1): 1–13.

11 Ji, B. and Nielsen, J. (2015). From next-generation sequencing to systematic modeling of the gut microbiome. *Front. Genet.* 6: 219. https://doi.org/10.3389/FGENE.2015.00219.

12 Methé, B.A., Nelson, K.E., Pop, M. et al. (2012). A framework for human microbiome research. *Nature* 486 (7402): 215–221.

13 Sanger, F. and Coulson, A.R. (1975). A rapid method for determining sequences in DNA by primed synthesis with DNA polymerase. *J. Mol. Biol.* https://doi.org/10.1016/0022-2836(75)90213-2.

14 Mardis, E.R. (2008). Next-generation DNA sequencing methods. *Ann. Rev. Genomics Hum .Genet.* 9: 387–402.

15 Lane, D.J., Pace, B., Olsen, G.J. et al. (1985). Rapid determination of 16S ribosomal RNA sequences for phylogenetic analyses. *Proc. Natl. Acad. Sci. USA* 82 (20): 6955.

16 Rinke, C., Schwientek, P., Sczyrba, A. et al. (2013). Insights into the phylogeny and coding potential of microbial dark matter. *Nature* 499 (7459): 431–437.

17 Greay, T.L., Gofton, A.W., Paparini, A. et al. (2018). Recent insights into the tick microbiome gained through next-generation sequencing. *Parasites. Vectors.* 11 (1): 1–14.

18 Rintala, A., Pietilä, S., Munukka, E. et al. (2017). Gut microbiota analysis results are highly dependent on the 16S rRNA gene target region, whereas the impact of DNA extraction is minor. *J. Biomol. Tech.* 28 (1): 19–30.

19 Sirichoat, A., Sankuntaw, N., Engchanil, C. et al. (2021). Comparison of different hypervariable regions of 16S rRNA for taxonomic profiling of vaginal microbiota using next-generation sequencing. *Arch. Microbiol.* 203 (3): 1159–1166.

20 Xia, Y., Sun, J., and Chen, D.-G. (2018). Statistical analysis of microbiome data with R. https://doi.org/10.1007/978-981-13-1534-3.

21 Schloss, P.D. (2021). Amplicon sequence variants artificially split bacterial genomes into separate clusters. *mSphere.* https://doi.org/10.1128/MSPHERE.00191-21.

22 Callahan, B.J., McMurdie, P.J., and Holmes, S.P. (2017). Exact sequence variants should replace operational taxonomic units in marker-gene data analysis. *ISME J.* 11 (12): 2639–2643.

23 Salipante, S.J., Kawashima, T., Rosenthal, C. et al. (2014). Performance comparison of Illumina and ion torrent next-generation sequencing platforms for 16S rRNA-based bacterial community profiling. *Appl. Environ. Microbiol.* 80 (24): 7583–7591.

24 Wensel, C.R., Pluznick, J.L., Salzberg, S.L. et al. (2022). Next-generation sequencing: insights to advance clinical investigations of the microbiome. *J. Clin. Invest.* https://doi.org/10.1172/JCI154944.

25 Liu, Y.X., Qin, Y., Chen, T. et al. (2021). A practical guide to amplicon and metagenomic analysis of microbiome data. *Protein Cell* 12 (5): 315–330.

26 Tian, S., Zeng, W., Fang, F. et al. (2022). The microbiome of Chinese rice wine (Huangjiu). *Curr. Res. Food Sci.* 5: 325–335.

27 Gorzelak, M.A., Gill, S.K., Tasnim, N. et al. (2015). Methods for improving human gut microbiome data by reducing variability through sample processing and storage of stool. *PLoS One.* https://doi.org/10.1371/JOURNAL.PONE.0134802.

28 Cuthbertson, L., Rogers, G.B., Walker, A.W. et al. (2014). Time between collection and storage significantly influences bacterial sequence composition in sputum samples from Cystic Fibrosis respiratory infections. *J. Clin. Microbiol.* 52 (8): 3011.

29 Salter, S.J., Cox, M.J., Turek, E.M. et al. (2014). Reagent and laboratory contamination can critically impact sequence-based microbiome analyses. *BMC Biol.* 12: 1–12.

30 Quince, C., Walker, A.W., Simpson, J.T. et al. (2017). Shotgun metagenomics, from sampling to analysis. *Nat. Biotechnol.* 35 (9): 833–844.

18

The Role of Probiotics and Prebiotics in Gut Modulation

Usman Atique[1], Muhammad Altaf[2], Dwaipayan Sinha[3], Shakira Ghazanfar[4], Md. Ayenuddin Haque[5], and Shahana Chowdhury[6]

[1] *Department of Bioscience and Biotechnology, Chungan National University, South Korea*
[2] *Department of Forestry, Range and Wildlife Management, The Islamia University of Bahawalpur, Pakistan*
[3] *Department of Botany, Government General Degree College, Mohanpur, Paschim Medinipur, India*
[4] *Pakistan Agricultural Research Council, Islamabad, Pakistan*
[5] *Bangladesh Fisheries Research Institute, Bangladesh*
[6] *Department of Biotechnology, German University Bangladesh, Bangladesh*

18.1 Introduction

Probiotics, a term derived from Latin, means 'for life.' More precisely, Fuller outlined it as a live microbial feed supplement, which beneficially affects the host animal by improving its intestinal microbial balance [1]. Probiotics is also defined as living microorganisms, ingested on purpose to alter the microflora of gastrointestinal tract, are beneficial for living beings [2]. Additionally, prebiotics is a substrate utilised by host microorganisms for health benefits [3]. Carl Wilhelm Scheele discovered that milk has lactic acid [4]. Elie Metchnikoff, a Russian scientist, is considered the 'father of probiotics,' as he recognised that lactic acid bacteria provide health advantages and promote durability; and he introduced a dairy product through milk fermentation utilising *Bulgarianbacillus* bacterium. Since then, the focus on probiotics has been increasing steadily.

The microbiome is associated with the organism's health, which means an imbalance could cause various diseases such as gastrointestinal tract (GIT) disorders (e.g., diarrhea), and obesity, outside of the GIT. Statistics show that the human body contains 90% bacteria. Scientists have realised that imbalance in microbiota concentration and alteration in their action gives birth to various disorders such as cancer, hypertension, oral health, and obesity. The marketing of probiotics on dairy products has shown a few health-improving features. Probiotic products are accepted worldwide due to their health benefits with no side effects [5]. Probiotics withstand all intestinal antimicrobial factors (i.e., reduce pH, gastric fluid, and other enzymes) as the host body endures heat shocks. Salt concentrations between 0.3% to 2% and pH of 2–5% are critical for probiotics [6]. Literature has shown that probiotic supplementation in healthy adults could increase the colonisation of probiotics [7].

The Gut Microbiota in Health and Disease, First Edition. Edited by Nimmy Srivastava, Salam A. Ibrahim, Jayeeta Chattopadhyay, and Mohamed H. Arbab.
© 2023 John Wiley & Sons Ltd. Published 2023 by John Wiley & Sons Ltd.

With the inevitable role of microbiota in gut modulation and other beneficial impacts on GIT, this chapter provides up-to-date knowledge on the background of pro- and prebiotics, their functions, different types and health benefits, their role in human health, and diet impact on gut microbiota (GM). We will discuss the role of probiotics and prebiotics in gut immunomodulation, neuroimmunology, and their effects on the immune system.

18.2 Probiotics and Prebiotics: A Functional Perspective

The Nobel Laureate Ilya Ilyich Mechnikov first proposed the probiotic concept in 1908 while researching the health benefits of yogurt on Bulgarian farmers [8]. Later, the term probiotics was described by the Food and Agriculture Organisation (FAO) and the WHO (World Health Organisation in 2001 as 'live microorganisms, which when administered in adequate amounts, exert a beneficial effect on the host's health' [9]. To be called a probiotic, an organism must meet specific criteria; these were specified in 2014 [10], and they must explicitly include:

- When microorganisms are administered, they must be thriving in adequate numbers.
- Genetically, strains must be recognised, classified, and labeled with numbers, letters, or names.
- Suitably scaled and planned investigations are essential to entitle a strain as a probiotic to fulfill the envisioned role.
- Strains helpful in one situation may not be probiotic in another.
- In experimental testing, probiotic strains for people used in various animal trials should be labeled as human probiotics.

Probiotic bacteria are predominantly gram-positive bacteria that live in the gut of humans. Probiotics might aid in the treatment of dysbiosis [11], cholesterol reduction [12], cancer prevention [13], allergy [14], and autoimmune illnesses [15]. A probiotic is only successful if the strain lives in a location thought to be active. It should be non-pathogenic, non-allergic, and non-mutagenic/carcinogenic [16]. Probiotics for humans should be classified as 'generally recognised as safe' [17], with a low risk of causing disease or being linked to its etiology. They must be able to sustain and flourish *in vivo* circumstances in the desired sites of their administration. This can be characterised by lower pH combined with higher levels of the conjugated and deconjugated bile acids. For optimal application, the probiotics utilised in foods must also be technologically compliant with the food manufacturing process. Furthermore, probiotic foods must retain the typical sensory characteristic [18]. The sources and benefits of prebiotics and probiotics are illustrated in Figure 18.1.

Gibson and Roberfroid originally defined prebiotics in 1995 [19], when they described a prebiotic as a 'non-digestible food ingredient that beneficially affects the host by selectively stimulating the growth and activity of one or a limited number of bacteria in the colon, thus improving host health.' Based on the definition, a few molecules of carbohydrates, namely short- and long-chain-fructans and lactulose, have been categorised as prebiotics. However, later in 2008, at the sixth meeting of the International Scientific Association of Probiotics and Prebiotics (ISAPP) they characterised them as 'dietary prebiotics' and 'a selectively fermented ingredient that results in specific changes in the composition and activity of the

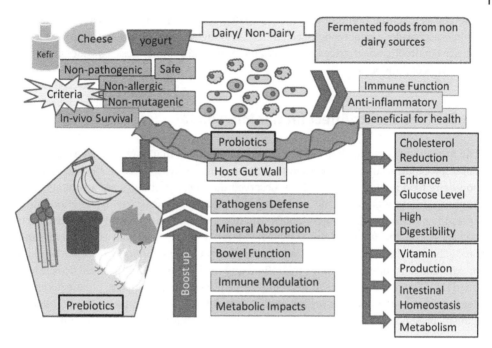

Figure 18.1 Sources and benefits of both the prebiotic and probiotic to the gastrointestinal tract.

gastrointestinal microbiota, thus conferring benefit(s) upon host health' [20]. Based on the available information, a substance to be classified as a prebiotic should satisfy the following conditions:

- It is resistant to the acidic pH inside the stomach, cannot be hydrolysed by the assembly of mammalian enzymes, and is incapable of being taken in the GIT. Gut microbes may ferment it.
- The compound may selectively enthuse intestinal bacterial growth and action, improving the host's well-being [21].

Later, in another meeting of the ISAPP in 2017 [22], prebiotics were defined as 'a substrate that is selectively utilised by host microorganisms, imparting a health advantage.' These agents must also possess the following qualities, which will be investigated *in vitro* and *in vivo* in various targets.

- Gastric acidity resistance, digestive enzyme hydrolysis, and gastrointestinal absorption.
- Intestinal microflora fermentation may be assessed *in vitro* by introducing appropriate carbohydrates to the colon substance formulations or bacterial cultures.
- Endurance to gastric acidity and hydrolysis by gastric enzymes; this definition appears to be the most comprehensive and widely used [23].

Most probiotics are oligosaccharide carbohydrates (OSCs), which form a subset of carbohydrate classifications [24]. The main prebiotics have long been inulin, Galactooligosaccharides, and Fructooligosaccharides. Additionally, other compounds and dietary fibres have emerged as potential prebiotics with variable degrees of health advantages [25]. The fructooligosaccharides, galactooligosaccharides, xylooligosaccharides, soybean oligosaccharides, isomaltooligosaccharides, fructans, guar gum, and pectinoligosaccharides constitute eight types of prebiotics.

18.3 Diet and its Effect on Gut Microbiota

The human gut contains many beneficial bacterial strains that may be used as probiotics. These probiotic strains may be used to prepare different types of cost-effective dairy and non-dairy food items [26]. It has been observed that these probiotics are advantageous in improving dietary patterns and increasing individuals' physical activity. The food influences the human intestinal microbiota's structure and function. Some of the several bacterial species in the intestine are shown in Figure 18.2. Several food components, milk products, and pharmaceutical products containing probiotics will increase when probiotic microorganisms' interaction with microflora and the human gastrointestinal tract is identified [27]. The crucial steps in understanding the physiology of probiotic organisms are the development of methods for *in vivo* and *in vitro* determination of the probiotic microorganism presence and activity in the host intestine, characteristics of the antibacterial

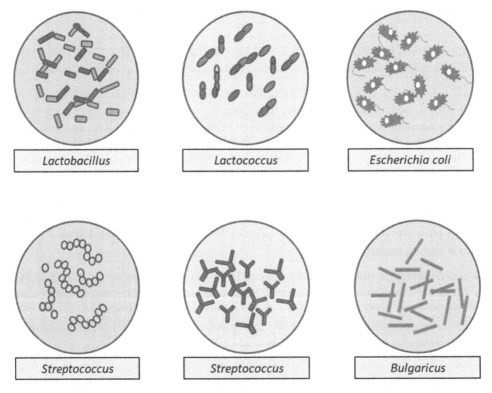

Figure 18.2 Morphological structure of some essential and beneficial probiotics of the gut microbiota.

properties of probiotic microorganisms, as well as the development of molecular methods to characterise probiotic microorganisms and resident intestinal microflora [28].

18.4 Modification of Intestinal Microbiota by the Application of Probiotics and Prebiotics

18.4.1 Dysbiosis and Human Diseases

Dysbiosis is an imbalance in the thousands of unique microbial operational taxonomic units (OTUs) present in each individual [29]. It is usually associated with the disease caused by the gut's gain or loss of a complex microbial community. Dysbiosis may generate chronic diseases in an individual in three significant ways; damage of beneficial microbes, a rapid increase in the number of potentially dangerous microbes, and deterioration of total microbial variety, which cause chronic inflammation, suppressed health-protective bacteria, and other bacterial infections [30]. Homeostatic imbalance in GM may also cause diseases in the central nervous, cardiovascular, and digestive systems. Furthermore, dysbiosis in GM is closely related to many metabolic ailments, including obesity and diabetes [31]. Dysbiosis and its associated common diseases may be controlled using nutraceuticals (prebiotics and probiotics), fecal microbial transplantation, and environmental changes in bacterial flora in the gut. Symbiotic interventions in GM are facilitated through biofilm formation, bacteriocin production, host immunity stimulation, and enhancement of gut barrier function of host epithelial cells [32].

18.4.2 How Probiotics Alter the Intestinal Microbiota

Introducing a probiotic into the mouse intestine alters the endogenous microbiota metabolic pattern. When germ-free mice monoassociated with *Bacteroides thetaiotaomicron* were challenged with *Bifidobacterium animalis* or *Lactobacillus casei*, both interventions generated changes in the *B. thetaiotaomicron* genome's gene expression pattern. These gene sets, which were differentially expressed (in response to the two probiotics), did not overlap, indicating that specific probiotics induce diverse responses. Many of the genes in *B. thetaiotaomicron*, which were affected by either probiotic strain, were connected to the growth of *B. thetaiotaomicron*'s carbohydrate metabolising capabilities. Thus, probiotics appear to affect the microbiota makeup by competing with them for substrate availability and modifying the dynamics of carbohydrate use by specific microbiota components. Recent research suggests that oral Bifidobacterium strains *B. adolescentis* reduce vitamin K content and compete with *Porphyromonas gingivalis* in the oral cavity, implying that this rivalry is not limited to the intestine [33, 34].

18.4.3 Probiotics and Intestinal Immunomodulation

The GM is the most important source of microbial stimulation, as it negatively and positively affects human well-being. The interaction of probiotics with enterocytes is the first step in immunomodulation and deserves special attention [35]. *Lactobacillus* and

Bifidobacterium are the most extensively utilised probiotic bacteria in the food and pharmaceutical industries, and various strains of these genera are valid. Other bacteria prevalent in the gut microbiome, such as *Faecalibacterium prausnitzii* and *Akkermansia muciniphila*, were isolated through animal and human studies and are known for health-promoting properties. Immunomodulation is the leading aspect of probiotic bacteria currently being researched. In particular, *lactobacilli* and *bifidobacteria* have been examined for their capacity to activate our immunological function, with some substances responsible for favorable actions (surface proteins and EPS) being identified. Several unique approaches allow researchers to look at probiotic-mediated immunomodulation from new angles. The modern tools employed in microbiome investigations [36], genomic editing such as CRISPR-Cas [37], and molecular techniques [38] elucidate the involvement of different pathways and molecules accountable for an effective mode of action of probiotics.

18.4.4 Probiotics and Prebiotics on Intestinal Neuroimmunology

Probiotics and prebiotics are the recent tools used to manage GM and improvement of the host's health [39]. The probiotics act via various processes, including the modulation of immune system functions, making antimicrobial compounds and organic acids, interacting with gut resident microbiota and the host, enhancing the enzyme creation, and maintaining the gut barrier integrity [40]. However, prebiotics are the substrates selectively used by the host microbiota giving a health advantage. Additionally, synbiotics are the blends of prebiotics and probiotics synergising to confer various health benefits [41]. Some probiotics augment cell phagocytosis processes, enhancing cellular activity and directly interacting with the dendritic cells [42]. They may upgrade the anti-inflammatory cytokine levels (e.g., tumor necrosis factor), to decrease colon cancer tissue and colitis [43]. Probiotics interact directly with GM in various ways, such as the compete for nutrient availability, cross-type feeding methods, opposition, and assistance for their stability [44].

Studies on various cell lines show probiotics improve the barrier functions by increasing the expression of the tight junction proteins of probiotic *Lactobacillus* and *Bifidobacterium* [45]. They may also upregulate the gene expression in mucus sections, reducing pathogens' binding to epithelial cells, and concomitantly improving the barrier functions. The microbial enzymes that help improve lactose digestion and human blood lipid profile are triggered and delivered by some probiotics [46]. Therefore, it is essential to know that gut microbes thrive in perpetual ecosystems with multitudes of roles, covering conversions of absorbed dietary carbohydrates, fats, and proteins into various metabolites [47]. As a measure of providing immunity to the pathogens, prebiotic administration may result in the decline of luminal pH level and inhibition of the propagation of pathogens [48]. Such developments will further reduce the availability of nutrients to new microorganisms to help curb their colonisation, and hence help in enhancing the host immunity [49]. Evidence has been reported that prebiotic introduction may suppress the responses of type 2 T helper cells [50].

Consequently, prebiotics help enhance the absorption of various elements in the host's intestine [51]. Some studies have reported the impact of prebiotics on improving bowel functions through the humectant water-binding capacity of carbohydrates; this includes simply bulking feces through dietary fibre consumption [52]. Furthermore, prebiotics regulate metabolic processes through intervention and positively impact glucose homeostasis, blood lipid profiles, and inflammation [53, 54], which is how the prebiotics increase satiety levels and reduce the body fat by decreasing the desire for higher energy sources daily.

18.5 Prebiotics and Gut Immunity

Gut immunity is impacted by a plethora of factors, including commensal bacteria and dietary components [55]. Food components such as prebiotics influence gut immunity, as they affect the microbiota composition, evolving as new therapeutic methods to heal various inflammatory diseases. The GM is also a super-organism integral to the digestive tract [56]. Prebiotics may stimulate the gut immune system directly or indirectly by enhancing the beneficial microbiota population, especially *bifidobacteria* and lactic acid bacteria [57]. One of the critical action mechanisms of prebiotics in strengthening immunity is altering cytokines' expression. Other impacts of prebiotics on improving the host gut immunity and overall health status include alteration to the populations and composition of GM, enhancing the production of fermentation products through gut microflora, stimulation of intestinal barrier functions, direct stimulation of the immune system, and improvements in the absorption of nutrients [57]. Furthermore, the SCFAs and similar microbial products affect gut immunity by attaching the G-protein-coupled receptors of immune cells in the gut-associated lymphoid tissues [58].

18.5.1 Effects (Direct and Indirect) of Prebiotics on the Immune System

The application of prebiotics may cause both direct and indirect effects. The most significant impact of prebiotics is the augmentation of beneficial bacteria populations, which enhance the release of their products in the gut. This shows that the enhancement of beneficial microbes is directly impacted while the production of the products is indirect. Another indirect effect of prebiotics is the change in the equilibrium of gut microbial populations to enhance the protective bacteria (*bifidobacteria* and *lactobacilli*) while decreasing the pathogenic microbes [59]. Furthermore, prebiotics may improve gut integrity and its desired functions by decreasing gut pH and reducing the nitrogenous metabolites [60]. Diet is strongly associated with the GM species [61]; consequently, the profile of predominant microbes in the gut may be altered by dietary intake, which also has other health consequences. For instance, the nutritional fibre may serve as an effective prebiotic and induce significant shifts in the human GM composition. It can directly affect the mucosal immune system, improving enteric inflammatory conditions and enhancing the systemic immune responses [55].

18.6 Conclusions and Future Research

The intestine is home to trillions of microorganisms (predominantly bacteria) exhibiting a symbiotic association as they co-evolve. A primary role assumed by the multitude of microbial populations (i.e., GM) is to safeguard the intestine against exogenous disease-causing and potentially harmful indigenous microbes. Despite having a complex configuration, the gut microbial population is very delicate, and slight disruptions in their thriving environment may lead to dysbiosis. Such imbalances result in the decline of disease resistance to pathogen colonies, expansion of pathobionts, and pathological responses. The collapse of a specific microbial population increases the infection risk by pathogens, inflammatory diseases, and the overgrowth of detrimental pathobionts in the host gut. The current research is exploring the environmental and genetic factors reshaping the GM; and the extent of the impact of such aspects and their mechanisms revealing the interactions leading to dysbiosis will remain the avenues of future investigations. Other questions that must be further investigated surround dysbiosis linked explicitly to particular disorders and the timing of dysbiosis in the host's lifetime. It is also essential to investigate further the direct immunomodulatory impacts of prebiotics by using them in a combination of varying degrees of polymerisation in various hosts.

References

1 McFarland, L.V. (2015 May). From yaks to yogurt: the history, development, and current use of probiotics. *Clin. Infect. Dis.* 60 (supp. 2): S85–90. https://doi.org/10.1093/cid/civ054.

2 Abatenh, E., Gizaw, B., Tsegay, Z. et al. (2018). Health benefits of probiotics. *J. Bacteriol. Infec. Dis.* 2 (1): 8–27.

3 Yahfoufi, N., Mallet, J.F., Graham, E. et al. (2018 April). Role of probiotics and prebiotics in immunomodulation. *Curr. Opi. Food Sci.* 20: 82–91. https://doi.org/10.1016/j.cofs.2018.04.006.

4 Manchester, K.L. (2007 September). Louis Pasteur, fermentation, and a rival: history of science. *S. African J. Sci.* 103 (9): 377–80.

5 Georgieva, M., Andonova, L., Peikova, L. et al. (2014). Probiotics–health benefits, classification, quality assurance and quality control–review. *Pharmacia* 61 (4): 22–31.

6 de Melo Pereira, G.V., de Oliveira Coelho, B., Júnior, A.I. et al. (2018 December). How to select a probiotic? A review and update of methods and criteria. *Biotech. Adv.* 36 (8): 2060–2076. https://doi.org/10.1016/j.biotechadv.2018.09.003.

7 Khalesi, S., Bellissimo, N., Vandelanotte, C. et al. (2019 January). A review of probiotic supplementation in healthy adults: helpful or hype? *Euro. J. Clin. Nut.* 73 (1): 24–37. https://doi.org/10.1038/s41430-018-0135-9.

8 Kareb, O. and Aïder, M. (2019 June). Whey and its derivatives for probiotics, prebiotics, synbiotics, and functional foods: a critical review. *Probiot. Antimicrob. Prot.* 11 (2): 348–369. https://doi.org/10.1007/s12602-018-9427-6.

9 Hill, C., Guarner, F., Reid, G. et al. (2014). Expert consensus document: the International Scientific Association for Probiotics and Prebiotics consensus statement on the scope and appropriate use of the term probiotic. *Nat. Rev. Gastroenterol. Hepatol.* https://doi.org/10.1038/nrgastro.2014.66.

10 Reid, G., Gadir, A.A., and Dhir, R. (2019 March). Probiotics: reiterating what they are and what they are not. *Front. Microbio.* 10: 424. https://doi.org/10.3389/fmicb.2019.00424.

11 Yoon, W., Park, S.H., Lee, J.S. et al. (2021 August). Probiotic mixture reduces gut inflammation and microbial dysbiosis in children with atopic dermatitis. *Australasian J. Derma.* 62 (3): e386–392. https://doi.org/10.1111/ajd.13644.

12 Cho, Y.A. and Kim, J. (2015 October). Effect of probiotics on blood lipid concentrations: a meta-analysis of randomized controlled trials. *Med. (Baltimore)* 94 (43): e1714. https://doi.org/10.1097/MD.0000000000001714.

13 Górska, A., Przystupski, D., Niemczura, M.J. et al. (2019 August). Probiotic bacteria: a promising tool in cancer prevention and therapy. *Curr. Microbio.* 76 (8): 939–949. https://doi.org/10.1007/s00284-019-01679-8.

14 Huang, J., Zhang, J., Wang, X. et al. (2022 February). Effect of probiotics on respiratory tract allergic disease and gut microbiota. *Front. Nutri.* 9: 821900. https://doi.org/10.3389/fnut.2022.821900.

15 Ferro, M., Charneca, S., Dourado, E. et al. (2021). Probiotic supplementation for rheumatoid arthritis: a promising adjuvant therapy in the gut microbiome era. *Front. Pharma.* 12. https://doi.org/10.3389/fphar.2021.711788.

16 Nagpal, R., Kumar, A., Kumar, M. et al. (2012 September). Probiotics, their health benefits and applications for developing healthier foods: a review. *FEMS Microbio. Lett.* 334 (1): 1–5. https://doi.org/10.1111/j.1574-6968.2012.02593.x.

17 Markowiak, P. and Śliżewska, K. (2017 September). Effects of probiotics, prebiotics, and synbiotics on human health. *Nutrients* 9 (9): 1021. https://doi.org/10.3390/nu9091021.

18 Gibson, G.R. and Roberfroid, M.B. (1995 June). Dietary modulation of the human colonic microbiota: introducing the concept of prebiotics. *J. Nutri.* 125 (6): 1401–1412. https://doi.org/10.1093/jn/125.6.1401.

19 Davani-Davari, D., Negahdaripour, M., Karimzadeh, I. et al. (2019 March). Prebiotics: definition, types, sources, mechanisms, and clinical applications. *Foods* 8 (3): 92. https://doi.org/10.3390/foods8030092.

20 Gibson, G.R., Scott, K.P., Rastall, R.A. et al. (2010 May). Dietary prebiotics: current status and new definition. *Food Sci. Tech. Bull. Func. Foods* 7 (1): 1–9.

21 Gibson, G.R., Hutkins, R., Sanders, M.E. et al. (2017 August). Expert consensus document: The International Scientific Association for Probiotics and Prebiotics (ISAPP) consensus statement on the definition and scope of prebiotics. *Nat. Rev. Gastroenterol. Hepa.* 14 (8): 491–502. https://doi.org/10.1038/nrgastro.2017.75.

22 Guarino, M.P.L., Altomare, A., Emerenziani, S. et al. (2020 April). Mechanisms of action of prebiotics and their effects on gastro-Iintestinal disorders in adults. *Nutrients* 12 (4): 1037. https://doi.org/10.3390/nu12041037.

23 Kaur, A.P., Bhardwaj, S., Dhanjal, D.S. et al. (2021 March). Plant prebiotics and their role in the amelioration of diseases. *Biomolecules* 11 (3): 440. https://doi.org/10.3390/biom11030440.

24 Carlson, J.L., Erickson, J.M., Lloyd, B.B. et al. (2018 January). Health effects and sources of prebiotic dietary fiber. *Curr. Devel. Nutri.* 2 (3): nzy005. https://doi.org/10.1093/cdn/nzy005.

25 Sabater-Molina, M., Larqué, E., Torrella, F. et al. (2009 September). Dietary fructooligosaccharides and potential benefits on health. *J. Phys. Biochem.* 65 (3): 315–328. https://doi.org/10.1007/BF03180584.

26 Saito, T. (2004 February). Selection of useful probiotic lactic acid bacteria from the Lactobacillus acidophilus group and their applications to functional foods. *Ani. Sci. J.* 75 (1): 1–3. https://doi.org/10.1111/j.1740-0929.2004.00148.x.

27 Sanders, M.E., Merenstein, D., Merrifield, C.A. et al. (2018 September). Probiotics for human use. *Nutri. Bull.* 43 (3): 212–225. https://doi.org/10.1111/nbu.12334.

28 Gueimonde, M. and Salminen, S. (2006 December). New methods for selecting and evaluating probiotics. *Diges. Liver Dis.* 38: S242-7. https://doi.org/10.1016/S1590-8658(07)60003-6.

29 Wilkins, L.J., Monga, M., and Miller, A.W. (2019 September). Defining dysbiosis for a cluster of chronic diseases. *Sci. Rep.* 9 (1): 1–10. https://doi.org/10.1038/s41598-019-49452-y.

30 DeGruttola, A.K., Low, D., Mizoguchi, A. et al. (2016 May). Current understanding of dysbiosis in disease in human and animal models. *Inflamm. Bowel Dis.* 22 (5): 1137–1150. https://doi.org/10.1097/MIB.0000000000000750.

31 Chen, Y., Zhou, J., and Wang, L. (2021 March). Role and mechanism of gut microbiota in human disease. *Front. Cell. Infec. Microbia.* 11: 86. https://doi.org/10.3389/fcimb.2021.625913.

32 Carlson, J.L., Erickson, J.M., Lloyd, B.B. et al. (2018 January). Health effects and sources of prebiotic dietary fiber. *Curr. Devel. Nutri.* 2 (3): nzy005. https://doi.org/10.1093/cdn/nzy005.

33 Sonnenburg, J.L., Chen, C.T., and Gordon, J.I. (2006 December). Genomic and metabolic studies of the impact of probiotics on a model gut symbiont and host. *PLoS Bio* 4 (12): e413. https://doi.org/10.1371/journal.pbio.0040413.

34 Hojo, K., Nagaoka, S., Murata, S. et al. (2007 November). Reduction of vitamin K concentration by salivary Bifidobacterium strains and their possible nutritional competition with Porphyromonas gingivalis. *J. App. Microbio.* 103 (5): 1969–1974. https://doi.org/10.1111/j.1365-2672.2007.03436.x.

35 Delcenserie, V., Martel, D., Lamoureux, M. et al. (2008 January). Immunomodulatory effects of probiotics in the intestinal tract. *Curr. Iss. Molec. Bio.* 10 (1–2): 37–54. https://doi.org/10.21775/cimb.010.037.

36 Douillard, F.P. and de Vos, W.M. (2019 November). Biotechnology of health-promoting bacteria. *Biotech. Ad.* 37 (6): 107369. https://doi.org/10.1016/j.biotechadv.2019.03.008.

37 Hidalgo-Cantabrana, C., Goh, Y.J., Pan, M. et al. (2019 August). Genome editing using the endogenous type I CRISPR-Cas system in *Lactobacillus crispatus*. *Proc.Nat. Acad. Sci.* 116 (32): 15774–83. https://doi.org/10.1073/pnas.1905421116.

38 Cross, K.L., Campbell, J.H., Balachandran, M. et al. (2019 November). Targeted isolation and cultivation of uncultivated bacteria by reverse genomics. *Nat. Biotech.* 37 (11): 1314–1321. https://doi.org/10.1038/s41587-019-0260-6.

39 Guinane, C.M. and Cotter, P.D. (2013 July). Role of the gut microbiota in health and chronic gastrointestinal disease: understanding a hidden metabolic organ. *Thera. Adv. Gastroent.* 6 (4): 295–308. https://doi.org/10.1177/1756283X13482996.

40 Edwards, P.T., Kashyap, P.C., and Preidis, G.A. (2020 September). Microbiota on biotics: probiotics, prebiotics, and synbiotics to optimize growth and metabolism. *Am. J. Physio.–Gastro. Liver Physio.* 319 (3): G382–390. https://doi.org/10.1152/ajpgi.00028.2020.

41 Klaenhammer, T.R., Kleerebezem, M., Kopp, M.V. et al. (2012 October). The impact of probiotics and prebiotics on the immune system. *Nat. Rev. Imm.* 12 (10): 728–734. https://doi.org/10.1038/nri3312.

42 Rowland, I., Gibson, G., Heinken, A. et al. (2018 February). Gut microbiota functions: metabolism of nutrients and other food components. *Euro. J. Nut.* 57 (1): 1–24. https://doi.org/10.1007/s00394-017-1445-8.

43 van Baarlen, P., Wells. J.M., and Kleerebezem, M. (2013 May). Regulation of intestinal homeostasis and immunity with probiotic lactobacilli. *Trends. Imm.* 34 (5): 208–215. https://doi.org/10.1016/j.it.2013.01.005.

44 La Fata, G., Weber, P., and Mohajeri, M.H. (2018 March). Probiotics and the gut immune system: indirect regulation. *Probio. Antimicro. Prot.* 10 (1): 11–21. https://doi.org/10.1007/s12602-017-9322-6.

45 Kotz, C.M., Furne, J.K., Savaiano, D.A. et al. (1994 December). Factors affecting the ability of a high β-galactosidase yogurt to enhance lactose absorption. *J. Dairy Sci.* 77 (12): 3538–3544. https://doi.org/10.3168/jds.S0022-0302(94)77296-9.

46 Kasubuchi, M., Hasegawa, S., Hiramatsu, T. et al. (2015 April). Dietary gut microbial metabolites, short-chain fatty acids, and host metabolic regulation. *Nutrients* 7 (4): 2839–2849. https://doi.org/10.3390/nu7042839.

47 Vulevic, J., Drakoularakou, A., Yaqoob, P. et al. (2008 November). Modulation of the fecal microflora profile and immune function by a novel trans-galactooligosaccharide mixture (B-GOS) in healthy elderly volunteers. *Am. J. Clin. Nutri.* 88 (5): 1438–1446. https://doi.org/10.3945/ajcn.2008.26242.

48 Vulevic, J., Juric, A., Walton, G.E. et al. (2015 August). Influence of galacto-oligosaccharide mixture (B-GOS) on gut microbiota, immune parameters and metabonomics in elderly persons. *Brit. J. Nutri.* 114 (4): 586–595. https://doi.org/10.1017/S0007114515001889.

49 Arslanoglu, S., Moro, G.E., Boehm, G. et al. (2012 July). Early neutral prebiotic Oligosaccharide supplementation reduces the incidence of some allergic manifestations in the first 5 years of life. *J. Bio. Regu. Homeo. Agen.* 26: 49–59.

50 Diaz de Barboza, G., Guizzardi, S., and Tolosa de Talamoni, N. (2015). Molecular aspects of intestinal calcium absorption. *W. J. Gastroenter.* 21 (23): 7142–7154. https://doi.org/10.3748/wjg.v21.i23.7142.

51 Lamsal, B.P. (2012 August). Production, health aspects and potential food uses of dairy prebiotic galactooligosaccharides. *J. Sci. Food Agri.* 92 (10): 2020–2028. https://doi.org/10.1002/jsfa.5712.

52 Kellow, N.J., Coughlan, M.T., and Reid, C.M. (2014 April). Metabolic benefits of dietary prebiotics in human subjects: a systematic review of randomised controlled trials. *Brit. J. Nutri.* 111 (7): 1147–1161. https://doi.org/10.1017/S0007114513003607.

53 Liu, F., Prabhakar, M., Ju, J. et al. (2017 January). Effect of inulin-type fructans on blood lipid profile and glucose level: a systematic review and meta-analysis of randomized controlled trials. *Euro. J. Clin. Nutri.* 71 (1): 9–20. https://doi.org/10.1038/ejcn.2016.156.

54 Vieira, A.T., Teixeira, M.M., and Martins, F.D. (2013 December). The role of probiotics and prebiotics in inducing gut immunity. *Front. Imm.* 4: 445. https://doi.org/10.3389/fimmu.2013.00445.

55 Qin, J., Li, R., Raes, J. et al. (2010 March). A human gut microbial gene catalogue established by metagenomic sequencing. *Nature* 464 (7285): 59–65. https://doi.org/10.1038/nature08821.

56 Shokryazdan, P., Faseleh Jahromi, M., Navidshad, B. et al. (2017 February). Effects of prebiotics on immune system and cytokine expression. *Med. Microbio. Imm.* 206 (1): 1–9. https://doi.org/10.1007/s00430-016-0481-y.

57 Brown, A.J., Goldsworthy, S.M., Barnes, A.A. et al. (2003 March). The Orphan G protein-coupled receptors GPR41 and GPR43 are activated by propionate and other short chain carboxylic acids. *J. Biolog. Chem.* 278 (13): 11312–11319. https://doi.org/10.1074/jbc. M211609200.

58 Roller, M., Rechkemmer, G., and Watzl, B. (2004 January). Prebiotic inulin enriched with oligofructose in combination with the probiotics *Lactobacillus rhamnosus* and *Bifedobacterium lactis* modulates intestinal immune functions in rats. *J. Nutri.* 134 (1): 153–156. https://doi.org/10.1093/jn/134.1.153.

59 Watson, R.R. and Preedy, V.R. (eds.). (2015). Probiotics, prebiotics, and synbiotics: bioactive foods in health promotion. In: *Probiotics, prebiotics, and synbiotics: Bioactive foods in health promotion*. Amsterdam: Academic Press. https://doi.org/10.1016/C2015-0-01023-1.

60 Gibson, G.R., Probert, H.M., Van Loo, J. et al. (2004 December). Dietary modulation of the human colonic microbiota: updating the concept of prebiotics. *Nutri. Res. Rev.* 17 (2): 259–275. https://doi.org/10.1079/NRR200479.

61 Gourbeyre, P., Denery, S., and Bodinier, M. (2011 May). Probiotics, prebiotics, and synbiotics: impact on the gut immune system and allergic reactions. *J. Leuk. Bio.* 89 (5): 685–695. https://doi.org/10.1189/jlb.1109753.

19

Probiotics, Prebiotics, and Synbiotics: A Potential Source for a Healthy Gut

Vandana Singh¹ and Bushra Shaida²

¹ *Assistant Professor, Department of Microbiology, School of Allied Health Sciences, Sharda University, Gr. Noida, U.P., India*
² *Assistant Professor, Department of Nutrition and Dietetics, School of Allied Health Sciences, Sharda University, Gr. Noida, U.P., India*
·

19.1 Introduction

The gut microbiota has an impact on human health through influencing the gut defence barrier, immunological function, and nutrition utilisation, as well as by potentially communicating directly with the gastrointestinal epithelium. The interaction of the host microbiota with external substances has the potential to disrupt or modify the natural microbial balance or activity in the GI tract. The pathophysiology of numerous illnesses has been linked to changes in microbiota. Several pathogens such as *E. coli*, *Salmonella* spp., *Shigella* and other food-borne pathogenic strains such as *Bacillus cereus*, *Staphylococcus aureus*, *Listeria monocytogenes*, and *Vibrio cholera* cause enteric illnesses. The potential of probiotics, prebiotics, and synbiotics has been recently explored and sparked a surge due to their use in healthy modification of the gut microbiota [1]. At first look, the only difference between these two words (prebiotics and probiotics) is the appearance of a single vowel, yet probiotics and prebiotics are actually significantly different. Probiotics are live organisms, whereas, prebiotics are indigestible fibres that feed the probiotics. The bacteria that live inside of us (the majority are dwell in our gut) provide us with an incredible array of life-supporting benefits, such as helping in synthesis of vital vitamins and enzymes which are required for supporting our digestion system, metabolic activity, moods, and immunity [2]. Unfortunately, numerous elements in our modern lifestyles are constantly threatening this bacterial balance, including antibiotics and pesticides in food, overzealous hygiene habits, use of antibacterial cleansers, and toxic pollutants in the environment. Along with that, stress and the ageing process are also part of reducing the quantity of these beneficial bacteria in our intestines [3]. The appropriate balance between probiotic and prebiotic supplements together, called synbiotic, may help one to restore their microbial gut custodian or flora and to maintain their dominance at a site where they can work at their best. Some spp. of *Coliform bacteria*, *Bifidobacterium* spp., and *Lactobacillus* spp. are example of the most promising probiotic microbial species, and

The Gut Microbiota in Health and Disease, First Edition. Edited by Nimmy Srivastava, Salam A. Ibrahim, Jayeeta Chattopadhyay, and Mohamed H. Arbab.
© 2023 John Wiley & Sons Ltd. Published 2023 by John Wiley & Sons Ltd.

their roles are well explored in the anticipation of various degenerative diseases; for instance obesity, cancer, diabetes, malignancy, cardiovascular diseases, liver disease, kidney diseases, and inflammatory bowel disease [4]. Whereas, banana, chicory root, garlic, dandelion greens, and onion are some organic prebiotic nourishments. As a result, incorporating probiotic and prebiotic supplements as synbiotics into a daily routine is essential for long-term healthy gut [5].

19.2   Prebiotics

The term prebiotic was first introduced by Gibson and Roberfroid in 1995. It is termed a non-digestible food element that enhances the health of the host by selectively boosting the growth activity of normal flora and limited number of pathogenic bacteria in the colon. These prebiotics generally do not participate in the food caloric value. Furthermore, the FAO and WHO defined the term prebiotics as a non-viable food component which enhances the health aids/benefits of the host by modulating the microbiota of gut. They also act as a support system for probiotics [3, 6].

At the strain or species level, different prebiotics are responsible for different changes. These non-digestible dietary supplements promote the growth and activity of 'good bacteria' such as *Lactobacilli* and *Bifidobacterium*, which act as probiotics. Prebiotics are not broken down by digestive enzymes as they transit through the gut, so they directly reach the large intestine of host in their whole form [5]. These provide nourishment for the probiotic microbial strains that live in the gut system. Prebiotics with established efficacy may thereby alter the gut microbiota by promoting the growth of beneficial gut microorganisms while reducing harmful (pathogenic) ones. Prebiotics help to maintain the proper pH of the GI, which is necessary for the probiotics strains to thrive [7].

Prebiotics boost the immune system by promoting the growth of probiotics, and prevent infections from reproducing and exhibiting their damaging effects by inhibiting their reproduction. They help to promote peristalsis and minimise gas production. The probiotics consume these prebiotics as supplemental food [8]. Any foodstuff that enters the large intestine has potential to work as a prebiotic, although a key factor is selective fermentation. Prebiotics have a selective effect on the microbiota, resulting in improved host health. Prebiotics such as low digestible saccharides (carbohydrates), have an osmotic impact in the intestinal tract if they are not fermented; but when fermented by the native normal microbial flora (i.e., at the site of prebiotic action), they increase the gas production [9]. Plant products such as inulin, lactulose, fructo-oligosaccharides, gums, and dietary fibre are the prebiotics most frequently used as food supplements [10]. Additionally, the trans-galactooligosaccharides (TOS) and inulin and are the two most prevalent prebiotics to be in use as prebiotics, and garlic, leeks, onions, shallots, spinach, peas, Jerusalem artichokes, asparagus, chicory, beans, oats, bananas, and lentils are some examples of foods that include the two. The most well-known and utilised prebiotics are oligosaccharides. Fructo-oligosaccharides (FOS), Inulin, Mannan-oligosaccharides (MOS), Xylo-oligosaccharides, and Lactulose are more regularly utilised prebiotics and are more commercially accessible [11].

19.2.1 Types of Prebiotics

Prebiotics come in a variety of forms; the majority of them are oligosaccharide carbohydrates (OSCs), which constitute a subset of carbohydrate groupings. The relevant articles focus primarily on OSCs, however there is some indication that prebiotics are more than just carbs [12].

- Fructans: Inulin and fructo-oligosaccharide, or oligofructose, fall within this category. Their structure is a fructose linear chain with a 21 linkage, which is frequently at the end of their glucose units. Inulin may have a degree of polymerisation (DP) of up to 60, whereas FOS has a DP of less than 10. Previously, some research suggested that fructans might specifically induce lactic acid bacteria. However, recent research has revealed that the chain length of fructans is a crucial factor for determining whether bacteria might ferment. As a result, fructans may support the growth of other bacterial species, either directly or indirectly [13].
- Galacto-oligosaccharides: (GOS) products are a form of lactose or an extension of lactose and are further divided into subgroups; GOS with extra galactose at C3, C4, or C6, and GOS made from lactose via enzymatic trans-glycosylation. Another type was formed by sucrose, and named the raffinose family of oligosaccharides (RFO). This reaction produces a mixture of tri- to pentasaccharides with galactose as the end-product. Trans-galacto-oligosaccharides, or TOS GOSs, are a form of GOS that may considerably increase *Bifidobacteria* and *Lactobacilli*. GOS has been found to be highly incorporated by *Bifidobacteria* in babies. GOS also stimulates Enterobacteria, Bacteroidetes, and Firmicutes, but to a lesser amount than Bifidobacteria. Some GOSs are made from lactulose, which is a lactose isomer. GOSs generated from lactulose are also termed prebiotics, and other forms of GOS exist in addition to these [14, 3].
- Starch and Glucose-Derived Oligosaccharides: Resistant starch (RS) is a type of starch that is resistant to digestion in the upper stomach. Because RS produces a high level of butyrate, it has been said that it should be categorised as a prebiotic. Firmicutes of various groups show the maximum incorporation with a large amount of RS. *Ruminococcus bromii* and *Bifidobacterium adolescentis* were found to break down RS in an in vitro research, as were Eubacterium rectale and Bacteroides, with taiotaomicron to a lesser extent. In the absence of *R. bromii*, however, RS breakdown is impossible in mixed bacterial and fecal incubations. Polydextrose is an oligosaccharide produced from glucose; it is made up of glucan with many branches and glycosidic connections. This is been observed to help in stimulation of *Bifidobacteria* but lack of research evidence has been found [8, 15].
- Other Oligosaccharides: Pectin, a polysaccharide, is the source of several oligosaccharides. Pectic oligosaccharide (POS) is the name for this sort of oligosaccharide. They are based on galacturonic acid (homogalacturonan) or rhamnose extension (rhamnogalacturonan). Methyl esterification may be used to replace the carboxyl groups, and the structure may be acetylated at C2 or C3. The side chains are connected to various sugars (such as arabinose, galactose, and xylose) or ferulic acid. The architecture of POSs differ greatly based on the POSs' source [16].
- Non-Carbohydrate Oligosaccharides: While carbohydrates are often more likely to meet the prebiotics defining criteria, some substances such as cocoa-derived flavanols, are not categorised as carbs but are recommended to be classed as prebiotics. Flavanols have been shown to boost lactic acid bacteria in both in vivo and in vitro tests [13] (see Figure 19.1).

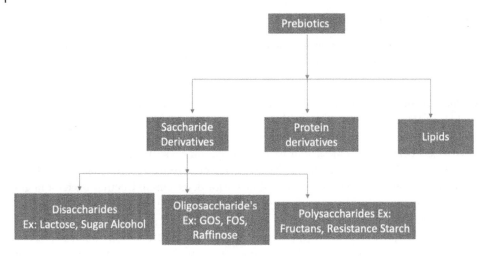

Figure 19.1 Types of probiotics.

19.2.2 Functioning of Prebiotics

Prebiotics are food components; non-digestible substances which favour in the growth of beneficial bacteria specially present on the membrane of the large intestine (colon) [3]. Prebiotics are helpful in the following ways:

1) Enhance production of fermentation products such as lactic acid and short chain fatty acids (SCFA).
2) Enhance growth of bacteria (probiotics) which help in increasing the level of minerals such as sodium, potassium, magnesium, and calcium in the large intestine (colon).
3) Enhance immunity of host by increasing the production of IgA, NK cells, and cytokine modulation [3].

Prebiotics have a role in modifying the gut's environment; the fermented products formed from prebiotics are generally acidic in nature and they decrease the gut pH. If there is any change in gut pH the composition of gut microbiota also changes. When the pH changes the quantity of some acid-sensitive species also change, such as that of Bacteroid, which then promote the formation of butyrate by the firmicutes; this process is called the butyrogenic effect. Many foodstuffs may be fortified with prebiotics; some examples are dairy products, health drinks, bread-spreads, infant formula, beverages, cereals, chocolates, bakery products, confectionery, chewing gum, soups, savoury products, meat products, canned foods, food supplements, dried instant foods, and animal feeds. These prebiotics have many nutraceutical properties such as being antimicrobial, anticarcinogenic, and hypolipidemic, with some health benefits in diabetic mellitus. They play a major role in the treatment of gut diseases such as constipation and inflammatory bowel syndrome (IBS). They also have a positive lipid absorption effect, thus promoting mineral absorption in the gut. Prebiotics have also been incorporated in infant's formula, thus helping in easy digestion. Prebiotics are thought to have no serious or life-threatening negative effects. Oligosaccharides and polysaccharides are not broken down by intestinal enzymes; they are transferred to the colon, where the gut microbiota ferment them. As a result, prebiotics' adverse effects are largely due to their

Table 19.1 Properties of ideal prebiotics.

Desirable Characteristics	Properties of Prebiotic (oligosaccharides)
Functional at low quantity/dosage	Selectively and commendably metabolised by probiotic strains (*Bifidobacterium*, *Lactobacillus* spp.)
No side effects	Efficient, selective, and no production of gas after metabolised by probiotics
Endurance throughout the colon	Have high molecular weight (MW)
Diverse viscosity	Available in various sizes (molecular weights) and linkages
Adequate storage and stable	Consist of 1–6 linkages and sugar rings (pyranosyl)
Ability to manage microbial normal flora modulation	Selectively processed by constrained microbial strains
Varying sweet taste	Different monosaccharide-based composition

osmotic activities. In this case, prebiotic recipients may have osmotic diarrhea, bloating, cramps, and gas [3, 6]. Some key properties of prebiotics are listed in Table 19.1.

19.3 Probiotics

In 1953, German scientist Werner Kollath coined the term probiotic from the Latin *pro* and the Greek word for *life*) to describe 'active substances that are required for a healthy development of life.' Further, in 1965 Lily and Stillwell coined the phrase for the description of probiotics as 'substances synthesised by the one organism that encourage the growth of the another one.' In 1992, Fuller also described probiotics as 'a live microbial feed additive that improves the host animal's intestinal microbial balance and so benefits the host animal.' The recent era of probiotics begins at the turn of the century with the pioneering research of former Nobel winner Elie Metchnikoff, a Russian research scientist at the Pasteur Institute in Paris. While Louis Pasteur discovered the microbes that induce fermentation, Metchnikoff focused on the potential impact of these microbes on human health [12]. In another words, a probiotic may be explained as a living or viable microbial (strain) food supplement that sup-portively affects the host gut system through its beneficial effects. The two most explored microbial strains as probiotics are *Lactobacillus* spp. and *Bifidobacterium*. However, Henry Tissier's work led to the breakthrough, as he discovered that the microbial strains' content of a specific type of bacteria in stool specimens of infected diarrhea infants was much lower than in healthy children. His recommendation that patients with diarrhea (infantile diar-rhea) take live organisms (*Bifidobacteria*) orally to help in restoration of healthy gut flora was the first of its kind. Havenaar and Huisint Veld further proposed the present definition of probiotics as a viable mono or mixed culture of microbes that, when given to an animal or a human, benefits the host by increasing the qualities of the native flora. Probiotics are described by the World Health Organisation (WHO) as 'microbial strains that bestow a health benefits to the host when introduced in sufficient concentrations.' In the context of food, the term might be tweaked to emphasise that microbes have a favourable impact, when taken in sufficient proportions as component of food [17].

Probiotics have evolved significantly in the last two centuries, with considerable break-throughs in the selection and characterisation of certain probiotic cultures, as well as significant health advantages when consumed. Understanding the importance of gut flora of humans, as well as the probiotic food concept and gastrointestinal tract (GIT) of each individual, have a different profile in terms of microbial species. These microbial flora can be classified as good and bad microbes [18]. The Probiotic strains fall in the category of good microbes. The microbial colonisation of the human gut begins from the time of birth when any newborns are exposed to a nonsterile environment. It then evolves and morphs over the course of a human's life, based on a diverse and complex interplay between the host's nutrition, lifestyle, and genome, as well as antibiotic exposure. The composition of the normal intestinal microflora of humans remains essentially consistent throughout adulthood. Consequently, developing a simple, low-cost, responsive, and intrinsic way to improve human gut health has become a significant concern. Additionally, probiotics act as a supplement to the host microbiota and give protection against a variety of enteric infections [19]. Probiotics have also been shown to increase gut mucosal integrity, in addition to their unique capacity to compete with microbial pathogens. Probiotics have become a preferred approach for improving digestive and immunological health, and medical professionals are increasingly endorsing these as an effective therapeutic approach [20].

Numerous bacteria, yeast, and mould strains are in use as probiotics; some examples are *Lactobacilli, Enterococci, Bifidobacterial, Streptococci, Saccharomyces* spp., and *Aspergillus* spp. Despite the extensive use of probiotics, the methods of obtaining them may provide certain challenges [21]. The microbes utilised are primarily anaerobic and cannot withstand temperature extremes. Probiotics have to be prepared in a viable form on a large level in order to be effective. The probiotic should be viable, safe, and stable throughout usage and storage, it should be able to live in the gastrointestinal ecology, and the host animal should benefit from harbouring the probiotic. Similarly, probiotic strains should able to cope with many physiochemical barriers in the digestive system of the host. Cheese, sour cream, yogurt, smoothies, fitness bars, soyabeans, and infant formulas are a few examples of current probiotic-containing food products commonly in use [22]. Some examples of probiotic strains are given in Table 19.2.

Table 19.2 Examples of probiotics strains along with species.

Probiotic strains	Species
Lactobacillus spp.	*L. acidophilus, L. plantarum, L. rhamnosus, L. paracasei, L. fermentum, L. reuteri, L. johnsonii, L. brevis, L. casei, L. lactis, L. delbrueckii*
Bifidobacterium spp.	*B. breve, B. infantis, B. longum, L. bifidum, L. thermophilum, L. adolescentis, L. animalis, L. lactis*
Bacillus spp.	*B. coagulans*
Streptococcus spp.	*S. thermophiles*
Enterococcus spp.	*E. faecium*
Saccharomyces spp.	*S. cerevisiae*

19.3.1 Characteristics of Probiotics

A good probiotic should have following features [23]:

- It has to be a commensal organism of a healthy gastrointestinal system.
- This must sustain the upper digestive tract and be capable of sustaining and growing in the intestine (hydrochloric acid and bile impermeable).
- It should also be safe to be consumed.
- It should emit antimicrobial substances such as bacteriocins, and have the ability to adhere to human gut wall and colonise.
- It should an isolate of the same species as its intended host.
- It should have no immunological response, the organism should remain genetically stable, and there should be no plasmid transfer.
- It should be non-pathogenic.
- It should be a normal flora/inhabitant of a healthy host's intestinal tract.
- It should have clear demonstrable beneficial synergetic effect on the host health.
- It should be able to sustain and survive within the transition through the gastrointestinal tract of the host.
- On storage and use, a large number of viable (living form) microbes must be able to survive for a prolonged span of time.

19.3.2 Mechanisms of Action of Probiotic Strains

In the gastrointestinal tract, about 10 trillion microbial strains and their species invade and maintain an intricate equilibrium. Some of these examples are *Bacteroides*, *Clostridium*, *LactobacillusiEubacterium*, *Fusobacterium*, *Peptococcus*, *Bifidobacterium Peptostreptococcus*, *Veillonella*, and *Escherichia coli*. The microbiome colonisation in the human gut begins by birth and eventually increases by exposure to a foreign microbial population, as well as antigens originating from ingested and digested food. As a result, the intestine serves as a barrier between the host and external agents including micro-organisms and allergens. The gut microbiota has an impact on human health through influencing the gut defence system, immunological function, and nutrition absorption, as well as by possible signaling directly with the gastrointestinal mucosa. The interaction of the host normal microbial flora with external agents (such as *Bacillus cereus*, *Clostridium* spp., *Listeria monocytogenes*, and *Vibrio cholera*) has the potential to disrupt or modify the natural microbial balance or activity in the GI tract, which ultimately leads to the numerous of enteric diseases. Generally pathogens cause infection by two approaches: by attachment at the surfaces of epithelial cells (intestine) through certain adhesive receptors such as glycoproteins or lipids, which then cause direct cytotoxic injury, intracellular migration, and finally disruption of epithelial tight junctions, resulting in mucosal infection; and by producing cytotoxic toxins and suppressing the normal flora, causing intracellular invasion, which leads to infection. Probiotics convalesce the GIT homeostasis and boost the growth of local beneficial gut microbial flora [20]. As a result, probiotics are suggested as an alternative biotherapeutic treatment for infections of the intestine. Furthermore, the mechanism of action of probiotics are antimicrobial compound synthesis, colonisation resistance with competition for nutritional substrates, competitive exclusion, improved intestinal barrier integrity, and immunomodulation.

19.3.2.1 Synthesis of Antimicrobial Tools

Probiotic stains, known for producing antimicrobial agents such as *lactobacilli* spp. are well known producers of antimicrobial substances such as ammonia, organic acids, H_2O_2, fatty free acids, biosurfactant, and bacteriocins, which inhibits the growth of Gram negative and Gram positive enteric pathogens. These probiotic strain-based antimicrobial agents exert a potent and steady effect on a pathogen in the right location at the intestinal tract. Similarly, certain probiotic bacteria create organic acids that reduce the external pH, causing acidification of the cell cytoplasm. Consequently, at lower pH values, these acids are partially undissociated. Organic acids that have not been dissociated are lipophilic and diffuse passively across the membrane, potentially causing intracellular acidification. They dissociate at high intracellular pH values, producing hydrogen ions, which interfere with critical bacterial metabolic activities. They also denature proteins and cause the electrochemical proton gradient to collapse, disrupting pathogenic bacteria's substrate transport systems. As a result, harmful bacteria's cell membrane permeability is altered. Another well-known antimicrobial agent produced by probiotic stains are H_2O_2. Free radicals, in combination with hydrogen peroxide (H_2O_2), serve as a precursor to DNA damage. The antibacterial activity of H_2O_2 is due to the oxidation of sulphydryl groups, which causes denaturation of a number of enzymes, which ultimately causes increased membrane permeability lipid membrane. Furthermore, CO_2 is another by-product of fermentative metabolism, which provides an anaerobic environment that may hinder the enzymatic decarboxylation reaction. Due to the significant concentration of CO_2 in the membrane lipid bilayer, it may cause permeability problems and cause death of pathogens. Similarly, some probiotic strains are known for production of biosurfactants such as *Lactobacillus paracasei*, which has bactericidal properties and inhibits the pathogen's growth. Bacteriocins are another antimicrobial agent that produces microbes and peptides in nature, and is synthesised. Bacteriocins are ribosomally synthesised low-molecular-weight antimicrobial peptides, which have therapeutic action against pathogens of the gastrointestinal tract. These bacteriocin generally alter the cell membrane's permeability of target pathogen and thus disturb the membrane transport system. Proton motive force is depleted because of cellular component leakage through these transmembrane pores system, which ultimately interferes with cellular biosynthesis and results in cell death. A few examples of bacteriocins are nisin, acidolin, lactocidin, and lactobrevin [19, 21].

19.3.2.2 Colonisation, Invasion Resistance, and Competitive Exclusion

The most significant attribute of probiotic strains for deactivating a pathogen in the colon is by not allowing them to attach to mucus glycoproteins called mucin, as well as competitive exclusion by depletion of nutrients or biogenic growth metabolites. The pathogen binds to intestinal epithelial cells via carbohydrate moieties in glycoconjugate receptor molecules, which starts the infection process. Generally, probiotic stains impede and prevent the invasion of pathogens by competing for glycoconjugate receptors at the infection site of intestinal epithelial cells, which can prevent infectious pathogen adherence and penetration to the gut cells. Probiotics also contend for receptors or adhere to intestinal epithelial cells, which could hinder pathogenic bacteria from colonising. One example is if probiotic strain *L. acidophilus* and *E. coli* have both exhibited similar adhesion to the epithelial cells thru mannose receptors at epithelial cells of human gut; this competitive property could limit pathogen colonisation at the same locations, hence protecting the host from infection. Probiotics may also vie for an ecological niche, making it difficult for invading pathogens to establish a foothold in the intestinal tract and limiting their potential to colonise. Gut microflora, probiotics, and pathogens all may combat for nutritional substrates and bioactive growth metabolites such as amino acids, vitamins, methylamines, fatty acids (short-chain), and bioactive peptides. An example of such competition is by competing for the growth factor, *Bifidobacterium adolescentis* (probiotic) may better utilise vitamin K and prevent the growth of *Porphyromonas gingivalis* (pathogen), and *Lactobacillus plantarum* (probiotic) may colonise to the intestinal epithelial cells by restricting the adherence of infective *Enterococcus faecalis* and *Clostridium sporogenes* [20, 2].

19.3.2.3 Improved Intestinal Barrier Integrity

Probiotics provide protection by guarding the epithelium from various hazardous antigenic components and prevent the penetration of microbial pathogens to the mucus layer. Probiotic stains sustain focal adhesion protein expression and promote host gut mucin synthesis, which enhances the mucus layer's potential to function as an antibacterial barrier by preventing the apoptotic ratio from rising [8].

19.3.2.4 Immunomodulation

Many researchers have explored and stated the unique physiological function of probiotic stains that impact or modulate the defence systems of hosts (both innate and acquired immune systems). Modulation of gastrointestinal immune systems by modifying inflammatory cytokine patterns and inhibiting proinflammatory pathways is amongst the most precise efficacies of probiotics. Probiotics also enhance the synthesis of natural killer (NK) cells along with serum IgA, secretory IgA, and phagocytosis, which plays a key role in enhancing the immunity of the intestine. They also impede apoptosis and suppress the proliferation of T cells, consequently preventing many inflammatory infirmities. By employing enzymatic pathways, probiotics may also modify toxin receptors and prevent toxin-mediated disease, for example, a well proven study states that *S. boulardii* produces polyamines that degrade *Clostridium difficile* toxin receptors and prevent cholera-induced secretion in the rat jejunum. Similarly, several probiotic bacteria regulate human-beta-defensin-2 of human host thru the cofactor NF-B, and boost gut defences [24, 25].

19.3.3 Applications of Probiotics

Consumers are more aware of the relationship between lifestyle, diet, and good health, which explains the growing desire for items that may improve health beyond basic nutrition. The number of health advantages attributed to functional food continues to grow, and probiotics are one of the fastest-growing dietary groups for which scientific research has shown therapeutic proof. The prevention of urogenital disorders, relief of constipation, protection against traveller's diarrhea, reduction of hypercholesterolaemia, protection against colon and bladder cancer, prevention of osteoporosis, and food allergy are only a few of the therapeutic uses of probiotics [26] (see Figure 19.2). Ingestion of probiotic strains has been also linked to a variety of health benefits, which include immune system modulation, steadily increasing resistance to cancer, and increased resistance to infectious disease.

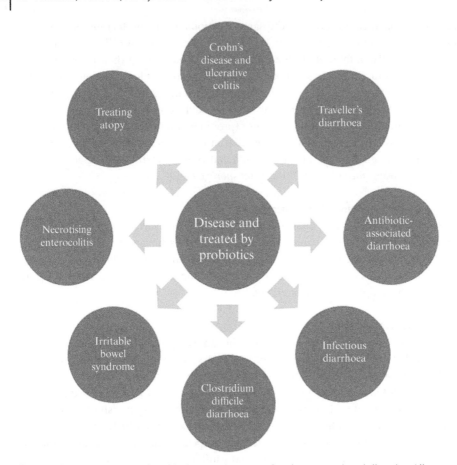

Figure 19.2 Application of probiotics as treatment of various gut related disorders/diseases.

The impact of *Lactobacillus casei* (probiotic strain) containing fermented milk, produces mucosal immune stimulation, strengthening the non-specific barrier, and modifying the innate immune response in the gut, preserving intestinal homeostasis [25, 23].

Infectious illnesses are still the world's most pressing public health issue. The leading causes of mortality are intestinal infections induced by the ingestion of harmful micro-organisms through contaminated water and food. In this instance, probiotics may help alleviate some foodborne illness. Similarly, an infant's diarrhea caused by rotavirus and *E. coli* might be reduced by dietary therapy with *B. lactis* (probiotic strain), potentially through a mechanism of increased immune-mediated protection. As a result, probiotic therapy may be a viable dietary option for avoiding or reducing diarrhea in human new-borns. The intestinal barrier protects the organism's epithelial integrity from bacterial or dietary antigens that might cause inflammatory pathways in the intestine, leading to IBD. Probiotic bacteria contend with harmful bacteria for epithelial binding sites, preventing *Salmonella* sp. and *E. coli* strains from colonising. Co-cultivation of intestinal bacteria with immunological and/or intestinal epithelial cells (IEC) has been performed to examine host–microbe interactions. Foods that contain some health-promoting component(s) beyond standard nutrients are characterised as functional foods. Designer foods, medical foods, nutraceuticals, therapeutic foods, superfoods, foodiceuticals, and Medi foods are all terms for functional foods. The word refers to a meal that has been altered in some way to become useful. The introduction of probiotics to meals is one technique to transform them into functional foods [27].

Since humans have shifted their focus entirely on moderating and enhancing their health, the commercial systems have also shifted their focus on manufacturing products that are related to human health. Population is focused on preparing home-cooked food, going vegan, and taking care of the gut with healthy bacteria. Part of the population is busy with work and tries to avoiding eating fast food but cannot fulfil the goal. In the end, an individual relies on keeping the gut running and healthy. Most probiotic drinks and foods are manufactured because the consumer demand is driving the production of probiotic bacteria-containing dairy and non-dairy products across the world. For direct or indirect human ingestion, probiotic cells are accessible in three different forms: fermented or non-fermented; dried or deep-frozen for industrial or residential usage; and medicines in powder, tablet, and capsule form [27], as shown in Figure 19.2.

19.4   Synbiotics

Synbiotics refers to the combination that consists of both the prebiotics and probiotics. The word denotes synergy, i.e., acting together. Gibson implemented a hypothesis about the potential advantages of prebiotics when paired with probiotics. He claims that compared with a prebiotic or probiotic functioning solo, the blending of both prebiotics and probiotics may have more effectiveness in preventing GIT disorders [12]. As a result synbiotics were developed, with the prebiotic component assisting the probiotic bacterium in growing and overcoming potential survival challenges. The probiotics utilise prebiotics as a nutritive source, allowing them to live in the GIT for longer periods than they would otherwise be able to. This is based on evidence that probiotic bacteria survive better when they pass through the upper digestive tract. H_2O_2, organic acids, pH, moisture, oxygen, and stress are just a few of the elements that have been linked to probiotic viability, particularly in dairy products such as yoghurt [28]. Synergism also aids in the proper implantation of dietary supplements, such as prebiotics in the colon, along with the growth of supplemented probiotic strains. For optimum survival in the GIT, a probiotic needs food and prebiotic fuel [8]. However, it is important that prebiotic compounds are selectively stimulating the growth metabolism of probiotic strains and have beneficial effects on human health, not on other pathogenic microorganisms. The combination of lactic acid bacilli, or *Bifidobacteria* and FOS (fructooligosaccharide) bacteria is the most common example of symbiotics [4, 5].

19.4.1   Selection Criteria

In the selection of synbiotics, the biggest challenge is to figure out the perfect combination of which prebiotic and probiotic will be optimal for the specific diseases for any specific person. If probiotics and prebiotics with distinct advantages are combined together, they will show an additive effect. To come up with the best combination, we first need to consider the specific properties that a prebiotic must have in order to be advantageous to the probiotic; as a result, synbiotic formula is formed. So for a synbiotic, a convenient probiotic and prebiotic must be chosen; the prebiotic employed should then have an improving effect on the probiotic strain, and the prebiotic must specifically enhance the growth of the probiotic microbiota [24].

19.4.2 Mechanism of Action

Synbiotics generally work by two different modes; they boost the effectiveness of the probiotics, and provide specific health advantages. When a prebiotic are combined with a probiotic, the probiotics are stimulated and metabolism in the intestine is regulated. This is characterised by an intact intestinal bio-structure, the expansion of the beneficial bacteria, and the incapacity of potential pathogens to proliferate in the gastrointestinal system [29]. Along with this, synbiotics promote the inactivation of nitrosamines and cancer-causing chemicals, as well as a reduction in the number of unwanted metabolites. Synbiotics also lower the level of SCFAs, ketones, methyl acetates, carbon disulphide, and many more, proving beneficial to the health of the host. These combinations also work in counter with the decay process within the gastro-intestine to prevent the constipation and diarrheal problems [7, 9].

19.4.3 Therapeutic Actions

Synbiotics have a variety of health benefits for humans, including antibacterial activity in pyogenic inflammation, as well as anti-cancerous, anti-allergenic, and antidiarrheal properties. They may be used to prevent osteoporosis, lower blood sugar levels, improve immunomodulatory abilities, control the immune system, brain functions, lower nosocomial infections after surgery, and improve hepatic function in patients with cirrhosis. These actions have already been documented in scientific studies. Research has also stated when metabolic products (such as lipopolysaccharides, SFCAs, and ethanol) cross the blood-barrier, they enter the liver and trigger synthesis along with storage of hepatic triacylglycerols (IHTG), which increases steatosis caused by fatty liver and may be reduced by using synbiotics containing five probiotic strains (*L. plantarum, L. delbrueckii, L. acidophilus, L. rhamnosus*, and *B. bifidum*) along with inulin as a prebiotic [30]. In similar context, synbiotics were also explored for reducing the generation of tumour necrosis factor (TNF), a factor that may contribute to insulin resistance and inflammatory cell uptake in non-alcoholic fatty liver disease [31, 32].

19.5 Conclusion

Probiotics are described as 'live microbial food supplements or components of bacteria that have been proved to have potential health benefits' in the context of human nutrition. Microorganisms from the genera *Lactobacillus* spp. and *Bifidobacterium* spp. have traditionally been proven as the properties to be used as probiotics. Probiotic strains improve the gut microbiota balance and pathogen defences, which is good for human health. Probiotics are also known for their immune system stimulation, blood cholesterol management, vitamin biosynthesis, anti-carcinogenesis, and anti-bacterial properties. Additionally, prebiotics are non-absorbable food components that beneficially stimulate one or more of the gut-beneficial microbe groups, and so has a good influence on human health. Furthermore, the term synbiotics was meant to describe the ingestion of specific probiotics and prebiotics in combination to deliver precise therapeutic effects through synergistic action. The perfect combination of prebiotics with probiotics in the form of synbiotics, may be beneficial for human gut health, and appropriate consumption may help in the treatment of many diseases such as diarrhea, IBD, gastric cancer, antibiotic induced diarrhea, and Crohn's disease. Along with these, Prebiotics, Probiotics, and Synbiotics are eco-friendly, economical, easily available, and have high health benefits. The capacity to influence the composition of the microbiota through the use of a synbiotic combination of prebiotic dietary substances and probiotic microbes is an intriguing approach to the prevention and treatment of gut illnesses.

References

1 Zheng, D.W., Li, R.Q., An, J.X. et al. (2020). Prebiotics-encapsulated probiotic spores regulate gut microbiota and suppress colon cancer. *Adv. Mater.* 32 (45): 1–11.

2 Sanders, M.E., Merenstein, D.J., Reid, G. et al. (2019). Probiotics and prebiotics in intestinal health and disease: from biology to the clinic. *Nat. Rev. Gastroenterol. Hepatol.* 16 (10): 605–616. https://doi.org/10.1038/s41575-019-0173-3.

3 Davani-Davari, D., Negahdaripour, M., Karimzadeh, I. et al. (2019). Prebiotics: definition, types, sources, mechanisms, and clinical applications. *Foods* 8 (3): 1–27.

4 Scaldaferri, F., Gerardi, V., Lopetuso, L.R. et al. (2013). Food components and dietary habits: keys for a healthy gut microbiota composition. *Nutrients* 11 (10): 2393.

5 Collins, M.D. and Gibson, G.R. (1999). Probiotics, prebiotics, and synbiotics: approaches for modulating the microbial ecology of the gut. *Am. J. Clin. Nutr.* 69 (5): 1052–1057.

6 Ng, Q.X., Loke, W., Venkatanarayanan, N. et al. (2019). A systematic review of the role of prebiotics and probiotics in autism spectrum disorders. *Medicina* 55 (5): 129.

7 Vyas, U. and Ranganathan, N. (2012). Probiotics, prebiotics, and synbiotics: gut and beyond. *Gastroenterol. Res. Pract.* 2012: 872716. https://doi.org/10.1155/2012/872716.

8 Adhikari, P.A. and Kim, W.K. (2017). Overview of prebiotics and probiotics: focus on performance, gut health and immunity – a review. *Ann. Anim. Sci.* 17 (4): 949–966.

9 Quigley, E.M.M. (2019). Prebiotics and probiotics in digestive health. *Clin. Gastroenterol. Hepatol.* 17 (2): 333–344. https://doi.org/10.1016/j.cgh.2018.09.028.

10 Yeo, S.K., Ooi, L.G., Lim, T.J. et al. (2009). Antihypertensive properties of plant-based prebiotics. *Int. J. Mol. Sci.* 10 (8): 3517–3530.

11 Slavin, J. (2013). Fiber and prebiotics: mechanisms and health benefits. *Nutrients* 5 (4): 1417–1435.

12 Pandey, K.R., Naik, S.R., and Vakil, B.V. (2015). Probiotics, prebiotics and synbiotics: a review. *J. Food Sci. Technol.* 52 (12): 7577–7587.

13 Panesar, P.S. and Bali, V. (2015). Prebiotics. *Encycl. Food Heal.* 18 (2): 464–471.

14 Huebner, J., Wehling, R.L., and Hutkins, R.W. (2007). Functional activity of commercial prebiotics. *Int. Dairy J.* 17 (7): 770–775.

15 Manigandan, T., Mangaiyarkarasi, S.P., Hemalatha, R., et al. (2012). Probiotics, prebiotics and synbiotics – a review. *Biomed Pharmacol. J.* 5 (2): 295–304.

16 Vieira, A.T., Teixeira, M.M.,and Martins, F.S. (2013 December). The role of probiotics and prebiotics in inducing gut immunity. *Front. Immunol.* 4: 1–12.

17 Roy, D. (2019). Probiotics. *Compr. Biotechnol.* 18 (2): 649–661.

18 Pearse Lyons, T. and Chapman, J.D. (2017). Probiotics. *Non-Trad. Feed Use Swine Prod.* 27: 315–326.

19 Lin, C.S, Chang, C.J., Lu, C.C. et al. (2014). Impact of the gut microbiota, prebiotics, and probiotics on human health and disease. *Biomed. J.* 37 (5): 259–268.

20 He, M. and Shi, B. (2017). Gut microbiota as a potential target of metabolic syndrome: the role of probiotics and prebiotics. *Cell. Biosci.* 7 (1): 1–14.

21 Schrezenmeir, J. and De Vrese, M. (2001 February). Probiotics, prebiotics, and synbiotics—approaching a definition. *Am. J. Clin. Nutr.* 73 (supp. 2): 361S–364S. https://doi.org/pubmed.ncbi.nlm.nih.gov/11157342.

22 Olveira, G. and González-Molero, I. (2016). An update on probiotics, prebiotics and symbiotics in clinical nutrition. *Endocrinol. Nutr. (English)* 63 (9): 482–494. https://doi.org/10.1016/j.endoen.2016.10.011.

23 Williams, N.T. (2010). Probiotics. *Am. J. Heal. Pharm.* 67 (6): 449–458.

24 Ducatelle, R., Eeckhaut, V., Haesebrouck, F. et al. (2014). A review on prebiotics and probiotics for the control of dysbiosis: present status and future perspectives. *Animal* 9 (1): 43–48.

25 Gill, H. and Prasad, J. (2008). Probiotics, immunomodulation, and health benefits. *Adv. Exp. Med. Biol.* 606: 423–54.

26 Miarons, M., Roca, M., and Salvà, F. (2021). The role of pro-, pre- and symbiotics in cancer: a systematic review. *J. Clin. Pharm. Ther.* 46 (1): 50–65.

27 Buckner, C.A., Lafrenie, R.M., Dénommée, J.A. et al. (2016). We are IntechOpen the worlds leading publisher of open access books built by scientists for scientists TOP 1%. *Intech* 11: 13. https://doi.org/intechopen.com/books/advanced-biometric-technologies/liveness-detection-in-biometrics.

28 Khan, S., Moore, R.J., Stanley, D. et al. (2020). The gut microbiota of laying hens and its manipulation with prebiotics and probiotics to enhance gut health and food safety. *Appl. Environ. Microbiol.* 86 (13).

29 Fooks, L.J., Fuller, R., and Gibson, G.R. (1999). Prebiotics, probiotics and human gut microbiology. *Int. Dairy J.* 9 (1): 53–61.

30 Gourbeyre, P., Denery, S., and Bodinier, M. (2011). Probiotics, prebiotics, and synbiotics: impact on the gut immune system and allergic reactions. *J. Leukoc. Biol.* 89 (5): 685–695.

31 Amitay, E.L., Carr, P.R., Gies, A. et al. (2020). Probiotic/synbiotic treatment and postoperative complications in colorectal cancer patients: systematic review and meta-analysis of randomized controlled trials. *Clin. Transl. Gastroenterol.* 11 (12): e00268.

32 Flesch, A.G.T, Poziomyck A.K., and Damin, D.C. (2014). The therapeutic use of symbiotics. *Arq. Bras. Cir. Dig.* 27 (3): 206–209.

20

Current Status and Efficacy of Fecal Microbiota Transplantation for Patients Suffering from Irritable Bowel Syndrome

Mohamed Hussein Arbab

Associate Professor of Medical Microbiology, Omdurman Ahlia University, Sudan

20.1 Introduction

Irritable bowel syndrome (IBS) is a chronic disorder affecting 11.2% of the world's population, with the highest prevalence in South America and the lowest prevalence in South Asia [1,2]. IBS is a benign disorder that is not associated with increased mortality, and it does not develop into a serious disease [3]. However, IBS reduces the quality of life of the affected patients considerably [1]. There is no effective treatment for IBS, with the available treatments being directed at symptom relief [4]. The etiology of IBS is unknown, but the intestinal microbiota seems to play a pivotal role in its pathophysiology [1]. The intestinal bacterial profile in IBS patients differs from that in healthy subjects [5–12]. IBS patients also have a lower diversity of gut bacteria (dysbiosis) than healthy subjects [5–10]. Fecal microbiota transplantation (FMT) has been applied to IBS patients in seven randomised controlled trials (RCTs) [13–19], four of which showed a positive effect [13,15,18,19], while the other three showed no effect [14,16,17]. At first, it appears to be challenging to compare these RCTs, due to variations in the criteria used to select the donors and patients, in the dose of the fecal transplant used, and in the FMT protocols. Furthermore, various measurements were used to assess efficacy of FMT in these RCTs. Thus, in the RCT of El-Salhy et al., the efficacy of FMT was measured by both IBS-symptom severity system (IBS-SSS), the rigorous requirements of the European Medicines Agency and (EMA), and the Food and Drug Administration (FDA) using a composite responder endpoint [20,21]. While reduction in IBS-SSS score was used in five RCTs to measure the efficacy of FM [13,14,16–18], relief of general IBS symptoms and abdominal bloating was used in one RCT [19]. Recommendations for consideration in future FMT studies in IBS concerning several topics of investigation have been suggested for improving the outcome of FMT in IBS [22,23].

Benech and Sokol considered that the application of FMT in gastrointestinal disorders represents the start of a new era [24]. All RCTs on FMT for IBS (regardless of their outcomes) provide crucial information that may be used to improve the efficacy of FMT in IBS patients. Hence, the present review includes an analysis of possible factors affecting the success or failure of these RCTs, with the aim of highlighting the gaps in our knowledge, and of sketching a possible model for successful FMT in IBS patients.

The Gut Microbiota in Health and Disease, First Edition. Edited by Nimmy Srivastava, Salam A. Ibrahim, Jayeeta Chattopadhyay, and Mohamed H. Arbab.

20.2 Donor Selection

The response to FMT in IBD appears to be donor-dependent, with variations in the study outcomes explainable by the differences between the donors [5,25]. This situation has led to the term super-donor being coined to describe a donor that induces desirable effects in recipients [5]. Since there are no clear criteria for the super-donor, predicting the clinical efficacy of the donor before FMT is impossible. Attempts to overcome this obstacle have led to suggestions that donors' feces should be pooled in order to increase the likelihood of patients receiving effective feces [26]. However, applying this approach did not increase the response rate to FMT, which is probably because the feces of the super-donor would be diluted, and consequently the recipients would not receive a sufficient dose from the super-donor [27].

The donors in all of the RCTs done on IBS patients were healthy and had a normal body mass index (BMI) [13–19]. The super-donor for the IBS patients was selected based either on clinical efficacy in a pilot trial or on clinical criteria and the fecal microbiota profile [15,17,19,28]. The RCT of Holvoet and colleagues used two donors who were effective in a pilot trial [19,28]. Another RCT selected two donors who had the highest fecal abundance of the butyryl-CoA CoA transferase gene [17]. El-Salhy et al. used both clinical criteria and the fecal bacterial profile when choosing a single donor [15]. The basis for choosing the clinical criteria and identifying the bacterial signature of their donor is explained next.

In the absence of clear criteria for a super-donor, El-Salhy and colleagues considered the factors that are known to affect the gut microbiota negatively or positively, and attempted to select a donor having the positive factors and lacking the negative factors. The factors that have negative effects on the gut microbiota and reduce the bacterial diversity include aging (>50years), smoking/smoking cessation, being born by cesarean section and/or being formula-fed, frequent treatment with antibiotics, and regular intake of non-antibiotic drugs [6,29]. On the other hand, regular exercise and consuming a sport-specific diet are associated with a favorable gut microbiota [30–32]. Furthermore, since the intestinal microbiota is affected by the genetic composition, the super-donor should not be a first-degree relative of any recipient, because genetic similarity may be associated with similarities in the fecal microbiota [33,34]. Applying these criteria resulted in the chosen donor being healthy with a normal BMI, a young male (37 years old), born via a vaginal delivery, breastfed, and a non-smoker, not taking any medication, having been treated only a few times with antibiotics, and regularly performing physical exercise. The donor's diet was within the normal range of those consumed by 35 healthy subjects as measured by the MoBa Food Frequency Questionnaire, but he also consumed a sport-specific diet that was richer in protein, fibre, minerals, and vitamins than average [35]. The donor was not related to any of the recipients [15]. Moreover, an examination of the fecal microbiota of this donor showed that he was normobiotic (i.e., having a high microbial diversity), but deviated from the normal abundance of 165 healthy subjects in 14 of 39 tested bacteria markers. Twelve of the bacteria were in the phylum Firmicutes, with one each in the phyla Proteobacteria and Verrucomicrobia [15]. The bacterial signature (deviation) included an abundance of *Streptococcus, Dorea, Lactobacillus,* and *Ruminococcaceae* spp. These four genera of bacteria have been reported to constitute favorable bacteria for a donor [5,28,36,37]. Holvoet et al. observed that the fecal bacterial composition of one of the two donors they used was stable over time, and that donor was more effective than the second donor whose fecal bacterial composition varied over time [19]. Based on these observations, those authors concluded that after a high bacterial diversity, stability of the bacterial composition over time is also an important factor when selecting an effective donor [19]. It is noteworthy that the fecal bacterial composition of the super-donor used in the RCT of El-Salhy et al. was stable over the 18-month period during which he donated his feces administering the fecal transplant to either the small or large intestine seems to be effective [13,15,17–19]. However, the placebo effect was higher in patients who received the fecal transplant into the large intestine via the working channel of a colonoscope (43%–44%) than in those received the fecal transplant into the small intestine via the working channel of a gastroscope or a naso-jejunal probe (23.6%–26%) [13,15,17–19]. The higher placebo response in those studies that used colonoscopy to administer the fecal transplant could be explained by the procedure itself, since colonoscopy requires bowel preparation, is often painful, takes more time than when using a gastroscope or nasojejunal probe, and the bowel cleansing required for colonoscopy has a positive effect on IBS symptoms [37]. Whether there is a difference in the efficacy of FMT administered to the small or large intestine remains to be determined in future studies. Administering a fecal transplant via capsules was not effective in IBS [14,16]. This is unfortunate given the ease of administration using this method and it being more acceptable to the patients. The lack of response in the RCTs that used capsules to administer donor fecal transplants could be due to other factors, such as the selected donors, a low transplant dose, and/or pooling of the donors [14,16]. The capsule administration route for fecal transplants has been successful in CDI [38]. Further studies exploring the effectiveness of administrating fecal transplant in capsule form to IBS patients are needed.

Frozen feces samples of donors appear to be effective in FMT for IBS, with storage at either −80°C or −20°C being equally efficacious [13,15,18,38–40]. This observation avoids the logistical problems associated with using fresh donor feces and facilitates the use of FMT in the clinic. Moreover, it makes it possible to establish feces banks for the routine clinical use of FMT.

20.3 Safety Issues of FMT for IBS

The adverse events reported in FMT for IBS patients after a 1-year observation time were mild, self-limiting, and only occurred during the first few days after FMT. Patients treated with FMT experienced more adverse events in the form of abdominal pain, cramping, tenderness, diarrhea, and constipation than did those in the placebo group. Moreover, a 52-year-old man and a 55-year-old woman developed diverticulitis at 2 and 3 months after FMT, respectively. However, these two patients had known diverticulosis and experienced several diverticulitis attacks before FMT, and so it is difficult to establish whether these new attacks were causally connected to FMT. Two patients were recently reported to have developed serious adverse events after FMT for other indications than IBS, which resulted in one fatality [41,42]. These events have started a discussion about safety issues around FMT for IBS, especially considering that IBS is a benign gastrointestinal condition [43,44]. The two patients involved in these events were immunosuppressed, 69 and 73 years old, with advanced liver cirrhosis and myelodysplastic syndrome. They received fecal capsules derived from a donor who had an antibiotic-resistant *Escherichia coli* strain [41,42]. It has been suggested that screening of FMT donors should include testing the donor feces for extended-spectrum-beta-lactase-producing *E. coli* and SARS-CoV-2, in order to reduce the risks of infection by known agents [44]. Furthermore, it has been suggested that the selection of IBS patients for FMT should be restricted to those without systemic disease, immune deficiency, treatment with immune-modulating medication, or severe illness in order to further reduce the risks [44].

20.4   Possible Mechanisms Underlying the Effects of FMT

While it is too early to definitively identify the mechanisms underlying the positive effects of FMT, several observations have been made that may shed light on such mechanisms. The fecal levels of total short-chain fatty acids (SCFAs) increased in IBS patients after 1 month and remained elevated at 1 year following FMT [37,45]. SCFAs regulate intestinal motility and the secretion and absorption of water and electrolytes [46,47]. These effects of SCFAs seem to be caused by increasing the secretion and up-regulating the gene expression of peptide YY,[48,49] which is a mediator of the ileal brake that stimulates the absorption of water and electrolytes in the large intestine [46,50,51].

The fecal level of the SCFA butyric acid was increased in IBS patients after 1month and remained elevated at 1year after FMT [37,45]. This increase could be explained by the increased levels of butyrate-producing *Eubacterium* and *Lactobacillus* spp. [15,51–53]. Butyrate is an important source of energy for colonic epithelial cells, and it affects the immune response, modulates the oxidative stress of the host, and decreases intestinal-cell permeability and intestinal motility. Moreover, butyrate modulates colonic hypersensitivity, and treatment with butyrate reduces abdominal pain in patients with IBS [54–56]. Interestingly, following FMT in IBS patients, the levels of butyric acid were found to be correlated inversely with the total score of both the IBS-symptom severity system and Fatigue Assessment Scale (FAS). Increased levels of the branched SCFAs isobutyric and isovaleric acids were observed in IBS patients at 1 year after FMT, suggesting a shift in microbial fermentation from a saccharolytic to a proteolytic pattern, which might be of pathophysiological relevance [37,57]. Moreover, the level of the straight SCFA acetic acid decreased significantly at 1 year after FMT [37], which could be important given that acetic acid induces visceral hypersensitivity in rodents [58].

20.5   Conclusion and Perspective

FMT appears to be a promising treatment for IBS. The outcome of FMT is donor-dependent, indicating the need for care when selecting donors. Clinical criteria that are associated with a favorable microbiota signature have been proposed. However, it is not yet clear whether some of these criteria are more important than others or whether all of the criteria should be satisfied in an effective (super) donor. Future studies should test the reliability of these criteria and compare the microbial signatures between the donor and healthy subjects.

The dose of the fecal transplant is important to the efficacy of FMT, with doses lower than 30g not showing any effect. Administering the fecal transplant to either the small or large intestine is effective, but further studies are needed to establish which route is optimal. Whether the effectiveness differs between single and repeated FMT also remains to be determined.

References

1 El-Salhy, M. (2015). Recent developments in the pathophysiology of irritable bowel syndrome. *W. J. Gastroenterol.* 21: 7621–7636.

2 Canavan, C., West, J., and Card, T. (2014). The epidemiology of irritable bowel syndrome. *Clin. Epidemiol.* 6: 71–80.

3 El-Salhy, M. (2012). Irritable bowel syndrome: diagnosis and pathogenesis. *W. J. Gastroenterol.* 18: 5151–5163.

4 El-Salhy, M. (2015). Recent advances in the diagnosis of irritable bowel syndrome. *Exp. Rev. Gastroenterol. Hepatol.* 9: 1161–1174.

5 Wilson, B.C., Vatanen, T., Cutfield, W.S. et al. (2019). The super-donor phenomenon in fecal microbiota transplantation. *Front. Cell. Infect. Microbiol.* 9: 2.

6 Maier, L., Pruteanu, M., Kuhn, M. et al. (2018). Extensive impact of non-antibiotic drugs on human gut bacteria. *Nature* 555 (7698): 623–628.

7 El-Salhy, M. and Mazzawi, T. (2018). Fecal microbiota transplantation for managing irritable bowel syndrome. *Exp. Rev. Gastroenterol. Hepatol.* 12 (5): 439–445.

8 Casén, C., Vebø, H.C., Sekelja, M. et al. (2015). Deviations in human gut microbiota: a novel diagnostic test for determining dysbiosis in patients with IBS or IBD. *Aliment Pharmacol. Ther.* 42 (1): 71–83.

9 Enck, P. and Mazurak, N. (2018). Dysbiosis in functional bowel disorders. *Ann. Nutr. Metab.* 72 (4): 296–306.

10 El-Salhy, M., Hatlebakk, J.G., and Hausken, T. (2019). Diet in irritable bowel syndrome (IBS): interaction with gut microbiota and gut hormones. *Nutrition* 11 (8): 1824.

11 Pozuelo, M., Panda, S., Santiago, A. et al. (2015). Reduction of butyrate- and methane-producing microorganisms in patients with Irritable Bowel Syndrome. *Sci. Rep.* 5: 12693.

12 Chong, P.P., Chin, V.K., Looi, C.Y. et al. (2019). The microbiome and irritable bowel syndrome–a review on the pathophysiology, current research and future therapy. *Front. Microbiol.* 10: 1136.

13 Johnsen, P.H., Hilpusch, F., Cavanagh, J.P. et al. (2018). Faecal microbiota transplantation versus placebo for moderate-to-severe irritable bowel syndrome: a double-blind, randomised, placebo-controlled, parallel-group, single-centre trial. *Lancet Gastroenterol. Hepatol.* 3 (1): 17–24.

14 Halkjær, S.I., Christensen, A.H., Lo, B.Z.S. et al. (2018). Faecal microbiota transplantation alters gut microbiota in patients with irritable bowel syndrome: results from a randomised, double-blind placebo-controlled study. *Gut* 67 (12): 2107–2115.

15 El-Salhy, M., Hatlebakk, J.G., Gilja, O.H. et al. (2020). Efficacy of faecal microbiota transplantation for patients with irritable bowel syndrome in a randomised, double-blind, placebo-controlled study. *Gut* 69 (5): 859–867.

16 Aroniadis, O.C., Brandt, L.J., Oneto, C. et al. (2019). Faecal microbiota transplantation for diarrhoea-predominant irritable bowel syndrome: a double-blind, randomised, placebo-controlled trial. *Lancet Gastroenterol. Hepatol.* 4 (9): 675–685.

17 Holster, S., Lindqvist, C.M., Repsilber, D. et al. (2019). The effect of allogenic versus autologous fecal microbiota transfer on symptoms, visceral perception and fecal and mucosal microbiota in irritable bowel syndrome: a randomized controlled study. *Clin. Transl. Gastroenterol.* 10 (4): e00034.

18 Lahtinen, P., Jalanka, J., Hartikainen, A. et al. (2020). Randomised clinical trial: faecal microbiota transplantation versus autologous placebo administered via colonoscopy in irritable bowel syndrome. *Aliment Pharmacol. Ther.* 51 (12): 1321–1331.

19 Holvoet, T., Joossens, M., Vázquez-Castellanos, J.F. et al. (2021). Fecal microbiota transplantation reduces symptoms in some patients with irritable bowel syndrome with predominant abdominal bloating: short- and long-term results from a placebo-controlled randomized trial. *Gastroenterology* 160 (1): 145–157.e8. https://doi.org/10.1053/j.gastro.2020.07.013.

20 European Medicines Agency. (2014). *Guideline on the evaluation of medicinal products for the treatment of irritable bowel syndrome, 1–18*. https://www.ema.europa.eu/en/documents/scientific-guideline/guideline-evaluation-medicinal-products-treatment-irritable-bowel-syndrome-revision-1_en.pdf.

21 Center for Drug Evaluation Research (CDER). (2012). *Guidance for industry: irritable bowel syndrome-clinical evaluation of drugs for treatment.* https://www.govinfo.gov/content/pkg/FR-2012-05-31/pdf/2012-13143.pdf.

22 Segal, J.P., Mullish, B.H., Quraishi, M.N. et al. (2020). Letter: faecal microbiota transplantation for IBS. *Aliment Pharmacol. Ther.* 52 (3): 556–557.

23 Ianiro, G., Porcari, S., Ford, A.C. et al. (2020). Letter: Faecal microbiota transplantation for irritable bowel syndrome-room for improvement. *Ali. Pharmacol. Ther.* 52 (5): 923–924.

24 Benech, N. and Sokol, H. (2020). Fecal microbiota transplantation in gastrointestinal disorders: time for precision medicine. *Gen. Med.* 12 (1): 58.

25 Moayyedi, P., Surette, M.G., Kim, P.T. et al. (2015). Fecal microbiota transplantation induces remission in patients with active ulcerative colitis in a randomized controlled trial. *Gastroenterology* 140 (1): 102–109.e6.

26 Kazerouni, A. and Wein, L.M. (2017). Exploring the efficacy of pooled stools in fecal microbiota transplantation for microbiota-associated chronic diseases. *PLoS One* 12 (1): e0163956.

27 Paramsothy, S., Kamm, M.A., Kaakoush, N.O. et al. (2017). Multidonor intensive faecal microbiota transplantation for active ulcerative colitis: a randomised placebo-controlled trial. *Lancet* 389 (10075): 1218–1228.

28 Holvoet, T., Joossens, M., Wang, J. et al. (2017). Assessment of faecal microbial transfer in irritable bowel syndrome with severe bloating. *Gut* 66: 980–982.

29 Capurso, G. and Lahner, E. (2017). The interaction between smoking, alcohol and the gut microbiome. *Best Pract. Res. Clin. Gastroent.* 31 (5): 579–588.

30 Biedermann, L., Brulisauer, K., Zeitz, J. et al. (2014). Smoking cessation alters intestinal microbiota: insights from quantitative investigations on human fecal samples using FISH. *Inflamm. Bowel Dis.* 20 (9): 1496–1501.

31 Korpela, K., Dikareva, E., Hanski, E. et al. (2019). Cohort profile: Finnish health and early life microbiota (HELMi) longitudinal birth cohort. *BMJ Open* 9 (6): e028500.

32 Yeung, O.Y., Ng, Y.F., Chiou, J. et al. (2019). A pilot study to determine the gut microbiota of Hong Kong infants fed with breast-milk and/or infant. *Curr. Dev. Nutr.* 3 (supp. 1): 11–101. https://doi.org/10.1093/cdn/nzz048.P11-101-19.

33 Jakobsson, H.E., Abrahamsson, T.R., Jenmalm, M.C. et al. (2014). Decreased gut microbiota diversity, delayed Bacteroidetes colonisation and reduced Th1 responses in infants delivered by caesarean section. *Gut* 63 (4): 559–566.

34 Rutayisire, E., Huang, K., Liu, Y. et al. (2016). The mode of delivery affects the diversity and colonization pattern of the gut microbiota during the first year of infants' life: a systematic review. *BMC Gastroent.* 16 (1): 86.

35 Ianiro, G., Tilg, H., and Gasbarrini, A. (2016). Antibiotics as deep modulators of gut microbiota: between good and evil. *Gut* 65 (11): 1906–1915.

36 Modi, S.R., Collins, J.J., and Relman, D.A. (2014). Antibiotics and the gut microbiota. *J. Clin. Invest.* 124 (10): 4212–4218.

37 Bibbò, S., Settanni, C.R., Porcari, S. et al. (2020). Fecal microbiota transplantation: screening and selection to choose the optimal donor. *J. Clin. Med.* 9 (6): 1757.

38 Murtaza, N., Burke, L.M., Vlahovich, N. et al. (2019). The effects of dietary pattern during intensified training on stool microbiota of elite race walkers. *Nutrition* 11 (2): 261.

39 Dalton, A., Mermier, C., and Zuhl, M. (2019). Exercise influence on the microbiome–gut–brain axis. *Gut Micro.* 10 (5): 555–568.

40 Motiani, K.K., Collado, M.C., Eskelinen, J.J. et al. (2020). Exercise training modulates gut microbiota profile and improves endotoxemia. *Med. Sci. Sports Exerc.* 52 (1): 94–104.

41 Pinn, D.M., Aroniadis, O.C., and Brandt, L.J. (2015). Is fecal microbiota transplantation (FMT) an effective treatment for patients with functional gastrointestinal disorders (FGID)? *Neurogastroent. Motil.* 27: 19–29.

42 Pinn, D.M., Aroniadis, O.C., and Brandt, L.J. (2014). Is fecal microbiota transplantation the answer for irritable bowel syndrome? A single-center experience. *Am. J. Gastroent.* 109: 1831–1832.

43 Ostgaard, H., Hausken, T., Gundersen, D.et al. (2012). Diet and effects of diet management on quality of life and symptoms in patients with irritable bowel syndrome. *Mol. Med. Rep.* 5: 1382–1390.

44 Bull, M.J. and Plummer, N.T. (2015). Part 2: Treatments for chronic gastrointestinal disease and gut dysbiosis. *Integr. Med. (Encinitas)* 14 (1): 25–33.

45 Chong, C.Y.L., Bloomfield, F.H., and O'Sullivan, J.M. (2018). Factors affecting gastrointestinal microbiome development in neonates. *Nutrition* 10 (3): 274.

46 El-Salhy, M., Kristoffersen, A.B., Valeur, J. et al. (2020). Long-term effects of faecal microbiota transplantation (FMT) in patients with irritable bowel syndrome. *Neurogastroent. Motil.* Submitted.

47 Dimidi, E. and Whelan, K. (2020). Food supplements and diet as treatment options in irritable bowel syndrome. *Neurogastroent. Motil.* 32 (8): e13951.

48 Barbara, G. and Ianiro, G. (2020). Faecal microbial transplantation in IBS: ready for prime time? *Gut* 69 (5): 795–796.

49 Ianiro, G., Maida, M., Burisch, J. et al. (2018). Efficacy of different faecal microbiota transplantation protocols for Clostridium difficile infection: a systematic review and meta-analysis. *United Euro. Gastroent. J.* 6 (8): 1232–1244.

50 El-Salhy, M., Hausken, T., and Hatlebakk, J.G. (2019). Increasing the dose and/or repeating faecal microbiota transplantation (FMT) increases the response in patients with irritable bowel syndrome (IBS). *Nutrition* 11 (6): 1415.

51 Chen, Q.Y., Tian, H.L., Yang, B. et al. (2020). Effect of intestinal preparation on the efficacy and safety of fecal microbiota transplantation treatment. *Zhonghua Wei Chang Wai Ke Za Zhi. (China)* 23 (Z1): 48–55.

52 Satokari, R., Mattila, E., Kainulainen, V. et al. (2015). Simple faecal preparation and efficacy of frozen inoculum in faecal microbiota transplantation for recurrent Clostridium difficile infection – an observational cohort study. *Ali. Pharm. Ther.* 41 (1): 46–53.

53 Mattila, E., Uusitalo-Seppälä, R., Wuorela, M. et al. (2012). Fecal transplantation, through colonoscopy, is effective therapy for recurrent Clostridium difficile infection. *Gastroenterol* 142 (3): 490–496.

54 Lahtinen, P., Jalanka, J., Hartikainen, A. et al. (2020). Letter: Faecal microbiota transplantation for irritable bowel syndrome-room for improvement. Authors' reply. *Ali. Pharmacol. Ther.* 52 (5): 925–926.

55 DeFilipp, Z., Bloom, P.P., Torres Soto, M. et al. (2019). Drug-resistant *E. coli* bacteremia transmitted by fecal microbiota transplant. *N. E. J. Med.* 381 (21): 2043–2050.

56 Blaser, M.J. (2019). Fecal microbiota transplantation for dysbiosis predictable risks. *N. E. J. Med.* 381 (21): 2064–2066.

57 Camilleri, M. (2020). FMT in IBS: A call for caution. *Gut* 70 (2): 431. https://doi.org/10.1136/gutjnl-2020-321529.

58 El-Salhy, M. (2020). FMT in IBS: how cautious should we be? *Gut* https://doi.org/10.1136/gutjnl-2020-322038.

Index

The Gut Microbiota in Health and Disease, First Edition. Edited by Nimmy Srivastava, Salam A. Ibrahim,
Jayeeta Chattopadhyay, and Mohamed H. Arbab.
© 2023 John Wiley & Sons Ltd. Published 2023 by John Wiley & Sons Ltd.